PHILOSOPHY
AND OCCUPATIONAL
THERAPY

Informing Education, Research, and Practice

PHILOSOPHY AND OCCUPATIONAL THERAPY

Informing Education, Research, and Practice

Editor

Steven D. Taff, PhD, OTR/L, FNAP, FAOTA
Associate Professor
Program in Occupational Therapy and
Department of Medicine
Director
Teaching Scholars Program
Washington University School of Medicine in St. Louis
St. Louis, Missouri

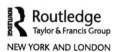

Routledge
Taylor & Francis Group
NEW YORK AND LONDON

First published in 2021 by SLACK Incorporated

Published 2024 by Routledge
605 Third Avenue, New York, NY 10158

and by Routledge
4 Park Square, Milton Park, Abingdon, Oxon OX14 4RN

Routledge is an imprint of the Taylor & Francis Group, an informa business

© 2021 by Taylor & Francis Group

Cover Artist: Lori Shields

Library of Congress Control Number: 2020949463

ISBN: 9781630916763 (pbk)
ISBN: 9781003525660 (ebk)

DOI: 10.4324/9781003525660

DEDICATION

This book is dedicated to everyone who views the world and asks, "What influenced it?" "How does it impact everyday life?" or "How could it be better?"

I would also like to dedicate the book to some thinkers who have been very influential in my work: Richard Rorty, Paul Ricoeur, Ted Brameld, Stanley Cavell, Cornel West, Herbert Marcuse, Maxine Greene, Gabriel Marcel, Jose Ortega y Gasset, Alfred Schutz, and Gert Biesta, among many others.

CONTENTS

Dedication .... *v*

Acknowledgments.. *xi*

About the Editor... *xiii*

Contributing Authors...*xv*

Foreword: Philosophy and Professional Reflection, Change, and Growth by
Barb Hooper, PhD, OTR/L, FAOTA..*xxi*

Chapter 1   What Is Philosophy? 1
                 Steven D. Taff, PhD, OTR/L, FNAP, FAOTA

Chapter 2   Reframing the Narrative on the Philosophies Influencing
                 the Development of Occupational Therapy................................... 7
                 Steven D. Taff, PhD, OTR/L, FNAP, FAOTA, and
                 Ganesh M. Babulal, PhD, OTD, MSCI, MOT, OTR/L

Chapter 3   Focus on the Mental and Spiritual:
                 Idealism and Occupational Therapy.. 23
                 Wanda J. Mahoney, PhD, OTR/L, and
                 Brad E. Egan, PhD, OTD, CADC, OTR/L

Chapter 4   Realism: Exploring the Divide Between What Exists and
                 What Humans Make of It.. 33
                 Jyothi Gupta, PhD, OTR/L, FAOTA, and
                 Bernard A. K. Muriithi, PhD, OTR/L

Chapter 5   A Teleological Perspective of Occupational Engagement:
                 Humanism Informing Occupational Therapy 45
                 Moses N. Ikiugu, PhD, OTR/L, FAOTA, and
                 Whitney Lucas-Molitor, PhD, OTD, MS, OTR/L, BCG

Chapter 6   Occupation and Meaningful Living:
                 An Existential Perspective... 53
                 Aaron M. Eakman, PhD, OTR/L, FAOTA, and
                 Moses N. Ikiugu, PhD, OTR/L, FAOTA

Chapter 7   Romanticism and Transcendentalism:
                 Ideas That Made Occupational Therapy Possible and
                 Holistic Practice Necessary.. 61
                 Charles H. Christiansen, EdD, OTR, FAOTA

Chapter 8   Slouching Toward Utopia:
Hope, Fear, and the Pursuit of the Unattainable 75
Richard L. Whalley, OTD, OTR/L;
Anna J. Neff, OTD, MSCI, OTR/L; and
Steven D. Taff, PhD, OTR/L, FNAP, FAOTA

Chapter 9   Pragmatic Foundations: Instrumentalism and
Transactionalism in Occupational Therapy 83
Moses N. Ikiugu, PhD, OTR/L, FAOTA, and
Ranelle M. Nissen, PhD, OTR/L

Chapter 10   Phenomenology: Returning to the Things Themselves
With Wonder and Curiosity 91
Valerie A. Wright-St Clair, PhD, MPH, DipProfEthics,
DipBusStud, DipOT, and Elizabeth Anne Kinsella,
PhD, MAdEd, BSc(OT)

Chapter 11   Tools, Thoughts, and Signs:
Sociocultural Perspectives on Mind and Occupation 101
Arun Selvaratnam, MS, OTR/L, and
Steven D. Taff, PhD, OTR/L, FNAP, FAOTA

Chapter 12   An African Philosophy of Personhood in
Southern Occupational Therapy 111
Thuli Mthembu, BSc OT, MPH, PhD, and Madeleine Duncan,
DipOT, BOT, BAHons(Psych), MSc OT, DPhil(Psych)

Chapter 13   Fundamental Impermanence:
Process Philosophy and Occupational Potential 127
Lauren Putnam, BS, and
Steven D. Taff, PhD, OTR/L, FNAP, FAOTA

Chapter 14   Analytic Philosophy: Guiding Method and
Adding Precision to Occupational Therapy 135
Marna Ghiglieri, OTD, MA, OTR/L;
Ronald R. Drummond, BA; Rose McAndrew, OTD, OTR/L, CHT;
and Steven D. Taff, PhD, OTR/L, FNAP, FAOTA

Chapter 15   Structuralism: Examining the Interrelationships
Around Occupation 145
Ganesh M. Babulal, PhD, OTD, MSCI, MOT, OTR/L, and
Jyothi Gupta, PhD, OTR/L, FAOTA

Chapter 16   Critical Theory: Resources for Questioning and
Transforming Everyday Life 155
Lisette Farias, PhD, MScOT, Reg. OT, and
Rebecca M. Aldrich, PhD, OTR/L

Chapter 17   Everyday Hermeneutics: Understanding (the Meaning of)
             Occupational Engagement..163
             Melissa Park, PhD, MA OT; Aaron Bonsall, PhD, OTR/L; and
             Don Fogelberg, PhD, OTR/L

Chapter 18   Deconstruction and the Institution of Occupation..........................181
             Ganesh M. Babulal, PhD, OTD, MSCI, MOT, OTR/L;
             Anil H. Chandiramani; and
             Steven D. Taff, PhD, OTR/L, FNAP, FAOTA

Chapter 19   Philosophical Influences on Occupational Therapy in Brazil:
             A Historical Timeline..189
             Daniel Marinho Cezar da Cruz, PhD, MSc, OT;
             Daniela da Silva Rodrigues, MSc, OT; and
             Helen Carey, PhD, MSc Adv OT, Dip COT, OTR/L

Chapter 20   Postmodernism: Foundations for Problematizing and
             Reimagining Conditions of Possibility..201
             Rebecca M. Aldrich, PhD, OTR/L;
             Debbie Laliberte Rudman, PhD, OT Reg. (ON); and
             Aaron Bonsall, PhD, OTR/L

Chapter 21   Intersectionality: Feminist Theorizing in the
             Pursuit of Justice and Equity 209
             Alison Gerlach, PhD, MSc (OT), and Lilian Magalhães, PhD, OT

Chapter 22   Capable *and* Occupied: How the Capabilities Approach
             Can Enrich the "Occupation" Discourse 221
             Ganesh M. Babulal, PhD, OTD, MSCI, MOT, OTR/L;
             Parul Bakhshi, PhD, DEA (MPhil); and
             Jean-Francois Trani, PhD, MSc, MPhil

Chapter 23   How Philosophy Can Support Occupational Therapy's
             Relevance in the 21st Century...233
             Steven D. Taff, PhD, OTR/L, FNAP, FAOTA;
             Moses N. Ikiugu, PhD, OTR/L, FAOTA; and
             Jyothi Gupta, PhD, OTR/L, FAOTA

Financial Disclosures 245
Index 247

ACKNOWLEDGMENTS

I would like to thank the talented and enthusiastic contributing authors who so willingly explored a host of philosophies and examined their potential impact on occupational therapy education, practice, and research. Here they have initiated the philosophizing in our profession that I deeply hope becomes commonplace as we move forward through the second century of occupational therapy.

I would also like to thank my colleagues and friends at SLACK Incorporated: Brien Cummings, Senior Acquisitions Editor, who recognized my passion for philosophy and nudged me to develop the book concept, Jennifer Cahill, and Allegra Tiver, and also Rashmi Malhotra at Westchester Publishing Services, the Production Project Manager. Thanks also to Ronald Drummond for his assistance with reviewing the formatting of in-text citations and references.

I would like to thank those who spurred my initial interest in philosophy while I was a doctoral student at the University of Missouri–St. Louis: Scot Danforth, Phil Ferguson, Chuck Fazzaro, Matt Keefer, Virginia Navarro, and Marvin Berkowitz all supported and challenged me to jump headlong into wide-ranging philosophies that transformed the way I view the world and shed critical light on how philosophical perspectives inform everyday practices in education and health care.

Thanks are also due to many students and colleagues at the Washington University School of Medicine Program in Occupational Therapy, Office of Education, and Academy of Educators who have been consistently supportive of my interest in applied philosophy and its impact on health professions education.

Last, but in no way least, I am thankful for the patience, love, and support of my wife, Helen, and sons, Aidan and Ryan.

ABOUT THE EDITOR

Steven D. Taff, PhD, OTR/L, FNAP, FAOTA, is Associate Professor in the Program in Occupational Therapy and Department of Medicine and Director of the Teaching Scholars Program at Washington University School of Medicine in St. Louis, Missouri. He is also co-founder of the Cross-Campus Educational Research Group, a multidisciplinary community of educational scholars and innovators at Washington University in St. Louis. Dr. Taff served as Chair of the Commission on Education of the American Occupational Therapy Association (AOTA) from 2016 to 2019 and is also a member of the leadership group of the AOTA Scholarship of Teaching and Learning Program. He is a co-author of the *AOTA Educational Research Agenda (Revised)* and the *Educator's Guide for Addressing Cultural Awareness, Humility, and Dexterity in Occupational Therapy Curricula*, and co-editor of the book *Perspectives on Occupational Therapy Education: Past, Present, and Future*. Dr. Taff was a recipient of the Emerson Excellence in Teaching Award in 2017.

CONTRIBUTING AUTHORS

Rebecca M. Aldrich, PhD, OTR/L (Chapters 16, 20)
Associate Professor of Clinical Occupational Therapy
Mrs. T. H. Chan Division of Occupational Science and Occupational Therapy
University of Southern California
Los Angeles, California

Ganesh M. Babulal, PhD, OTD, MSCI, MOT, OTR/L (Chapters 2, 15, 18, 22)
Assistant Professor
Department of Neurology
Washington University School of Medicine in St. Louis
St. Louis, Missouri

Parul Bakhshi, PhD, DEA (MPhil) (Chapter 22)
Assistant Professor
Program in Occupational Therapy
Washington University School of Medicine in St. Louis
St. Louis, Missouri

Aaron Bonsall, PhD, OTR/L (Chapters 17, 20)
Assistant Professor
Department of Occupational Therapy
A. T. Still University of Health Sciences
Mesa, Arizona

Helen Carey, PhD, MSc Adv OT, Dip COT, OTR/L (Chapter 19)
Professional Lead/Principal Lecturer
Department of Occupational Therapy
Wrexham Glyndwr University
Wrexham, Wales, United Kingdom

Anil H. Chandiramani (Chapter 18)
Independent Researcher
Minneapolis, Minnesota

Charles H. Christiansen, EdD, OTR, FAOTA (Chapter 7)
Clinical Professor
Department of Occupational Therapy
The University of Texas Medical Branch
Galveston, Texas

Daniel Marinho Cezar da Cruz, PhD, MSc, OT (Chapter 19)
Adjunct Professor
Department of Occupational Therapy/Occupational Therapy Graduate Program
Universidade Federal de São Carlos–UFSCar
São Carlos, São Paulo, Brazil

Ronald R. Drummond, BA (Chapter 14)
Doctoral Student
Program in Occupational Therapy
Washington University School of Medicine in St. Louis
St. Louis, Missouri

Madeleine Duncan, DipOT, BOT, BAHons(Psych), MSc OT, DPhil(Psych)
(Chapter 12)
Emeritus Associate Professor
Division of Occupational Therapy
Department of Health & Rehabilitation Sciences
Faculty of Health Sciences
University of Cape Town
Cape Town, South Africa

Aaron M. Eakman, PhD, OTR/L, FAOTA (Chapter 6)
Associate Professor
Department of Occupational Therapy
Colorado State University
Fort Collins, Colorado

Brad E. Egan, PhD, OTD, CADC, OTR/L (Chapter 3)
Associate Professor and Site Coordinator
Department of Occupational Therapy
Lenoir-Rhyne University
Columbia, South Carolina

Lisette Farias, PhD, MScOT, Reg. OT (Chapter 16)
Assistant Professor
Division of Occupational Therapy
Department of Neurobiology
Care Sciences and Society
Karolinska Institutet
Stockholm, Sweden

Don Fogelberg, PhD, OTR/L (Chapter 17)
Associate Professor
Department of Rehabilitation Medicine
University of Washington
Seattle, Washington

Alison Gerlach, PhD, MSc (OT) (Chapter 21)
Assistant Professor
School of Child & Youth Care
University of Victoria
British Columbia, Canada

Marna Ghiglieri, OTD, MA, OTR/L (Chapter 14)
Assistant Clinical Professor
Occupational Therapy Doctoral Program
University of the Pacific
Sacramento, California

Jyothi Gupta, PhD, OTR/L, FAOTA (Chapters 4, 15, 23)
Chair and Program Director
Department of Occupational Therapy
A. T. Still University of Health Sciences
Mesa, Arizona

Barb Hooper, PhD, OTR/L, FAOTA (Foreword)
Division Chief and Program Director
Occupational Therapy Doctorate Division
Duke University
Durham, North Carolina

Moses N. Ikiugu, PhD, OTR/L, FAOTA (Chapters 5, 6, 9, 23)
Professor
Department of Occupational Therapy
University of South Dakota
Vermillion, South Dakota

Elizabeth Anne Kinsella, PhD, MAdEd, BSc(OT) (Chapter 10)
Institute of Health Sciences Education
Faculty of Medicine & Health Sciences
McGill University
Montreal, Quebec, Canada

Whitney Lucas-Molitor, PhD, OTD, MS, OTR/L, BCG (Chapter 5)
Assistant Professor
Department of Occupational Therapy
University of South Dakota
Vermillion, South Dakota

Lilian Magalhães, PhD, OT (Chapter 21)
Adjunct Professor
Faculty of Occupational Therapy
Federal University of São Carlos
São Carlos, São Paulo, Brazil
Professor Emeritus
Western University
London, Ontario, Canada

Wanda J. Mahoney, PhD, OTR/L (Chapter 3)
Associate Professor of Occupational Therapy and Medicine
Program in Occupational Therapy
Washington University School of Medicine in St. Louis
St. Louis, Missouri

Rose McAndrew, OTD, OTR/L, CHT (Chapter 14)
Lecturer
Program in Occupational Therapy
Washington University School of Medicine in St. Louis
St. Louis, Missouri

Thuli Mthembu, BSc OT, MPH, PhD (Chapter 12)
Senior Lecturer
Department of Occupational Therapy
University of the Western Cape
Bellville, Cape Town, South Africa

Bernard A. K. Muriithi, PhD, OTR/L (Chapter 4)
Assistant Professor
Department of Occupational Therapy
A. T. Still University of Health Sciences
Mesa, Arizona

Anna J. Neff, OTD, MSCI, OTR/L (Chapter 8)
Occupational Therapist
St. Louis, Missouri

Ranelle M. Nissen, PhD, OTR/L (Chapter 9)
Associate Professor
Department of Occupational Therapy
University of South Dakota
Vermillion, South Dakota

Melissa Park, PhD, MA OT (Chapter 17)
Associate Professor
School of Physical & Occupational Therapy
Faculty of Medicine
McGill University
Montréal, Québec, Canada

Lauren Putnam, BS (Chapter 13)
Doctoral Student
Program in Occupational Therapy
Washington University School of Medicine in St. Louis
St. Louis, Missouri

Daniela da Silva Rodrigues, MSc, OT (Chapter 19)
Assistant Professor
School of Occupational Therapy
Universidade de Brasília
Brasília, Distrito Federal, Brazil

Debbie Laliberte Rudman, PhD, OT Reg. (ON) (Chapter 20)
Professor
School of Occupational Therapy & Occupational Science Field
Health and Rehabilitation Sciences Graduate Program
The University of Western Ontario
London, Ontario, Canada

Arun Selvaratnam, MS, OTR/L (Chapter 11)
Occupational Therapist
Making Strides of Virginia
Richmond, Virginia

Jean-Francois Trani, PhD, MSc, MPhil (Chapter 22)
Associate Professor
George Warren Brown School of Social Work
Institute of Public Health
Washington University in St. Louis
St. Louis, Missouri

Richard L. Whalley, OTD, OTR/L (Chapter 8)
Occupational Therapist
Lang Hand Therapy and Theralympic Speech, PLLC
New York, New York

Valerie A. Wright-St Clair, PhD, MPH, DipProfEthics, DipBusStud, DipOT (Chapter 10)
Professor
Department of Occupational Science & Therapy
Auckland University of Technology
Auckland, New Zealand

FOREWORD: PHILOSOPHY AND PROFESSIONAL REFLECTION, CHANGE, AND GROWTH

The first time I met Dr. Steven Taff, his interest in philosophy was clear. Steve first attended the Center for Occupational Therapy Education's summer teaching and learning institute in 2011. As the discussion at the institute moved to epistemology and to how teaching can challenge students' assumptions about the nature of knowledge and knowing, Steve's enthusiasm was palpable. That first meeting led to several shared projects related to philosophy. The next few years, Steve returned to the summer institute as a presenter on educational philosophies and on creating a personal teaching philosophy. We collaborated on a paper titled "Balancing Efficacy and Effectiveness With Philosophy, History, and Theory-Building in Occupational Therapy Education Research" (Hooper et al., 2018). Under Steve's direction, we also collaborated on—more like labored over—a paper using Ricoeurian hermeneutics as an analytic frame for analyzing education research data (Taff et al., 2018). My personal collaborations with Steve pertaining to philosophy, however, represent only a fraction of his larger body of work. Many of Steve's collaborations and publications attest to his passion for re-engaging the philosophical conversation in occupational therapy (Taff & Babulal, 2016; Taff et al., 2014). That passion is especially evident in this book, *Philosophy and Occupational Therapy: Informing Education, Research, and Practice.*

In the chapters herein, the authors offer several ways to help us think about the relationship between occupational therapy and philosophy. First, the authors suggest we recognize that philosophy is omnipresent in occupational therapy education, research, and practice, even though its influence is often hard to recognize. This book helps us trace the murky path outward from philosophical foundations to their expression in occupational therapy's education, research, and practice. For example, the authors argue that the field's key concept, *client-centeredness*, is grounded ultimately in philosophical beliefs about knowledge: knowledge is shared, is situated between the therapist and the client, and is constructed through dialogue. This concept of client-centeredness also stems from beliefs about values and right action: therapists enter into respectful, participatory relationships with clients in order to jointly solve occupational problems. Thus, the book illustrates that although the concepts used frequently by educators, researchers, and practitioners are prominent, the supporting philosophies behind those concepts typically are not. The authors explain that the relegation of philosophy to its current background status is due, in part, to the rise of a culture of evidence, where evidence and research became separated from philosophy. However, just because the philosophical foundations are in the background, this should not be taken to mean that these foundations are unimportant. To the contrary: as this book argues, philosophy matters, and teaching, research, and practice without philosophy are incomplete and inadequate.

Divorced from philosophy, not only are teaching, research, and practice inadequate, they can also actually stymie the growth of the profession. This is the second strong argument that the authors in this book make about the relationship between occupational therapy and philosophy. As teaching, research, and practice go forward without their philosophical backings (as noted earlier), they can proliferate dominant Western worldviews that remain unquestioned. Unquestioned worldviews, or habitual ways of perceiving and thinking, limit the growth of a field to only what can be imagined within those accepted views. Newer philosophies (and reinterpretations of older ones), however, can break open and illuminate occupational therapy's accepted and unquestioned perspectives and practices, thereby allowing change and growth. For example, chapter authors Gerlach and Magalhães explain "feminisms" as philosophies at the intersections of race, gender, ethnicity, and sexual identity and expression. These philosophies, they argue, help illuminate how Western-derived knowledge has prevailed in occupational therapy, keeping the teaching, research, and practice in this field focused predominantly on individuals within majority groups. Once these views are brought to light, educators, researchers, and practitioners can perceive how their methods may "(re)produce social relations of power and represent sites of occupational agency or oppression." So informed, teaching, research, and practice can then grow toward critical, socially transformative approaches that were previously unseen. Keeping philosophy alive is, therefore, critical in the sense that such aliveness prompts the profession to deepen its self-reflectivity and expand its teaching, research, and practice.

Third, the authors emphasize that the relationship between occupational therapy and philosophy is an important consideration for the specific and important roles that educators, researchers, and practitioners alike play. By considering each of these roles as its own craft with particular skills, language, concepts, and methods, members of the profession apply their craft to problems of learning, knowledge development, and practice, respectively. This book suggests that just below the skills, language, concepts, and methods used in the everyday artistries of teaching, research, and practice there is a deep well. That well is philosophy. Each craft is performed as inspired by notions of a desired future for the profession. From where do such notions of desired futures arise? Each craft is performed from notions of why the profession exists. From where do notions of existence and reality arise? Each craft is performed from notions of the most important actions to take. From where do the values for right actions arise? Each craft is performed in response to particular questions and problems. From where do particular questions arise and particular problems become problems? For each of the preceding questions—questions examining the very essence of occupational therapy—answers arise from the philosophical level.

Further, the authors suggest that we think about occupational therapy and philosophy by remembering this: Although sometimes opaque, sometimes overshadowed by the evidentiary discourse, and sometimes hegemonic, occupational therapy and occupational science *do* value philosophy. This value is apparent early in the profession in Meyer's 1922 paper, "The Philosophy of Occupational Therapy," and more recently in Hooper's and Wood's 2019 chapter, "The Philosophy of Occupational Therapy." In that chapter, we argued that occupational therapy has a distinctive philosophy; we distilled the ontological, epistemological, and axiological commitments of occupational therapy from historical texts in the field. We recognized, however, that the distinctive philosophy of occupational therapy draws from many philosophical influences. Those multiple influences are the substance of this book.

This book, *Philosophy and Occupational Therapy: Informing Education, Research, and Practice,* provides a valuable resource for educators, researchers, and practitioners reality by chiefly speculative rather than observational means" ("Philosophy," 2019). That simple definition, however, does not accurately portray the much deeper descriptions and implications that have surfaced intermittently throughout history. Once revered as a source of wisdom and rational alternative to myth and religion in the age of ancient Greece and Rome, more recent descriptions of philosophy are often less flattering. Bertrand Russell (1912/2016) noted that many are "inclined to doubt whether philosophy is anything better than innocent but useless trifling, hair-splitting distinctions, and controversies on matters concerning which knowledge is impossible" (p. 135). More than a century later, Catapano (2016) echoed Russell's concern that philosophy was perceived as cryptic and out-of-touch with modern circumstances, and therefore "somehow deficient, an impractical, even indulgent intellectual pursuit" (p. xiv). Despite such criticisms, others have made more earnest efforts to explore the essence and potential purposes of philosophical thought. American pragmatist philosopher William James (1911) viewed the core of philosophy as its ability to "fancy everything different from what it is. . . . It rouses us from our native dogmatic slumber and breaks up our caked prejudices" (p. 7). In other words, James asserts that philosophy arouses the curiosity in us, and as a result opens our minds. Kwasi Wiredu (1980) describes philosophy as ranging from a "guide to the living of life to the narrower concept . . . as a theoretical discipline devoted to detailed and complicated argument" (p. 32). Both identities, he suggests, help us understand the world and (it is hoped) change it for the better. Channeling Gramsci, Cornel West (1989) defines the task of philosophy as "nourishing and being nourished by the philosophical views of oppressed people themselves for the aims of social change and personal meaning" (p. 231). More broadly, West defines philosophy as a "form of cultural criticism . . . a continuous cultural commentary" (p. 5). In *The Claim of Reason*, Stanley Cavell (1979) frames philosophy as a learning process comprised of change and growth, which denotes the "education of grownups" (p. 125). The anxiety and effort required in this education—for ourselves and as we teach others—are what constitute the essence and value of philosophy as both an individual and communal enterprise.

APPROACHES TO ANSWERING THE QUESTION

Each of the preceding descriptions of philosophy falls within a much larger, varied, and dynamic conversation centered on the purposes and value of philosophy. Here I briefly explore four approaches to answering the question "What is philosophy?" One method of addressing the *what* of philosophy is to separate it into its constituent elements. Scholars have consistently delineated at least three significant divisions of philosophy: epistemology, ontology, and axiology (Ahmad et al., 2015; Payne, 2015; Pritchard, 2016). *Epistemology* is "concerned with the nature, sources, and limits of knowledge" (Klein, 2000, p. 246). As the study of knowledge, epistemology seeks to answer questions such as: What is knowledge? What are its sources? How much can be known? What are the different ways of knowing? Definitions of knowledge tend to fall into the basic distinction between conceptual and active knowledge, or *knowing that* and *knowing how* (Ryle, 1949/2009). Exploring the different aspects of epistemology is critical for occupational therapy, because how knowledge is defined and used is fundamental to the identity and evolution of professions. *Ontology* refers to the philosophical exploration of being or existence. More specifically, ontology explores what things exist and the general features of those things that do exist (Hofweber, 2017). It is part of a larger branch of philosophy known as *metaphysics*, which dwells on formal aspects (or first principles) of being, or attempts to answer questions such as: What is reality? What is time itself? How are the present, past, and future related? Metaphysics and ontology, taken together, constitute what for a long time used to be known as *natural philosophy* (Massimi, 2009). Best known for his work in ethics, Immanuel Kant (1787/1999) also contributed to ontological studies through contrasting the world as it actually exists independent of perception (*noumenal*) and the world as the totality of our perceptions (*phenomenal*). Discussions of ontology are central to guiding the therapeutic relationships and research agendas that are the core of occupational therapy practice. *Axiology* explores questions surrounding value (what is good or right), in particular, the aesthetic and ethical dimensions of philosophy. Ethics, or moral philosophy, focuses on how humans act in their everyday lives. Questions that moral philosophy asks include: What values guide a good life? What actions are right and wrong? In other words, what ought we to do or not do under prescribed circumstances? Ethical considerations are the roadmap for guiding the enactment of occupational therapy principles in client interaction, teaching, and research: that which does no harm and promotes individual capabilities.

A second approach to explaining the *what* of philosophy is to compare and contrast it with science. Pritchard (2016) portrays the difference by suggesting that philosophical problems tend to deal with generalities in contrast to the specificity characteristic of scientific subject specialties. Philosophers *ask* questions whereas scientists *answer* them (Russell, 1912/2016). That said, Russell is quick to point out that acts of asking are influential and "increase the interest of the world, and show the strangeness and wonder lying just below the surface even in the commonest things in life" (p. 9). Deleuze and Guattari (1994) offer a similar perspective and claim that philosophy *creates* concepts, whereas science *tests* them. These concepts are neither found ready-made nor discovered by science, but instead are constructed through philosophical introspection and critique. Regardless of the possible distinctions, philosophy and science share a long and close history; indeed, philosophy has been credited with providing the elemental pool from which the sciences arose. Over time, the apparent rigor and prestige of science superseded philosophy as the accepted means of investigating questions in the natural and social worlds. The longstanding legitimization of science as the path to progress and an increasing anti-intellectualism (Hofstadter, 1963) have combined to paint philosophy with a broad brush as a discipline and process that has no pragmatic value and is (or should be) relegated to within the walls of academia. In *The Story of Philosophy*, Will Durant (1926/1991) laments how philosophy withdrew from its role as coordinator of the sciences as human knowledge and technology overwhelmed its capacity. In this context, philosophy

> hid itself in recondite and narrow lanes, timidly secure from the issues and responsibilities of life. Human knowledge had become too great for the human mind. All that remained was the scientific specialist, who knew more and more about less and less and the philosophical speculator, who knew less and less

about more and more. . . . Facts replaced understanding; and knowledge, split into a thousand isolated fragments, no longer generated wisdom. Every science, and every branch of philosophy, developed a technical terminology intelligible only to its exclusive devotees; as men learned more about the world, they found themselves ever less capable of expressing to their educated fellow-men what it was that they had learned. (p. vi)

By abdicating its role in informing science, the withdrawal of philosophy led to the loss of soul in science and possible closing of the mind to new possibilities (Payne, 2015). Within occupational therapy, the dichotomization between science and philosophy is clear. The primacy of science as a foundation of the profession, and the perception that philosophy and its subjective paradigm are of limited use as we move forward through the 21st century, seems prevalent in the profession. Accordingly, any discussion of the "what" of philosophy necessitates an accompanying justification of its value in a gestalt view, as well as debates surrounding which particular philosophical schools best represent the traditions and increasing needs of the occupational therapy profession.

Yet another way to describe philosophy is to distinguish it from its close analogue, ideology. Philosophy is a mode of inquiry, question-asking, and critique. Regardless of which philosophical school one adheres to, positions can be stated, debated, and clarified, but are never beyond criticism. With philosophy, skepticism is typical; however, an openness, a space for even vastly opposing dialogues to inch ever closer, is always present. Philosophy, then, is not a zero-sum game. Ideology, in contrast, is typically composed of values, beliefs, and underlying assumptions about reality that are frequently inaccurate but underpin identity and help adherents make sense of the world (Eagleton, 2007). Ideologies can serve a pragmatic purpose by providing a "shorthand guide to action, intellectual equipment designed to be portable and simple" (Keohane, 1976, p. 82). All too often, though, ideology becomes a "distorted, if only because unilateral and partial, view of reality which comes to supersede and substitute for the real world" (Bartlett, 1986, p. 4). As such, ideologies can be alienating and dangerous, frequently subtly so. Indeed, Bartlett (1986) noted that "the strength of an ideology lies in its status being unrecognized . . . its grip on a population is weakened if its members are made aware of the pluralism of values and beliefs" (p. 7). Philosophy illuminates alternative positions and thus serves as a buffer or antidote to ideology. Given the recent sociopolitical climate, it is critical for us not only to distinguish philosophy from ideology but also, more importantly, to employ ongoing cultural conversations that detail how philosophy can counteract the damaging impacts of ideological thinking on policy, science, and our engagement with one another in a democratic society.

The work of Richard Rorty (1979, 1989, 1999) provides a fourth dimension from which to differentiate philosophy on two very different levels, both of which are necessary as humans navigate the modern world. This perspective is the one on which I wish to focus as a foundational lens for this text. "Upper-case" philosophy is defined as the variant of philosophy most prevalent in academia and similar intellectual circles. In such contexts, philosophy typically focuses on big questions, such as: What is knowledge; what is good, just, or right; and what is the purpose of life? These questions of epistemology, axiology, and ontology are fundamentally essential to ask. However, the ensuing discussions frequently boil down to debates surrounding representations of reality or truth that do not address the dilemmas facing societies today (Saarinen, 2013). Upper-case philosophy therefore risks affirming Rorty's suggestion that "philosophers have given their subject a bad name by seeing difficulties nobody else sees" (Rorty, 1989, p. 12). Such a conception of philosophy makes it an easy target for standard charges that it is a discipline so esoteric that it completely misses the opportunity to affect everyday life. Nonetheless, we see the value that philosophy can bring into the profession when we ponder dilemmas faced in practice regarding the legitimate tools and scope of occupational therapy (the ontology of the profession) and ethical dilemmas that practitioners face every day due to productivity and insurance reimbursement restrictions. In these cases, we can see the need to employ the methods of philosophy to create a deep understanding of our essence in occupation-based practice (ontology) and the values that inform what we do in practice every day (axiology).

In stark contrast, "lower-case" philosophy is not concerned with abstract reflection, but instead an in-depth examination of life with a singular goal of making life better for as many people as possible. Lower-case philosophy explores the "life-enhancing application of philosophical thinking in action" (Saarinen, 2013, p. 152). Rorty strongly reminds us that although philosophy has value as a purely intellectual exercise, it would be a critical mistake to leave it or limit it to that alone. The true value of philosophy lies in grappling with its opaqueness, discussing it, arguing over it, exploring it, critiquing it, and, most importantly, *using* it for the potential value it holds for everyday life. Saarinen (2013) suggests that Rorty's distinctly lower-case pragmatism "is a call for the better . . . a philosophy of a better life as a practical art" (p. 146).

Catapano (2016) harkens to Rorty's lower-case philosophy with his "naturally-occurring philosopher," suggesting that perhaps a philosopher is "anyone who thinks about existence and takes a whack at trying to explain it" (p. xix). Philosophers maintain a close congruency with journalists in how they approach their craft (Catapano, 2016). In their roles, they both can serve as investigators or watchdogs whose efforts hopefully result in practical action to address the problems they discover. Charges that philosophy does not solve practical problems (as science does) misses an immensely important point: philosophy serves a critical role in societies by assessing and pressing public opinion (Catapano, 2016), which can have an "educative or even emancipatory effect" (p. xxii). In this way, philosophy is not merely for intellectuals and academics; instead, it engages the public and influences "how a culture converses with itself, understands itself, talks to other cultures and seeks to understand them" (Catapano, 2016, p. xxii). These cultural conversations are essential to ethical and equitable living, and at the heart of Rorty's hopes for philosophy to be a means for everyone to use to shape a better world.

Perhaps the *what* of philosophy is not so much the point after all, and its true value is in *how* it is integrated into professional consciousness as a viable guide to serving our clients as they pursue occupational engagement in a more just and equitable global context. Toward this end, *Philosophy and Occupational Therapy: Informing Education, Research, and Practice* offers glimpses of multiple philosophical variants, each of which offers new possibilities for supporting lives lived well.

REFERENCES

Ahmad, A. A., Musa Singhry, I. M., Adamu, H., & Abubakar, M. M. (2015). Ontology, epistemology and axiology in quantitative and qualitative research: Elucidation of the research philosophical misconception. *Proceedings of The Academic Conference: Mediterranean Publications & Research International on New Direction and Uncommon, 2*(1), 1–26.

Bartlett, S. J. (1986). Philosophy as ideology. *Metaphilosophy, 17*(1), 1–13. https://doi.org/10.1111/j.1467-9973.1986.tb00840.x

Catapano, P. (2016). Introduction. In P. Catapano & S. Critchley (Eds.), *The stone reader: Modern philosophy in 133 arguments* (pp. xiii–xxii). Livewright.

Cavell, S. (1979). *The claim of reason: Wittgenstein, skepticism, morality, and tragedy.* Oxford University Press.

Deleuze, G., & Guattari, F. (1994). *What is philosophy?* (H. Tomlinson & G. Burchell, Trans.). Columbia University Press.

Durant, W. (1991). *The story of philosophy.* Pocket Books. (Original work published 1926)

Eagleton, T. (2007). *Ideology: An introduction.* Verso.

Hofstadter, R. (1963). *Anti-intellectualism in American life.* Alfred A. Knopf.

Hofweber, T. Logic and ontology. (2017). In E. N. Zalta (Ed.), *The Stanford encyclopedia of philosophy* (Summer 2018 ed.). https://plato.stanford.edu/entries/logic-ontology/#Ont

James, W. (1911). *Some problems of philosophy: A beginning of an introduction to philosophy.* Longman's, Green.

Kant, I. (1999). *Critique of pure reason* (P. Guyer and A. Wood, Trans.). Cambridge University Press. (Original work published 1787)

Keohane, N. O. (1976). Philosophy, theory, and ideology: An attempt at clarification. *Political Theory, 4*(1), 80–100. https://doi.org/10.1177/009059177600400107

Klein, P. D. (2000). Epistemology. In E. Craig (Ed.), *The concise Routledge encyclopedia of philosophy* (pp. 246–249). Routledge.

Massimi, M. (2009). Philosophy and the sciences after Kant. *Royal Institute of Philosophy Supplement, 65,* 275–311. https://doi.org/10.1017/S1358246109990142

Payne, W. R. (2015). *An introduction to philosophy.* https://open.umn.edu/opentextbooks/textbooks/an-introduction-to-philosophy

Philosophy. (2013). In *The Free Dictionary.* https://encyclopedia2.thefreedictionary.com/philosophy

Philosophy. (2019). In *Merriam-Webster's online dictionary* (11th ed.). https://www.merriam-webster.com/dictionary/philosophy

Pritchard, D. (2016). *What is this thing called philosophy?* Routledge.

Rorty, R. (1979). *Philosophy and the mirror of nature.* Princeton University Press.

Rorty, R. (1989). *Contingency, irony, and solidarity.* Cambridge University Press.

Rorty, R. (1999). *Philosophy and social hope.* Penguin Books.

Russell, B. (2016). *The problems of philosophy.* Enhanced Media. (Original work published 1912)

Ryle, G. (2009). *The concept of mind.* http://s-f-walker.org.uk/pubsebooks/pdfs/Gilbert_Ryle_The_Concept_of_Mind.pdf (Original work published 1949)

Saarinen, E. (2013). Kindness to babies and other radical ideas: Rorty's anti-cynical philosophy. In A. Groschner, C. Koopman, & M. Sandbothe (Eds.), *Richard Rorty: From pragmatist philosophy to cultural politics* (pp. 145–164). Bloomsbury.

West, C. (1989). *The American evasion of philosophy.* The University of Wisconsin Press.

Wiredu, K. (1980). *Philosophy and an African culture.* Cambridge University Press.

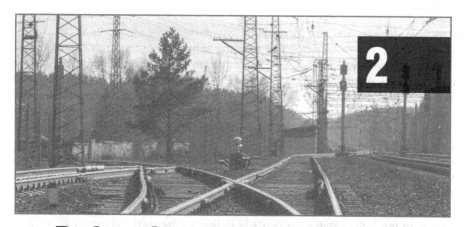

Reframing the Narrative on the Philosophies Influencing the Development of Occupational Therapy

Steven D. Taff, PhD, OTR/L, FNAP, FAOTA
Ganesh M. Babulal, PhD, OTD, MSCI, MOT, OTR/L

INTRODUCTION

The Progressive Era (roughly 1890–1920) in the United States was a time of high flux in the thoughts, attitudes, politics, and ways of living in a radically altered social landscape. The Progressive Era ushered in many pressures and social problems brought on by the daunting combination of industrialization, urbanization, mass immigration, class struggle, and capitalist expansion (Diner, 1998; Hofstadter, 1955; Rodgers, 1982; Wiebe, 1967). During this period, philosophy, while still seen as relevant in some quarters, also experienced the coda of a transition where science supplanted it as the basis for intellectual thought and the desired instrument for modern progress. Multiple philosophies were fashionable in the United States during the late 1800s and early 1900s, mostly European imports, particularly the utilitarianism of John Stuart Mill and Hegel's neo-idealism (Hall, 1879). Comtean positivism, as filtered through Mill and appropriated by

Taff, S. D. (Ed.). *Philosophy and Occupational Therapy:*
Informing Education, Research, and Practice (pp. 7-22).
© 2021 Taylor & Francis Group.

American thinkers, was also increasingly prominent, as we expand upon later in this chapter. Influential to a lesser extent were the fading ideas of Scottish commonsense realism, particularly Hamilton's (1852) conception of the limits of knowledge, a type of "philosophical humility" (Pearce, 2015, p. 449). Utilitarianism's core tenets meshed well with American ideals of efficiency, democratic liberalism, and the new science of evolution. Hegelianism was less embraced but established a foothold in the Midwest, mainly due to the efforts of William Torrey Harris, superintendent of the St. Louis public schools (Hall, 1879; Kuklick, 2001). This potpourri of philosophies also included the lingering presence of transcendentalism and the more distinctly American pragmatism born and nurtured in the Metaphysical Club of Cambridge, Massachusetts, in the 1870s (Menand, 2001; Pearce, 2015).

In the three decades before the origination of occupational therapy, the scholarly climate in the United States (particularly in the Northeast, the epicenter of intellectualism at the time) was influenced by both the reaction to multiple social changes and a spirit of progress in using science and technology to advance American society. The development of entire professions, including occupational therapy, was one significant outcome of Progressivism (Hofstadter, 1955; Taff, 2005). Professions rely upon philosophy and theory to establish and guide the goals, structure, values, knowledge, and methods of their practitioners, scholars, and educators (Breines, 1986; Ikiugu & Schultz, 2006; Payne, 2015). However, the initial philosophical influences of occupational therapy are vague and ill-defined at best if judged by explicit mentions in the literature. Breines (1987) noted that occupational therapy's

> foundational principles were never clearly defined, not even by the founders of the profession. The foundational beliefs of the profession were not clearly stated in the early literature. The only exception is the paper published by Meyer in 1922, but even Meyer's paper offers no citations and therefore no support for his position. (p. 522)

Nonetheless, scholars have suggested multiple philosophical influences on the development of occupational therapy; the most commonly cited include Moral Treatment, Deweyan pragmatism, and the Mental Hygiene, Arts and Crafts, and Settlement House Movements (Andersen & Reed, 2017; Bockoven, 1971; Breines, 1987; Cohen, 1983; Hooper & Wood, 2019; Quiroga, 1995; Serrett, 1985). Though certainly informed by philosophies, these five major influences were, aside from pragmatism, not formal schools of philosophy at all, but rather social movements. In this chapter, we identify and distinguish the philosophies underpinning the origin of occupational therapy from the movements they catalyzed. To this end, we suggest that transcendentalism, pragmatism, positivism, and Christian socialism were the most significant influences that catalyzed Progressive Era reform and provided the pivotal philosophical foundation for the development of the profession of occupational therapy. In the absence of explicit reference from the founders, more recent literature has retrospectively posited Deweyan pragmatism as a central philosophical foundation of occupational therapy (Breines, 1986; Cutchin, 2004; Ikiugu & Schultz, 2006; Morrison, 2016). Although it is clear that pragmatism (as forwarded by Dewey, James, and Peirce) informed many of the fundamental principles of occupational therapy, we suggest that there is more to the story and that additional philosophies were at play. The reality is that there has always been a polytomous network of schools that provided fertile ground for occupational therapy to take root and flourish. Here we explore how transcendentalists (Henry David Thoreau, Margaret Fuller, and Ralph Waldo Emerson), other pragmatists (Charles Sanders Peirce and William James), positivists (Auguste Comte, John Stuart Mill, Chauncey Wright, and Ernst Mach), and Christian socialists (W. D. P. Bliss, Shailer Mathews, and Jane Addams) had a significant role in shaping the intellectual landscape that nourished the origins of occupational therapy.

TRANSCENDENTALISM AND THE AMERICAN INTELLECTUAL TRADITION

The early 19th century in the United States saw unparalleled growth in agriculture, global migration, westward expansion, and the origins of American politics and ideology (Gura, 2007). This epoch also saw the birth of several philosophical schools of thought that innervate American ideals to this day. One such school was transcendentalism, described as a religious, philosophical, literary, artistic, and social movement (Honderich, 2005). Transcendentalism sought a conscious perspective that embraced nature, spirituality, subjective experiences, and intuition. This came as an organic response to the prevalence and dominance of scientific empiricism and rationalism and Calvinism's predestination from the previous century. Transcendentalism is a philosophy that was directly influenced by Romanticism and thinkers and artists such as Johann Wolfgang von Goethe, Friedrich Schelling, Friedrich Schiller, William Wordsworth, and Lord Byron, among others. Transcendentalism was also heavily influenced by Unitarianism, and by Hinduism through sacred texts such as the Bhagavad Gita and Upanishads (Goodman, 2019).

Transcendentalism was an intentional response to rationalism and empiricism and a departure from the Age of Reason/Enlightenment, which was the dominant intellectual discourse and perspective based on work by Locke and Rousseau, among others (Myerson, 2000). Objectivity, abstraction, order, and deductive reasoning propelled advances in material science, industrialism, and societal growth in the 19th century. However, this perspective and practice created knowledge inaccessible to many and belonging only to a gifted few. Transcendentalism emerged as a new perspective to go beyond or "transcend" the limits of logical and rational thinking to seek a holistic view of the world and one's place in it (Goodman, 2019; Thoreau, 2004). It posited that humans have access to a holistic knowledge of the world and themselves that extends beyond mere sensations and perceptions. A basic tenet of transcendentalism argues that knowledge of life and its relationships is gleaned from intuition and imagination. The institutions within a society were viewed as obstacles that interfered with and often corrupted one's purity. People can be self-reliant and independent, and should trust themselves as an authority about morality/ethics, expression, and purpose. Humans were seen as inherently good and, by reflecting on the divinity of nature and art and through everyday work, one could surmount many of life's challenges (Myerson, 2000). This movement strengthened the neophyte American identity; notable transcendentalist Ralph Waldo Emerson urged his fellow Americans to avoid imitating their European counterparts and conforming to their thought and lifestyle, calling for them instead to be authentic and create their own identity (Gura, 2007).

Prominent transcendentalist thinkers included Henry David Thoreau, Margaret Fuller, and Ralph Waldo Emerson, among others. These poets, leaders, and philosophers are notably recognized for their contributions to literature and art through the Transcendental Club and publications like *The Western Messenger* and *The Dial* (Goodman, 2019). However, these scholars are less recognized for grounding the progressivism of 19th-century America in morality and self-reflection. Progress in any society is always balanced by the sacrifice of some ideals, expenditure of some precious resources, the subjugation of a group or groups, and ultimately loss of life. The unprecedented growth and wealth accumulation in America in this era was accompanied by documented historical injustices like the continued expansion of slavery, gender inequity, and displacement of Native American tribes. Emerson vocally opposed the forced movement of more than 16,000 Cherokees in a letter to then-President Van Buren, "for how could we call the conspiracy that should crush these poor Indians our Government, or the land that was cursed by their parting and dying imprecations our country, any more?" (Emerson, 1995, p. 3). Margaret Fuller renounced the election of James Polk as president and slave owner, "You see the men, how they are willing to sell shamelessly, the happiness of countless generations of fellow-creatures, the honor of their country, and their immortal souls for a money market and political power" (Fuller, 1998, p. 98). Finally, Thoreau denounced legislation concerning slavery: "I cannot for an instant recognize that political organization as my government which is the slave's government also" (Thoreau, 1973, p. 67). These three examples of transcendentalists directly addressing political and moral failings are among many others that served to give a voice to the disenfranchised, marginalized, and subjugated groups. This focus on humanitarian reform and critical opposition to immoral and unethical practices are embedded in the foundation of transcendentalism.

As the Americanized version of Romanticism, transcendentalism represents many of the cultural values ingrained in American society. Accordingly, it also informed pragmatism and can be considered an element of the artistic influence in our profession. Historically, transcendentalism preceded pragmatism by many decades and contributed directly to its democratic ideals (Dewey, 1903). The rich social tapestry of occupational therapy that reflects revered concepts such as client-centeredness, meaningful occupations, lived experience, autonomy, choice, and control all derive from transcendentalism. Even occupational justice as a concept and practice is reflected in the transcendentalists' fight for the abolition of slavery, women's suffrage, and equality/access for all. It is not by chance that classic American ideals, which include "pull yourself up by your bootstraps," independence, living a meaningful life, and the health-promoting benefits of nature, are also present in one form or another in modern-day rehabilitation and occupational therapy. These terms used in the occupational therapy vernacular were common constructs used in transcendentalism, but were labeled self-reliance (independence), individualism (autonomy), morality/purpose (meaningful life), and embracing nature (health benefits). There is little concrete peer-reviewed evidence enshrining transcendentalism in the philosophical pantheon of occupational therapy. However, the thoughts and writings of Thoreau, Emerson, and Fuller (among other scholars) contributed directly to the founders (e.g., Slagle, Barton, Dunton, Johnson, Kidner, Newton), to the overall intellectual collective of early-1900s America, to the birth of pragmatism, and indirectly to concepts in occupational therapy's practice milieu.

PRAGMATISM: THE CONTRIBUTIONS OF PEIRCE AND JAMES

As conventional wisdom considers Socrates to be the father of modern Western philosophy, in a similar vein, pragmatism is celebrated as a uniquely American contribution to philosophy, with John Dewey as its iconic progenitor. Originating in the late 1870s, pragmatism reified the practical application and utility of ideas, axioms, and theories as valid and truthful through experience and testing through rigorous experimentation (Goodman, 1995). These foci were counter to traditional philosophical schools that dealt with the abstractions and fixed principles that often remained inaccessible, esoteric, and untestable (Honderich, 2005). Notably, Dewey expanded the application of pragmatism to the areas of politics, education, and societal development for improvement. Unsurprisingly, occupational therapy has long embraced and identified with Deweyan pragmatism (Hooper & Wood, 2002). Though Dewey's mantle shoulders much of the recognition and acclaim, the roots of pragmatism are owed to members of the Metaphysical Club, including Charles Sanders Peirce, William James, Chauncey Wright, and George Herbert Mead (Menand, 2001). In this section, we limit the discussion to exploring the role of Peirce and James in shaping the form that is today known as *classic pragmatism.*

Charles Sanders Peirce is credited as the progenitor of pragmatism because he formulated and operationalized the foundation of pragmat[ic]ism (to distinguish his from James's pragmatism) in *The Fixation of Belief* (1877) and *How to Make Our Ideas Clear* (1878). His contributions extended beyond philosophy to mathematics, chemistry, semiotics, and research methods. By training and employment, Peirce was a physical scientist, and he believed that logic and philosophy were also sciences. He read philosophy voraciously and examined works of Aristotle and Hegel, but was a particular admirer of Kant (Scheffler, 1974). Peirce's approach to philosophy was based on logic, and his intent for pragmatism was to create a technique to find solutions to both scientific and philosophical problems. He proposed three phenomenological categories: firstness, secondness, and thirdness (Peirce, 1931). *Firstness* is the purest presentation of phenomena, one that exists in isolation or absence of influence. *Secondness* is a reaction to the phenomena in a relationship with something else, and there are always two objects/parties. *Thirdness* is the connection or mediation between two objects/ parties. This work on triadic structures extended into his three levels of clearness. The basic level is an idea that is universally familiar and easily recognizable without much thought or development. The second level is establishing criteria (free of ambiguity) on parts of an idea or concept. Peirce observed that philosophers and erudite teachers assume they each understand the definition of axioms, but most time and effort are spent in pedantic discussion clarifying gray areas or slivers of difference. Peirce conjectured this third level of clearness, called the *pragmatic maxim,* thus: "Consider what effects, that might conceivably have practical bearings, we conceive the object of our conception to have. Then, our conception of these effects is the whole of our conception of the object" (Peirce, 1931, p. 23). Though there have of course been multiple interpretations of this rule, it is generally accepted as stipulating that any concept, and its meaning and value, should be evaluated and anchored in its utility/action and experience. The pragmatic maxim sought to remove the subjectivity associated with conceptual definitions that lack uniformity or guidelines. These beliefs about what philosophy should do and ideas about verification laid the foundation for classical pragmatism.

William James is renowned as the founder of contemporary psychology in the United States. His notable contribution was *The Principles of Psychology,* published in 1890, which espoused the fluid nature of consciousness, proposed a new theory on emotion and the formation and purpose of habits, and gave a definition of free will (James, 1890). Many intellectual purists were influenced by his extensive readings and study of philosophy, discussions with colleagues, and the examination of daily life and his personal experiences. James was a colleague and contemporary of Peirce and is recognized for further developing and making pragmatism more accessible to a lay audience. In *Pragmatism: A New Name for Some Old Ways of Thinking,* James adeptly explores and discusses with resounding clarity the nature of pragmatism and its charge to resolve longstanding metaphysical debates, such as monism vs. pluralism, common sense, truth, humanism, and religion (James, 1907).

Pragmatism for James was a keystone that not only upheld the empiricist scientific standards of the time, but also could also support faith and human values. James was drawn to pragmatism for numerous reasons, chief among them the treatment of truth, and he used Peirce's pragmatic maxim to further shape his understanding of it (Scheffler, 1974). However, there is a fundamental difference in how truth was understood between the two philosophers. Peirce viewed truth as a monistic objective method to understand a concept vital for the scientific method, which then becomes real. This perspective is captured in his maxim "truth is the end of inquiry," where *end* means the purpose or goal. James embraced the plurality that can be the truth, an idea heavily influenced by his views of religion. For James (1909), truth inheres in an idea or belief that can be experienced, validated, and has some usefulness. James (1907) further posited, "True ideas are those that we can assimilate, validate, corroborate and verify. False ideas are those that we cannot" (p. 201). This embraced the universal pragmatist perspective on the purpose of striving for truth. However, he also recognized that truth could take many forms, including faith and religion, and could change over time. Nevertheless, James insisted that truth must have some practical impact, benefit, and consequence and should serve the greater good. This view was aptly extended across pragmatism as a whole when James (1907) wrote,

> Pragmatism is willing to take anything, to follow either logic or the senses, and to count the humblest and most personal experiences. She will count mystical experiences if they have practical consequences. She will take a God who lives in the very dirt of private fact—if that should seem a likely place to find him. (p. 80)

The utility of pragmatism as a philosophy, perspective, and paradigm has a long tradition in occupational therapy practice, education, and research. However, as James firmly held to the pluralism of truth, so too should the profession hold to the pluralism and utility of other philosophies' contributions to addressing the diversity of challenges facing the field.

The influence of a sole philosophy—specifically, John Dewey's pragmatism in the case of occupational therapy—is dogmatic (Cutchin, 2004). However, the seminal work of Deweyan pragmatism is owed in large part to Peirce and James; the former developed and the latter expounded on pragmatism while popularizing its utility in the late 19th and early 20th centuries. Peirce's pragmatic maxim sought to supplant subjectivity by anchoring reasoning to service and experience. This principle is highlighted by one of Dunton's tenets of occupational therapy, which emphasized the need to create structure, organize time, and engage in purposeful occupation. The practice of the profession had to be tethered to a unifying structure and relate to the tasks associated with the treatment a person receives. James's predilection for searching and striving for truth (which can take many different forms) also spoke to the multiple meanings that an occupation can have for different individuals, given that life experiences, culture, and goals are all different parts of a person's dimensionality (Townsend & Polatajko, 2013). Both Peirce and James established what came to be classic pragmatism, which Dewey later explored in greater detail, expanded within a frame of democracy, and applied in various ways in educational contexts.

POSITIVISM AND ITS IMPACT ON PROGRESSIVISM AND NASCENT PROFESSIONS

In contemporary thought, the term *positivism* is used more as a pejorative to condemn a rigid, quantitative, and in some cases colonialist, scientific paradigm than to identify a definite school of philosophy. Perhaps an even less likely use would be to associate positivism with the origins of occupational therapy, yet that is precisely what we suggest in this section. Positivism, along with Marxism, is considered to be one of the most influential philosophical streams of thought of the 19th century (Fillafer et al., 2018). Certainly, its influence lingered into the first two decades of the 20th century, after which it morphed into the logical positivism of the Vienna Circle.

Auguste Comte's vision was for positivism to serve as the science of society, using observation, comparison, and experimentation as its primary methods (Pickering, 1993). Positivism recognized empirical facts and observable phenomena while taking a robust anti-metaphysical stance. Lenzer (1998) noted that it was Comte "who effectively bridged the gulf that separated the study of natural phenomena from the study of human phenomena by providing a methodology that would allow for the application of the positive-scientific method to the analysis of social phenomena as well" (p. xxviii). In post-revolution France, Comte was once secretary to the utopian socialist Henri de Saint-Simon, but later broke with his mentor and developed a new positive philosophy that was meant to "cure the ills of society: it was to guarantee stability and spiritual authority in an age of untrammeled political radicalism and capitalism" (Fillafer et al., 2018, p. 6). The climate in Europe that gave rise to positivism in the early and mid-1800s was a time of significant sociopolitical disruption, not unlike the Progressive

Era in the United States a few decades later. As a novel way to address the challenges of mid-19th-century Europe, positivism was extraordinarily influential; Comte's work was considered by John Stuart Mill to be "very nearly the grandest work of the age" (Mill, 1963). Comtean positivism was designed to be a universally applied scientific paradigm and was purposefully exported to England, Germany, Turkey, Poland, and Brazil (Fillafer et al., 2018).

Positivism came to the United States via England, where Mill refined it to be complementary to his renewed version of utilitarianism. Mill shared Comte's beliefs regarding the primacy of "scientific objectivity that did not amount to impartiality, to a detachment from political life, but instead envisaged scholars as pacesetters of sociopolitical progress, as they developed panaceas to cure the moral, economic, and spiritual ills of their age" (Fillafer et al., 2018, p. 10). Mill's (1865) philosophical outlook and specifically his book *Auguste Comte and Positivism* were very influential in the United States and introduced positivism as the most significant intellectual device for social reform in the Progressive Era. The intellectual circles of New England in the late 1800s held Mill in particularly high regard, and his influence was enormous among scholars and popularizers such as John Fiske, Chauncey Wright, and Francis Ellingwood Abbot (Pearce, 2015).

Mill's (1865) work *Auguste Comte and Positivism* made quite an impact on the American philosophy community, notably Chauncey Wright (Pearce, 2015). Wright was a respected philosopher of science, leader of the Metaphysical Club, and frequently cited as one of the founders of pragmatism (Menand, 2001; Schneider, 1946). Madden (1953) argues that Wright was, in actuality, a "positivistic empiricist" (p. 62) who was greatly influenced by Mill's modified version of Comtean positivism (Pearce, 2015). Wright moved even further into the positivist ethos in 1870 when he joined the faculty at Harvard, which was then under the new leadership of C. W. Eliot, a strong proponent of positivism (Pearce, 2015). An avowed empiricist first and foremost, Wright saw positivism's most valuable role as that of organizing the sciences: "Positivism . . . must be a system of the universal methods, hypotheses and principles which are founded on them" (Thayer, 1878, pp. 140–142). This consilience amounted to a framework for the philosophy of science, which focused on methods rather than results (or "truth"). Wright was certainly skeptical of metaphysics, but as a wide-ranging thinker, he valued philosophy for its emotional and practical utility (Pearce, 2015). Wright was perhaps the leading American scholar in the 1860s and 1870s and was held in high esteem by Charles Sanders Peirce, William James, and George Herbert Mead, all members of the Metaphysical Club. In particular, his intellectual conversations (he rarely published) with Peirce and James influenced the development of pragmatism, which may explain the many similarities between Millean utilitarian positivism and the new American philosophy.

As evidenced by the cases of Chauncey Wright, Charles Sanders Peirce, and William James, positivism and pragmatism show many similarities. Interestingly, scholars and historians of occupational therapy have not highlighted the role positivism has played in the ongoing development of the profession, although it is clear that the quest for professional legitimacy led to the adoption of the positivist paradigm to match the status of medicine (Andersen & Reed, 2017). Serrett (1985) mentions the "structuralism" of the Machine Age as an early influence in the development of occupational therapy, asserting that "[s]tructuralism aligned with the predominant scientific modes . . . reductionism, analysis, cause-and-effect determinism" (p. 12). By that definition, it is possible that the intended reference was positivism, and Serrett (1985) frames structuralism as something against which pragmatism and functionalism rebelled. Most historical accounts of the early stages of occupational therapy stress the primacy of pragmatism in its development, despite its apparent tension with professional values, training, research, and practice. Pragmatism is frequently linked to the art side of the art-science debate in occupational therapy's intellectual history (Hooper & Wood, 2002; Peloquin, 1989; Wood, 1995). The literature, therefore, appears to indicate a chasm between pragmatic and positivistic thought when they actually are quite comparable and similar in several important ways. Positivism and pragmatism were both scientifically oriented philosophies that viewed science as the way to achieve progress for humanity (Nekrasas, 2001). Both schools of thought also placed great significance on the role of experience in developing knowledge and the practicality of theories and concepts (Nekrasas, 2001). William James (1907) himself stated that pragmatism shared with positivism "its disdain for verbal solutions, useless questions and metaphysical abstractions" (p. 21). The credo of the Metaphysical Club, *How to Make Our Ideas Clear*, was prepared by Peirce (1876) with the intent of including positivist concepts that were highly influential in the 1870s.

Ernst Mach was a progenitor of the Vienna Circle, where logical positivism arose (Frank, 1938). He represented one of the critical characteristics of positivism in that he advocated for "the unification of science and the elimination of metaphysics" (Frank, 1938, p. 250). Mach was a fervent empiricist whose ideas were very influential in the late 1800s, and as one of the "seminal figures in the shaping of the modern world view . . . [h]is work came to be read, debated and used not only by physicists but also by major thinkers in mathematics, logic, biology, physiology, psychology, economics . . . and education" (Holton, 1992, p. 29). Mach's work was especially salient in the United States, even among laypeople (Blackmore, 1973; Holton, 1992). Paul Carus and the pragmatist philosopher William James were the two most prominent popularizers of Mach in America (Holton, 1992). An "amateur philosopher and indefatigable author who sought to develop an agnostic, monistic, and evolutionist world view" (Holton, 1992, p. 30), Carus was also editor of the intellectual journals *Open Court* and *The Monist*, as well as leader of the Open Court Publishing Company, all of which became avenues for wide dissemination of Mach's ideas in English translation. James viewed Mach as a kindred empiricist and first visited him in Prague in 1882, initiating a professional correspondence that would continue until James's death in 1910 (Holton, 1992). It is no coincidence, then, that Machian positivism and pragmatism (and later, behaviorist psychology) share the same anti-metaphysical stance and proclivities toward empiricism and experiential phenomena.

A positivist paradigm of science defined most scholars and professions during the Progressive Era, most critically medicine, with which occupational therapy aligned itself early in its existence (Andersen & Reed, 2017; Hilton & Southgate, 2007). With the influences—both scholarly and mainstream—of Comte, Mill, Wright, Mach, and others, positivism became well-known and enthusiastically accepted in the United

States during the Progressive Era, hailed as a scientific path forward in a contemporary society where traditional metaphysical philosophy was no longer the answer to the advanced problems of the Industrial Age. Thus, positivism and its associated characteristics and variations (reductionism, empiricism) defined modern medicine and guided the development of fledgling disciplines and professions such as psychology, social work, and occupational therapy.

CHRISTIAN SOCIALISM AND THE
SPIRIT OF PROGRESSIVE REFORM

Karl Marx and Friedrich Engels introduced the term "utopian socialism" in their seminal work *The Communist Manifesto* (1848/2002), where they distinguished it from the scientific socialism they proposed. Marx and Engels noted the influence of early utopian socialists such as Henri de Saint-Simon, Charles Fourier, and Robert Owen in the development of their socioeconomic philosophy. While acknowledging these utopian socialist thinkers, Marx and Engel were critical of that version of socialism, deeming it naïve, too focused on the leadership of the elite and lacking in the radical action required to resolve the struggle between the working and owning classes. Utopian socialism (specifically the versions championed by Fourier and Owen) was exported to the United States in the early to mid-19th century (Sargent, 2010). While varying in significant ways, these two perspectives shared many ideas and aims, among them using science to address modern class conflict through social progress, establishing a "religion of humanity" (as influenced by Comte's later positivism), and emphasizing a novel outlook on a collective social bond that was critical of individualism (Picon, 2003).

Mainly through the progressive ideas and experimental communities of Fourier (Brook Farm, Massachusetts) and Owen (New Harmony, Indiana), utopian socialism secured a broad influence in American lives and minds (especially in the intellectual and reform core of the Northeastern United States). However, this influence was not limited to academics and scientists: works such as Edward Bellamy's (1888/2007) *Looking Backward* were wildly popular with the public and thus entered the consciousness of mainstream American thought. A proliferation of muckrakers soon followed, as the people demanded to be informed of hidden agendas, business monopolies, and poor working conditions. Muckrakers often had immigrant origins and championed social reform as members of the "popular press and the socially conscious elements of the U.S. literary establishment" (Kaminsky, 1992, p. 190). Though they did not often explicitly advocate utopian socialism, muckrakers played a significant role in exposing the corruption and lack of attention to worrisome social issues such as industrialization, child labor, immigration, education, and basic human rights. Combined with an existing sense of moral improvement held by the Unitarians and other denominations, social reform became the phenomenon that gave the Progressive Era its name. Thus, a wide stratum of American society—from intellectuals to factory workers—was very aware of the troubles of modern society, and religious leaders were no exception. They tethered social reform to a growing Protestantism, driving the expansion of a Christian national identity that combined religion with science, politics, and a socially aware humanism that approached problems from a perspective most Americans understood and supported.

In the Progressive Era United States, utopian socialism was most clearly represented by a specific offshoot known as Christian socialism, and the accompanying movement referred to as the Social Gospel. Bliss (1890) defined Christian socialism as "Christianity applied to Social Order" (p. 15), where "we must apply the Sermon on the Mount, the spirit of the cross to the construction of society" (p. 14). Bliss (1890) went on to explicitly state what Christian socialism is *not*:

> Much so called socialism is vague, negative, denunciatory. This is not the case with Christian socialism. It sees gigantic evils in the present conditions of society, but it believes that the best way, and the scientific way, to overcome those evils is not by denunciation and destruction, but by gradual reform and by construction. Christian socialists believe in progress. (p. 4)

Similarly, the movement directly inspired by Christian socialism, the Social Gospel, stated its goals as "the application of the teaching of Jesus and the total message of Christian salvation to society, the economic life, and social institutions . . . as well as to individuals" (Mathews, 1921, p. 416). Evans (2017) identifies the Social Gospel as "an offshoot of theological liberalism that strove to apply a progressive theological vision to engage American social, political, and economic structures" (p. 2).

Bliss's and Mathews's narratives display an important overall theme, namely the complementary nature of positivist science, secular reform, scholarly philosophy, and Social Gospel. Members of these constituent groups held a classic Progressive Era vision of progress and possibility in a new age and viewed other lines of thought as partners, rather than ideological rivals, in achieving that goal. A second theme arising here is Christian socialism: a philosophical perspective that not only bridged religious and secular concerns but also spawned a movement which "can be best understood as a more or less continuous attempt by American Protestantism to Christianize America first through revivalism and then through the social gospel" (White & Hopkins, 1976, p. xiv).

In America (initially in the Northeast), Christian socialism grew steadily in presence and power throughout the 1870s and 1880s with the founding in Boston of the Christian Labor Union and the Society of Christian Socialists, led by W. D. P. Bliss (Morgan, 1969). Nationally, Christian socialism spread through various channels, including numerous periodicals with extensive subscriber lists, such as *The Dawn, Equity, The Kingdom, The Social Gospel, Social Service, Social Progress,* and the Christian Social Union's *Bulletin.* The Social Gospel was also widely disseminated through traveling national lecturers and a summer institute at Lake Chautauqua in Western New York state (White & Hopkins, 1976). Throughout the 1890s, a who's-who of Christian socialist leaders, politicians, and reformers appeared at or wrote textbooks for Chautauqua study courses, including Washington Gladden, Theodore Roosevelt, Graham Taylor, Jacob Riis, Josiah Strong, and Jane Addams (White & Hopkins, 1976). White and Hopkins (1976) noted that Graham Taylor, a friend of Jane Addams, and eventually a national Social Gospeler, founded the first professorship of Christian Sociology at the Chicago Theological Seminary in 1892, and followed this by establishing Chicago Commons, an affiliated settlement house, in 1894. By securing traction in academia, Christian socialism gained both legitimacy and publicity. The Social Gospel movement gained further momentum after the turn of the 20th century, and by 1908, most mainline Protestant denominations had signed the *Social Creed of the Churches*, a collection of 11 principles which reflected the essence of the Social Gospel's merger of faith, advocacy, and reform (Gorrell, 1988).

Christian socialism (and, by association, the Social Gospel) was a sizeable socio-intellectual phenomenon that attracted many proponents, including Jane Addams, W. D. P. Bliss, Washington Gladden, Francis Peabody, Walter Rauschenbusch, and Josiah Strong. For purposes of this section, we briefly focus on the thought and work of occupational therapy founder Jane Addams as an exemplar of how the Christian socialist paradigm, as informed by science, was enacted in real reform. Primarily portrayed as a social worker, settlement house founder, and early pragmatist philosopher, Addams as reformer addressed many of the same issues as Social Gospelers such as Washington Gladden and Walter Rauschenbusch (Villadsen, 2018). Perhaps less explored is Addams's "new social ethics," which called for a shift from the American ideal of individualism "towards a society based on cooperation and fellowship" (Villadsen, 2018, p. 224). This ethical perspective displayed a Christian humanitarianism not conspicuous in her more philosophical writings. Thyer (2008) notes that a biography of Addams states that "Positivism, the outgrowth of the speculation of Auguste Comte, had begun to interest her; she saw in it a connection between the democracy she loved and the Christianity she longed to understand" (Linn, 1935, p. 77). For Addams (1912), the church did not grant redemption, which was instead constructed through meaningful activities that imparted the skills necessary for daily living in a humanistic democracy: "Christianity must seek a simple and natural expression in the social organism itself" (p. 228). Agnew (2004) framed Addams's approach as "an effort to resuscitate the New Testament notion of caritas, or love, and do away with charity in its debased and familiar form of almsgiving" (p. 73). Thus, Addams is perhaps the archetype for Progressive Era reform with her combined use of the humanism of the transcendentalists, pragmatism, positivism, and Christian socialism to address the ills of modern society.

Advocates of the Social Gospel were more than comfortable with the pairing of science and religion in the name of social reform. Indeed, Harp (1991) suggested that "positivism legitimized science without destroying religious fervor or traditional morality. Also, it provided a scientific answer to the 'social question' that sounded both orderly and humane" (p. 519). They were assisted in this endeavor by a group of intellectuals in the Northeast, which included John Fiske and Francis Ellingwood Abbot, among others (Pearce, 2015). John Fiske, a historian, philosopher, and colleague of members of the Metaphysical Club, was a vocal supporter of a broad interpretation of positivism and the major popularizer of the utilitarian ideas of Herbert Spencer (Pearce, 2015). Fiske also played a prominent role in fusing positivism and theology (Cashdollar, 1989), and he "early dedicated himself to the task of reconciling evolution with orthodox Christianity" (Commager, 1941, p. 334). Morgan (1969) notes that Fiske had shown that "there was no necessary contradiction between the teachings of the new science and the idea of the creative God" (p. 48). In 1868, a group of Comtists formed the First Positivist Society of New York, comprised mostly of comfortably middle-class professionals, as was typical of reformers during the Progressive Era (Harp, 1991). Fiske was an occasional participant in that society and helped bring a theological element into their discussions. Fiske thereby united both sides of the science-religion divide and made them allies in the Progressive reform movement. Similarly, Abbot, a member of the Metaphysical Club, wanted to refashion both philosophy and theology (as "spiritual science") into a positivist framework (Pearce, 2015).

Christian socialism and the Social Gospel movement were key catalysts for reform in the Progressive Era. Their partnership (either implied or very real in many circumstances) with positivist science, pragmatism, and the humanist elements of transcendentalism made for a potent force that was accepted and utilized by all sectors of American society to address the troubles of a modern, urbanized, and industrialized age. The history of occupational therapy has not explicitly focused on the role of theological liberalism in the origins and early growth of the profession, but it is apparent that this type of thought, as manifested through the Social Gospel, was a facilitator on the sociopolitical level and a source of inspiration and action for many of the founders.

CONCLUSION

The period from the late 19th to the early 20th century was a time of significant upheaval in all aspects of American society. Occupational therapy was one of the many professions (social work, clinical psychology, and others) that developed largely in response to the needs of this newly industrialized and urbanized society. In March 1917, the founders established the National Society for the Promotion of Occupational Therapy at a meeting in Clifton Springs, New York (Andersen & Reed, 2017). The founders came from a variety of disciplines, including architecture, medicine, psychiatry, social work, and nursing. Despite these disparate areas of expertise, they were all drawn together in a time and place where American thought was thoroughly immersed in an intricate miscellany of philosophical influences that merged science, social conscience, efficiency, ethics, and religion. The often-contradictory forces of social reform and professional legitimacy created an art-science dichotomy, the intricate dynamics of which have been both an inspiration and a challenge for occupational therapy since its inception (Hooper & Wood, 2002). The tension between art and science has existed for a century because, although we wholeheartedly believe in the art and potentiality of occupational engagement as a means and end to well-being, we have not always been very successful in enacting that art in the context of health care systems based upon reductionist science. Given this sophisticated professional contrast, the philosophical context of the Progressive Era in the United States that forged the development of occupational therapy must be acknowledged as multifaceted, and cannot be distilled into Deweyan pragmatism alone (Kuklick, 2001). In this chapter, we have proposed that the socio-intellectual movements that influenced the birth of occupational therapy were directly informed by at least four major strands of philosophy that permeated American thought and reform efforts at the time: transcendentalism, classic pragmatism, positivism, and Christian socialism. Although the founders made no explicit mention of specific philosophies as drivers for originating occupational therapy, history suggests that certain schools of philosophy were deeply entrenched in the thought of American scholars, reformers, muckrakers, and the general public. Jane Addams, in particular, is documented to have had impactful encounters and partnerships with both positivist and Christian socialist thinkers and reformers (Thyer, 2008; Villadsen, 2018; White & Hopkins, 1976). We also know that, in the Northeast, where occupational therapy originated, the paths of positivists, latter-day transcendentalists, Social Gospelers, and pragmatists often crossed, so the core ideas that were held in common were therefore most certainly known to the founders. Although some of those influences have faded over the past century, the pull of both pragmatism and positivism (framed as varieties of post-analytic realism) remains strong in the profession, particularly in North America. Simultaneously, however, the global development of occupational therapy has brought alternative, refreshing, and varied philosophical perspectives to light, enriching and adding to the complexity of what education, research, and practice look like in response to local needs and the new challenges of 21st-century living.

REFERENCES

Addams, J. (1912). *The Christian register*. Cornell University Press.

Agnew, E. N. (2004). *From charity to social work: Mary E. Richmond and the creation of an American profession*. University of Illinois Press.

Andersen, L. T., & Reed, K. L. (2017). *The history of occupational therapy: The first century*. SLACK Incorporated.

Bellamy, E. (2007). *Looking backward: 2000–1887*. Oxford University Press. (Original work published 1888).

Blackmore, J. (1973). *Ernst Mach: His life, work and influence*. University of California Press.

Bliss, W. D. P. (1890). *What is Christian socialism?* Wildside Press.

Bockoven, J. S. (1971). Occupational therapy—a historical perspective: Legacy of moral treatment, 1800s to 1910. *American Journal of Occupational Therapy, 25*, 223–225.

Breines, E. (1986). *Origins and adaptations: A philosophy of practice*. Geri-Rehab.

Breines, E. (1987). Pragmatism as a foundation for occupational therapy curricula. *American Journal of Occupational Therapy, 41*(8), 522–525. https://doi.org/10.5014/ajot.41.8.522

Cashdollar, C. D. (1989). *The transformation of theology, 1830–1890: Positivism and Protestant thought in Britain and America*. Princeton University Press.

Cohen, S. (1983). The mental hygiene movement; the development of personality and the school: The medicalization of American education. *History of Education Quarterly, 23*(2), 123–149. https://doi.org/10.2307/368156

Commager, H. S. (1941). John Fiske: An interpretation. *Proceedings of the Massachusetts Historical Society, 66*, 332–345.

Cutchin, M. P. (2004). Using Deweyan philosophy to rename and reframe adaptation-to-environment. *American Journal of Occupational Therapy, 58*(3), 303–312. https://doi.org/10.5014/ajot.58.3.303

Dewey, J. (1903). Emerson—The philosopher of democracy. *The International Journal of Ethics, 13*(4), 405–413. https://doi.org/10.1086/intejethi.13.4.2376270

Diner, S. J. (1998). *A very different age: Americans of the Progressive Era*. Hill and Wang.

Emerson, R. W. (1995). *Emerson's antislavery writings*. (J. Myerson & L. Gougeon, Eds.). Yale University Press.

Evans, C. H. (2017). *The social gospel in American religion: A history*. New York University Press.

Fillafer, F. L., Feichtinger, J., & Surman, J. (2018). Introduction: Particularizing positivism. In F. L. Fillafer, J. Feichtinger, & J. Surman (Eds.), *The worlds of positivism: A global intellectual history, 1770–1930* (pp. 1–27). Palgrave Macmillan.

Frank, P. (1938). Ernst Mach: The centenary of his birth. *Erkenntnis, 7*, 247–256.

Fuller, M. (1998). *Woman in the nineteenth century* (L. J. Reynolds, Ed.). W. W. Norton and Co.

Goodman, R. B. (Ed.). (1995). *Pragmatism: A contemporary reader.* Routledge.

Goodman, R. (2019). *Transcendentalism.* In E. N. Zalta (Ed.), *The Stanford encyclopedia of philosophy* (Winter 2019 ed.). https://plato.stanford.edu/entries/transcendentalism

Gorrell, D. K. (1988). *The age of social responsibility: The social gospel in the Progressive Era, 1900–1920.* Mercer University Press.

Gura, P. H. (2007). *American transcendentalism: A history.* Hill and Wang.

Hall, G. S. (1879). Philosophy in the United States. *Mind, 4*(13), 89–105.

Hamilton, W. (1852). *Discussions on philosophy and literature, education and university reform.* Longman, Brown, Green and Longmans.

Harp, G. J. (1991). "The church of humanity": New York's worshipping positivists. *Church History, 60* (4), 508–523. https://doi.org/10.2307/3169031

Hilton, S., & Southgate, L. (2007). Professionalism in medical education. *Teaching and Teacher Education, 23*, 265–279. https://doi.org/10.1016/j.tate.2006.12.024

Hofstadter, R. (1955). *The age of reform.* Vintage Books.

Holton, G. (1992). Ernst Mach and the fortunes of positivism in America. *Isis, 83*(1), 27–60. http://nrs.harvard.edu/urn-3:HUL.InstRepos:37903228

Honderich, T. (Ed.). (2005). *The Oxford companion to philosophy.* Oxford University Press.

Hooper, B., & Wood, W. (2002). Pragmatism and structuralism in occupational therapy: The long conversation. *American Journal of Occupational Therapy, 56*(1), 40–50. https://doi.org/10.5014/ajot.56.1.40

Hooper, B., & Wood, W. (2019). The philosophy of occupational therapy: A framework for practice. In B. Schell, G. Gillen, & M. Scaffa (Eds.), *Willard and Spackman's occupational therapy* (13th ed., pp. 35–46). Wolters Kluwer.

Ikiugu, M. N., & Schultz, S. (2006). An argument for pragmatism as a foundational philosophy of occupational therapy. *Canadian Journal of Occupational Therapy, 73*(2), 86–97. https://doi.org/10.2182/cjot.05.0009

James, W. (1890). *The principles of psychology* (Vol. 1). Henry Holt.

James, W. (1907). *Pragmatism: A new name for some old ways of thinking.* Harvard University Press.

James, W. (1909). *The meaning of truth.* Harvard University Press.

Kaminsky, J. S. (1992). A pre-history of educational philosophy in the United States: 1861 to 1914. *Harvard Educational Review, 62*(2), 179–198. https://doi.org/10.17763/haer.62.2.g387n7j15n70x180

Kuklick, B. (2001). *A history of philosophy in America, 1720–2000.* Oxford University Press.

Lenzer, G. (1998). *Auguste Comte and positivism.* Transaction.

Linn, J. W. (1935). *Jane Addams: A biography.* Appleton-Century.

Madden, E. H. (1953). Pragmatism, positivism, and Chauncey Wright. *Philosophy and Phenomenological Research, 14*(1), 62–71. https://doi.org/10.2307/2218263

Mathews, S. (1921). Social gospel. In S. Mathews & G. B. Smith (Eds.), *A dictionary of religion and ethics.* Kessinger.

Marx, K., & Engels, F. (2002). *The communist manifesto.* Penguin Classics. (Original work published 1848).

Menand, L. (2001). *The Metaphysical Club: A story of ideas in America.* Farrar, Straus and Giroux.

Mill, J. S. (1865). *Auguste Comte and positivism.* N. Trubner.

Mill, J. S. (1963). *Collected works of John Stuart Mill.* University of Toronto Press.

Morgan, J. G. (1969). The development of sociology and the social gospel in America. *Sociological Analysis, 30*(1), 42–53. https://doi.org/10.2307/3709933

Morrison, R. (2016). Pragmatist epistemology and Jane Addams: Fundamental concepts for the social paradigm of occupational therapy. *Occupational Therapy International, 23*, 295–304. https://doi.org/10.1002/oti.1430

Myerson, J. (Ed.). (2000). *Transcendentalism: A reader.* Oxford University Press.

Nekrasas, E. (2001). Pragmatism and positivism. *Problemos, 59,* 41–52.

Payne, W. R. (2015). *An introduction to philosophy.* Bellevue College, Creative Commons. https://commons.bellevuecollege.edu/wp-content/uploads/sites/125/2017/04/Intro-to-Phil-full-text.pdf

Pearce, T. (2015). "Science organized": Positivism and the Metaphysical Club, 1865–1875. *Journal of the History of Ideas, 76*(3), 441–465. https://doi.org/10.1353/jhi.2015.0025

Peirce, C. S. (1876). How to make our ideas clear. In P. Wiener (Ed.), *C. S. Peirce: Selected writings* (pp. 113–136). Dover.

Peirce, C. S. (1877). The fixation of belief. *Popular Science Monthly, 12,* 1–15.

Peirce, C. S. (1878). How to make our ideas clear. *Popular Science Monthly, 12,* 286–302.

Peirce, C. S. (1931). *Collected papers of Charles Sanders Peirce.* Harvard University Press.

Peloquin, S. M. (1989). Sustaining the art of practice in occupational therapy. *American Journal of Occupational Therapy, 43*(4), 219–226. https://doi.org/10.5014/ajot.43.4.219

Pickering, M. (1993). *Auguste Comte: An intellectual biography* (Vol. 1). Cambridge University Press.

Picon, A. (2003). Utopian socialism and social science. In T. M. Porter & D. Ross (Eds.), *The Cambridge history of science* (pp. 71–82). Cambridge University Press.

Quiroga, V. A. M. (1995). *Occupational therapy: The first 30 years, 1900–1930.* American Occupational Therapy Association.

Rodgers, D. (1982). In search of progressivism. *Reviews in American History, 10*(4), 113–132. https://doi.org/10.2307/2701822

Sargent, L. T. (2010). *Utopianism: A very short introduction.* Oxford University Press.

Scheffler, I. (1974). *Four pragmatists: A critical introduction to Peirce, James, Mead, and Dewey.* Routledge & Kegan Paul.

Schneider, H. W. (1946). *A history of American philosophy.* Columbia University Press.

Serrett, K. D. (1985). *Philosophical and historical roots of occupational therapy.* The Haworth Press.

Taff, S. D. (2005). *The phenomenology of the "backward" child: A history of school failure in progressive era America, 1890–1930* (Unpublished doctoral dissertation). University of Missouri-St. Louis, St. Louis, MO.

Thayer, J. B. (1878). *Letters of Chauncey Wright: With some account of his life.* John Wilson and Son.

Thoreau, H. D. (1973). *Reform papers.* (W. Glick Ed.). Princeton University Press.

Thoreau, H. D. (2004). *Walden.* (J. S. Cramer Ed.). Princeton University Press.

Thyer, B. A. (2008). The quest for evidence-based practice?: We are all positivists! *Research on Social Work Practice, 18*(4), 339–345. https://doi.org/10.1177/1049731507313998

Townsend, E., & Polatajko, H. (2013). *Enabling occupation II: Advancing an occupational therapy vision for health, well-being, & justice through occupations* (2nd ed.). CAOT.

Villadsen, K. (2018). Jane Addams' social vision: Revisiting the gospel of individualism and solidarity. *The American Sociologist, 49*(2), 218–241. https://doi.org/10.1007/s12108-018-9369-1

White, R. C., & Hopkins, C. H. (1976). *The social gospel: Religion and reform in changing America.* Temple University Press.

Wiebe, R. H. (1967). *The search for order, 1877–1920.* Hill and Wang.

Wood, W. (1995). Weaving the warp and weft of occupational therapy: An art and science for all times. *American Journal of Occupational Therapy, 49*(1), 44–50. https://doi.org/10.5014/ajot.49.1.44

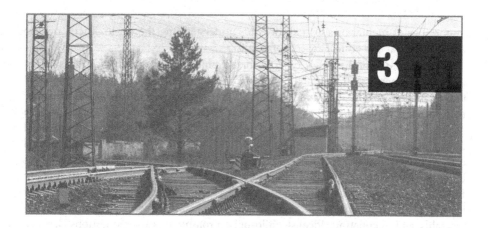

Focus on the Mental and Spiritual

Idealism and Occupational Therapy

Wanda J. Mahoney, PhD, OTR/L
Brad E. Egan, PhD, OTD, CADC, OTR/L

INTRODUCTION

When someone mentions idealism in a typical conversation, they are usually referring to extreme optimism and unrealistic consideration of ideal situations. Philosophical idealism is different from this. Philosophical idealism focuses on *ideas* rather than *ideals*.

Philosophy sets out to answer three major types of questions (Craig, 2002):

1. What is reality? (metaphysics or ontology)

2. How do we know? (epistemology)

3. What should we do? (ethics or axiology)

Idealism is most often considered a metaphysical, ontological philosophy; it describes what reality is. Idealism's answer to this question about reality is "ideas." The diverse ways of conceptualizing these ideas have changed over time; the key underpinning that categorizes a philosopher as an idealist is the emphasis on the

Taff, S. D. (Ed.). *Philosophy and Occupational Therapy:*
Informing Education, Research, and Practice (pp. 23-31).
© 2021 Taylor & Francis Group.

importance of mental or spiritual ideas for understanding the world. There are also epistemological and ethical aspects of idealism.

Idealism is one of the oldest types of formal philosophy. Idealism describes reality in terms of ideas with the mental or spiritual realm as primary. Because occupational therapy recognizes the dual and equal importance of the mental and physical, rather than focusing on the mental as primary, pure or true idealism is less consistent with occupational therapy. However, idealist philosophy was popular when occupational therapy began in the United States, and this classic Western philosophy likely informed early conceptualizations in the profession. One may certainly question the applicability of Plato, Kant, Hegel, and other idealist philosophers to occupational therapy. However, philosophy is a dialogue that builds on previous arguments. Exploring the ideas of these White, European, male philosophers can still enrich our understanding of reality and occupation. Idealist philosophy prompts us to ask questions that can deepen our understanding of occupation and inform occupational therapy.

IDEALISM: PHILOSOPHERS AND KEY CONCEPTS

Plato (427 BCE–347 BCE), the famous ancient Greek philosopher, is often cited as one of the earliest idealists, although his theory of ideas is quite different from those of modern idealist philosophers (Vesey, 1982). The "idea" that Plato emphasized was *forms*, universal ideas or characteristics that transcended experience. Plato viewed objects as imperfect representations of ideal forms, and the ultimate, most valued forms were beauty, truth, and goodness. Plato's explanation of the world and subsequent religious interpretations of it underpinned and dominated Western philosophy until the modern era, when other prominent idealists proposed new conceptualizations of the world. Although modern philosophers may have rejected Plato's views of forms, the emphasis on the mental rather than the physical to explain the world persisted, as did Plato's assertion that "the unexamined life is not worth living" (Plato, 1891/2008).

René Descartes (1596–1650) was a French mathematician and philosopher who initiated modern Western philosophy after centuries of Christianity-interpreted Platonic and Aristotelian thought (Burman, 2009). Rather than accepting church dogma as the starting point for knowledge, Descartes advocated doubt and the acceptance of something as truth only if one could be certain of it. He explained that sensation could be deceptive, reminding us that vivid dreams, for instance, could result in the perception of being awake and interacting with the world. He concluded that thought (reason) was a reality, and he started with his fundamental truth: "I think, therefore I am." (Descartes, 1637/2009, pt. 4). Descartes recognized the primacy of ideas as what is real. He did not deny the existence of matter; instead, he recognized both the interconnectedness and the distinctness of mind, body (matter), and God.

George Berkeley (1685–1753) was an Irish philosopher and Anglican cleric. He recognized the primacy of spirit (perceiver) and ideas (perception) as reality, describing matter only in terms of perceptions (Berkeley, 1710/2009). He attempted to reconcile scientific ideas with religious ideas and saw God as the universal connection of human spirits. Berkeley asserted that mental ideas are the only reality, and that the existence of objects outside of conceptual perception was impossible because that existence is dependent upon one having a mental conception of an object. This immaterialism is the main critique of his philosophy that led subsequent idealist philosophers to distance themselves from Berkeley's philosophy (Hoernlé, 1927).

Immanuel Kant (1724–1804) was a German philosopher whose ideas on the relationship between mind and matter continue to influence the writings and ideas of many contemporary philosophers (Bayne, 1994). Kant founded transcendental idealism, which distinguishes experience as separate from reality. His most famous writing, *Critique of Pure Reason*, explored the difference between things of the outside world and actions of the mind (Kant, 1787/1998). Kant's epistemological idealism recognized that things that exist in the world are indeed "real"; nevertheless, the human mind is needed to provide order and explain the relationships among the experience, things in the world, and their spatial and temporal components. For example, a person is only able to see a few walls of a house at any given moment, yet the mind mentally builds a complete house. That is, although one can only see part of a whole, the mind can create the whole. Thus, Kant reasoned that we only know what we can initially gather through our senses, and pure reason requires some reference to the outside world. Sensory experiences provide the mind with content that is actively formed into a system of knowledge through the mind's innate ways of working.

Georg Wilhelm Friedrich Hegel (1770–1831) was a German idealist philosopher whose work is notorious for being difficult to understand (Craig, 2002; Inwood, 1982). The essence of his philosophy is that the mental or spiritual (*Geist*) is a reality (Hegel, 1807/1910). Hegel did not deny the existence of matter, but he considered matter subordinate to the mental and spiritual. In his view, an idea can exist only if something embodies it; the idea and the embodiment are versions of each other. He used a dialectical method of logic to explain the world. This dialectical method involves a cyclical process of recognizing thesis, antithesis, and synthesis, with each synthesis leading to a new thesis; he called this highly structured system "the idea." For example, a thesis may begin as existence or being which one can only understand by considering its opposite: non-existence or nothing (the antithesis). The synthesis concept that merges existence and non-existence is "becoming" (Hegel, 1892). Becoming—the spirit's movement toward self-awareness—is the purpose of reality and life, according to Hegel.

In Hegel's philosophy, the way for the spirit to achieve self-understanding is not by thinking or reflecting, but by doing something (Craig, 2002; Inwood, 1982). The way to learn about oneself is to produce something and then reflect on the product that one created. Although the connections between Hegel's philosophy and occupational therapy may appear evident from this example, there is one component of his system that can make direct application difficult. Hegel negates the importance of any individual mind or spirit; in his philosophy, the reality is the process of the idea, spirit, or *Geist* working toward self-consciousness. The individual is not real; each person is part of the process of a vast idea seeking to understand itself and its significance.

Francis Herbert (F. H.) Bradley (1846–1924) was a British idealist who was highly influenced by the works of Hegel. F. H. Bradley's philosophy similarly argues that there is one ultimately real thing, the Absolute, which has a spiritual, not material, nature (absolute idealism). Absolute idealists recognize that perceptions and laws of nature are unable to fully explain the connectedness of the world. Bradley's reflections address this issue by suggesting that the world is an expression of a single universal spirit of which each of us is a part. Bradley (1897) suggested that all "real" things must be abstractions from a single higher unity (*cosmic Nunc Stans*). Bradley explained the relationship between wholes and their parts by claiming that the relationship between them was mere appearance not grounded in reality. His stance makes it impossible to analyze an ordinary object based on its properties because an object is more than just its properties. The determination of what is real cannot simply be derived from distinguishing objects and properties (Nielsen, 1994). For example, sugar is more than white, sweet, and hard.

Idealism often involves the intertwining of philosophy and theology. Idealism contends that every individual is part of a larger collective spirit or greater life force, often named as God. This greater spirit is the source of individuals' search for personal understanding and self-identity (Velasquez, 2008). Individuals understand how the cosmos is ordered, their places within that system, and their overall purpose through experience, a subjective phenomenon that only the individual can discern (Velasquez, 2008).

Idealist Epistemology

Idealist philosophers endorse different epistemologies or ways of knowing. Plato and Descartes believed that knowledge was gained through intellect or reason rather than through the senses, because what one could sense was imperfect, incomplete, and misleading. Berkeley was an empiricist; he purported that the only way to know was through sensation and perception. Other idealist philosophers, such as Kant and Hegel, attempted to merge these divergent epistemologies, recognizing scientific laws of nature, thought, and personal experience as sources of knowledge.

Idealist Ethics

According to idealist ethical tenets, humans should consistently examine their lives, seek knowledge, and work to understand themselves. Additionally, Kant extensively wrote about ethics. Kant asserted that ethics are not situation-dependent; goodwill and duty are universal constructs (Hoernlé, 1927). However, individuals need to personally analyze what goodwill and duty are and construct their lives accordingly.

The consistent theme across these diverse ideas in idealism is the focus on the mental or spiritual realm, individual subjectivity, and the interconnectedness of humanity. These core principles of idealism are relevant to occupational therapy.

IMPACT ON UNDERSTANDING OF OCCUPATION AND OCCUPATIONAL ENGAGEMENT

Occupational therapy recognizes the importance of both physical and mental aspects of reality. Idealist philosophy requires prioritizing the mental aspects, which would likely be a source of contention in occupational therapy. Although occupational therapy is unlikely to incorporate idealism into its philosophy directly, idealism can deepen our understanding of the mental aspects of occupation and prompt questions about our practices to ensure that we do not minimize the importance of the mental or spiritual realm, subjectivity, or human interconnectedness.

Doing, Being, Belonging, Becoming

Occupational therapy practitioners focus on the observable elements of occupation, as this is essential for clinical documentation. However, this has the likely consequence of prioritizing physical occupations over mental occupations. Process skills provide an example of how occupational therapy practitioners attempt to make mental aspects of doing occupation observable; nevertheless, mental occupations, such as contemplation or learning, may be insufficiently represented in categorizations of occupation (American Occupational Therapy Association [AOTA], 2020).

One conceptualization that incorporates a more comprehensive view of occupation is that of doing, being, belonging, and becoming (Wilcock & Hocking, 2015). All of these have explicit mental components that connect with idealism. A key aspect of *being*, "contemplation about the self," is intricately connected with the mental and spiritual aspects of occupation (Wilcock & Hocking, 2015, p. 135). *Doing* explicitly includes internal, mental, and spiritual occupations in addition to observable, physical ones. This duality of doing has been present from the beginning of the profession, as reflected in the Credo: "That every human being should have both physical and mental occupation" (Dunton, 1919, p. 10). *Belonging* is an internal sense of connection with others that focuses on one's mental perceptions (Wilcock & Hocking, 2015). *Becoming* involves a process of self-actualization and is such a key concept in idealism that Hegel used becoming as the synthesis to understand existence. One could argue that the conceptualization of occupation as being, doing, belonging, and becoming prioritizes the mental realm in a way consistent with idealism. Three of the four ways occupation is conceptualized are mental. The fourth, doing, is both mental and physical, and physical doing leads to and enacts the mental being, belonging, and becoming. The arguments idealist philosophers have made about mental understanding of the world and how these link with our understanding of occupation could be used to inform the profession's assertion of the fundamental importance of occupation in the world.

Meaning and Purpose

Meaning and purpose are fundamental aspects of occupation; without them, occupation does not exist (AOTA, 2020). Occupations are considered to be distinct from other activities because they are personally meaningful and provide a sense of purpose to one's life. Because meaning and purpose are both mental phenomena, the necessity of meaning and purpose for occupation denotes the potential usefulness of idealism in exploring these mental ideas. Idealist philosophy provides a framework for distinguishing how meaning and purpose are derived from personally interpreted experiences of doing (mental), rather than merely from the physical performance of doing (physical). Such a stance allows for the prioritization of outcomes related to participation, engagement, and other factors that lead to a sense of meaning and purpose in life, rather than simply recognizing the physical performance of doing.

Holistic View of the Person

Occupational therapy was founded on the principles of holism, a view that describes people as complex beings with interconnected mind, body, and spirit (Quiroga, 1995). This holistic view supports occupation as a way to enable healing and engage the mind and spirit in addition to the body. Moreover, this holistic view necessitates that the occupational therapy process assess and address the mental, spiritual, and physical dimensions of clients and their performance. Valuing mind and spirit is consistent with idealism, and idealist philosophy may prompt us to ensure that we are not valuing the body/physical aspects over the mental and spiritual aspects of the person.

Mental and Physical Dualism

Idealist philosophy argues that the mind and body are not identical; in fact, Descartes proposed a dualism holding that the mind and spirit have a nonphysical nature which can be distinguished or "separated" in some categorical way from the body, which has a material or physical nature (Descartes, 1687/2009). Idealism holds that the truest understanding of the mind–body relationship lies in prioritizing how the mind affects the body and recognizing that matter is based on mental perception. Occupational therapy practitioners routinely consider how the mind influences the body and vice versa, yet generally reject prioritizing the mental over the physical. In fact, in his 2017 Slagle lecture, Smith (2017) addressed the metaphysical divide between the emotive (mental) and physical dimensions of reality and proposed a metaphysical physical-emotive theory of occupation. Rather than prioritizing one dimension over the other, Smith (2017) suggested that healthy participation in occupation is predicated on the two dimensions being balanced and working harmoniously with one another. The emotive is consistent with idealism; however, since both are essential, it is not an application of true idealism.

Communities of Individuals

Idealism does more than consider the primacy of mental or spiritual realms of individuals; it also recognizes the connectedness of individuals (Ozmon, 2011). Idealism postulates that the Absolute idea manifests as virtues, unity, and social consciousness, which is discerned through self-and social awareness (Hoernlé, 1927). This acknowledgment of the importance of social connections is consistent with occupational therapy's assessment of the social and cultural influences on performance, as well as its consideration of groups and populations as occupational therapy clients. Further, exploring the mental realm of communities could be a useful way to challenge how occupations can perpetuate unjust power dynamics that result in broad social issues related to occupational therapy, such as health access disparities, societal violence, and structural racism (Ramugondo, 2018). The pairing of this classic Western idealist philosophy with challenges to hegemonic social norms is unusual, though not unique, especially as it relates to examining social consciousness (Ozmon, 2011). Idealism may prompt questions and considerations related to internal mental subjectivity and interconnectedness that other philosophies do not.

Occupation: Idea and Experience

Occupational therapy differentiates between the "idea" of an occupation and the experience or performance of occupation in a way consistent with idealism. Pierce (2001) described this in terms of distinguishing activity (the idea) from occupation (the experience). Both are important for occupational therapy, and both have idealist philosophical underpinnings.

Making this distinction between the idea of occupation and the doing of occupation is important for activity analysis, an essential aspect of the occupational therapy process. Activity analysis involves analyzing how an occupation is typically performed and what is required; it involves breaking down the expected components of the *idea* of an occupation (AOTA, 2020; Schell et al., 2019). Occupational therapy practitioners use the mental process of activity analysis to determine the detailed requirements of an abstract idea of an activity. This analysis informs evaluation to determine occupational supports and barriers by comparing the abstract to the person's actual performance. Activity analysis also informs intervention through the selection of appropriate therapeutic activities whose abstract components are expected to elicit needed changes when performed.

The experience of doing occupation includes both objective, observable components of physical actions and subjective, mental experience. Occupational therapy practitioners value both, but we may not sufficiently stress or demonstrate the value of the mental experience of doing.

Subjective Perspective

Clients' subjective perspectives are of primary importance in guiding occupational therapy services and ensuring client-centered practice. The occupational therapy process starts with developing an occupational profile, narrative, or occupational formulation of clients' sense of their situations (AOTA, 2020; Bass et al., 2015; Forsyth, 2017). Consistent with idealist philosophy that identifies subjective thought and experience as reality, occupational therapy practitioners recognize that how a person perceives a situation can be more important than an outside description of the situation. Yerxa (1967) asserted that a goal of authentic occupational therapy is to examine and help change clients' perceptions of their environments and sense of self. Prompting such examination of one's life and changing internal views of situations may entail a foundation in idealist philosophy.

Although occupational therapy is unlikely to incorporate idealist philosophy wholly, idealism prompts questions that can deepen our understanding of occupation and challenge our practice. Idealism reminds us not to overemphasize the body at the expense of the mental and spiritual: to focus on the client's subjective experience, and to consider the spiritual and mental connectedness of individuals and communities. The following section synthesizes idealism and its connections to occupational therapy as key questions for education, research, and practice.

KEY IMPLICATIONS FOR OCCUPATIONAL THERAPY EDUCATION, RESEARCH, AND PRACTICE

Education

- How do we teach about mental occupations and being, belonging, and becoming?
- How do we teach about the mental and spiritual aspects of experience?

Research

- How do we study the mental and spiritual realms of doing, being, belonging, and becoming?
- How do we study mental occupations with populations who have cognitive impairments and may not be able to share their in-depth perspectives via traditional methods?

Practice

- To what extent do occupational therapy assessments and interventions adequately capture and influence the mental dimension of occupation?
- Do assessing and intervening to change clients' process skills sufficiently address mental doing?
- How do we document intervening to change mental occupations?

RECOMMENDED READINGS

Craig, E. (2002). *Philosophy: A very short introduction*. Oxford University Press.

Hoernlé, R. F. A. (1927). *Idealism as a philosophy*. George H. Doran.

Ozmon, H. A. (2011). Idealism and education. In H. A. Ozmon & S. M. Craver (Eds.), *Philosophical foundations of education* (9th ed., pp. 7–24). https://www.pearson-highered.com/assets/samplechapter/0/1/3/2/0132540746.pdf

REFERENCES

American Occupational Therapy Association (AOTA). (2020). Occupational therapy practice framework: Domain and process (4th ed.). *American Journal of Occupational Therapy, 74*, 7412410010. https://doi.org/10.5014/ajot.2020.74S2001

Bass, J. D., Baum, C. M., & Christiansen, C. H. (2015). Interventions and outcomes: The person-environment-occupation-performance (PEOP) occupational therapy process. In C. H. Christiansen, C. M. Baum, & J. D. Bass (Eds.), *Occupational therapy: Performance, participation, and well-being* (4th ed., pp. 57–79). SLACK Incorporated.

Bayne, S. (1994). Objects of representations and Kant's second analogy. *Journal of the History of Philosophy, 32*(3), 381–410. https://doi.org/10.1353/hph.1994.0059

Berkeley, G. (2009). A treatise concerning the principles of human knowledge. In A. Haines (Ed. & Trans.), *The project Gutenberg ebook of a treatise concerning the principles of human knowledge*. http://www.gutenberg.org/ebooks/4723 (Original work published 1710)

Bradley, F. H. (1897). *Appearance and reality*. http://krishnamurti.abundanthope.org/index_htm_files/Appearance-and-Reality-by-FH-Bradley.pdf

Burman, R. (2009). *Descartes: An introduction* [Audiobook]. Naxos.

Craig, E. (2002). *Philosophy: A very short introduction*. Oxford University Press.

Descartes, R. (2009). Discourse on the method of rightly conducting one's reason and of seeking truth in the sciences. In J. Veitch (Ed. & Trans.), *The project Gutenberg ebook of discourse on the method of rightly conducting one's reason and of seeking truth in the sciences*. https://www.gutenberg.org/ebooks/59 (Original work published 1687)

Dunton, W. R. (1919). *Reconstruction therapy*. W. B. Saunders.

Forsyth, K. (2017). Therapeutic reasoning: Planning, implementing, and evaluating the outcomes of therapy. In R. Taylor (Ed.), *Kielhofner's model of human occupation* (5th ed., pp. 159–172). Wolters Kluwer.

Hegel, G. W. F. (1892). The logic of Hegel. In W. Wallace (Ed. & Trans.), *The logic of Hegel*. https://www.gutenberg.org/ebooks/55108 (Original work published 1812)

Hegel, G. W. F. (1910). *Phenomenology of mind* (J. B. Baillie, Trans.). https://ia800504.us.archive.org/29/items/cu31924097557171/cu31924097557171.pdf (Original work published 1807)

Hoernlé, R. F. A. (1927). *Idealism as a philosophy*. George H. Doran.

Inwood, M. (1982). Hegel on action. In G. Vesey (Ed.), *Idealism: Past and present* (pp. 141–154). Cambridge University Press.

Kant, I. (1998). *Critique of Pure Reason* (P. Gyer & A. Wood, Trans.). http://strangebeautiful.com/other-texts/kant-first-critique-cambridge.pdf (Original work published 1787)

Nielsen, K. (1994). Jolting the career of reason: Absolute idealism and other rationalisms reconsidered. *Journal of Speculative Philosophy, 8*(2), 113–140. https://www.jstor.org/stable/25670101

Ozmon, H. A. (2011). Idealism and education. In H. A. Ozmon & S. M. Craver (Eds.), *Philosophical foundations of education* (9th ed., pp. 7–24). https://www.pearsonhighered.com/assets/samplechapter/0/1/3/2/0132540746.pdf

Pierce, D. (2001). Untangling occupation and activity. *American Journal of Occupational Therapy, 55*(2), 138–146. https://doi.org/10.5014/ajot.55.2.138

Plato. (2008). Apology. In B. Jowett (Ed. & Trans.), *The project Gutenberg ebook of apology*. https://www.gutenberg.org/ebooks/1656 (Original work published 1891)

Quiroga, V. (1995). *Occupational therapy: The first 30 years, 1900 to 1930*. American Occupational Therapy Association.

Ramugondo, E. L. (2018). Healing work: Intersections for decoloniality. *World Federation of Occupational Therapists Bulletin, 74*(2), 83–91. https://doi.org/10.1080/14473828.2018.1523981

Schell, B. A. B., Gillen, G., Crepeau, E. B., & Scaffa, M. E. (2019). Analyzing occupations and activity. In B. A. B. Schell & G. Gillen (Eds.), *Willard & Spackman's occupational therapy* (13th ed., pp. 320–334). Wolters Kluwer.

Smith, R. O. (2017). Technology and occupation: Past, present, and the next 100 years of theory and practice. *American Journal of Occupational Therapy, 71*, 7106150010p1–7106150010p14. https://doi.org/10.5014/ajot.2017.716003

Velasquez, M. (2008). *Philosophy: A text with readings* (13th ed.). Cengage Learning.

Vesey, G. (1982). Foreword: A history of "ideas." In G. Vesey (Ed.), *Idealism: Past and present* (pp. 1–18). Cambridge University Press.

Wilcock, A. A., & Hocking, C. (2015). *An occupational perspective of health* (3rd ed.). SLACK Incorporated.

Yerxa, E. J. (1967). 1966 Eleanor Clarke Slagle lecture: Authentic occupational therapy. *American Journal of Occupational Therapy, 21*(1), 1–9.

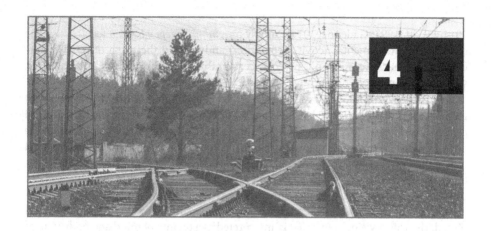

Realism

Exploring the Divide Between What Exists and What Humans Make of It

Jyothi Gupta, PhD, OTR/L, FAOTA
Bernard A. K. Muriithi, PhD, OTR/L

INTRODUCTION

Realism is one of the oldest forms of philosophy, dating back to Plato in 400 BCE. Its central tenet is that reality exists independent of the human mind; therefore, what we know at any point in time is only an approximation of true reality. Realist philosophers hold diverse views about realism, and there is no consensus regarding what specifically constitutes the philosophy. Regardless of the differences in perspectives, scholars do agree on two general aspects of realism: a claim about existence and a claim about mind-independence (A. Miller, 2016; C. Miller, 2002). The claim about existence or being relates to ontological questions and takes a stance on the need to acknowledge that there is a world, facts, or entities that exist. The second claim of mind-independence responds to epistemological questions and claims that the existence of the world, facts, or entities is not affected by our conceptual schemes such as theories, values, and language (Brock & Mares,

Taff, S. D. (Ed.). *Philosophy and Occupational Therapy:*
Informing Education, Research, and Practice (pp. 33-44).
© 2021 Taylor & Francis Group.

2014; Devitt, 1991; Gadenne, 2014). Simply put, *mind-independence* refers to existence outside of human mental activity (cognition) and beyond the reach of sensory perception. Just because we do not perceive certain things (e.g., black holes, dark matter, viruses, proteins) does not mean that they do not exist.

In his theory of knowledge, Plato described the world as a world of Forms and eternal truths. The world we live in is a world of becoming, and the unchanging and eternal "world of Forms" is the world of being. In this theory, beauty, for instance, is not a property of one particular entity, but a changeless and eternal reality exemplified in less than perfect ways in a particular entity (Hale, 2017). Plato believed in the existence of two worlds: (1) the unobservable spiritual or mental world, which is eternal, permanent, orderly, regular, and universal; and (2) the observable world as experienced through our senses of sight, touch, smell, taste, and sound that is imperfect and disorderly. This division is often (mis)interpreted as a duality of mind and body (Guyer & Horstmann, 2018). Plato's realism embraces *universals before things,* meaning that universals (characteristics, properties, attributes, and ideas) can exist in a free-standing manner independent of forms, objects, entities, or things that embody these attributes or ideas. An example is the notion that beauty can exist without a beautiful object. Plato's own student Aristotle broke away from this ideal, also known as "extreme realism," and instead supported a "moderate realism," which states the existence of *universals in things.* Universals are not free-standing, but can exist only in particular things that exemplify them (Hale, 2017). Aristotle would argue, for example, that beauty exists only when embodied in beautiful things. Aristotle, a biologist and physicist, saw metaphysics as the study of nature or physics (Solomon, 2008). Because he defined reality as only that which is perceptible by human senses, his form of metaphysics later inspired empiricism (Sgarbi, 2013).

Individuals choose when to accept or reject realism based on the nature of the reality examined (Brock & Mares, 2014; Williamson, 2005). Disagreements over a specified reality may relate to how we know the reality (epistemology). Thus, epistemological realism holds to the claim that we know the world as it is in itself; that is, what we know about reality is not simply the appearances of things, as Kant and neo-Kantians believe (Allison, 2004; Tegtmeier, 2014). Kant and other *idealists* hold that we know everything that exists because "nothing exists except minds and ideas in minds" (Brock & Mares, 2014, p. 48). Because an individual's mind is perceived as "a part of the greater mind: the mind of God" (Brock & Mares, 2014, p. 48), all reality is understood as known to the collective mind. Disagreements also arise over questions of existence, or ontology, though this is less contentious. Realists hold that being (ontology) and knowing (epistemology) are not the same. There is a possibility of reality being in existence that is as yet unknown. By arguing that nothing exists except minds and their ideas, antirealists have been described as wrongly subsuming ontology under epistemology (Brock & Mares, 2014). To conflate these two dimensions is, according to Bhaskar (1989), to commit the "epistemic fallacy." The great variations of perspectives about realism from antiquity to the present day make it impossible to do full justice to the subject in a single chapter. Hence, here we limit our focus to forms of realism that are of particular significance to the foundational disciplines of occupational therapy and those that bear relevance to the conceptual models that guide practice.

THE VARIETIES OF REALISM

Scientific realism endorses the belief in observable and unobservable realities that are amenable to inquiry through accepted scientific theories and models of a given point in time and to scientific experimentation (Psillos, 2018). Chakravartty (2017) distinguishes scientific realism when he states that "scientific realism is a positive epistemic attitude towards the content of our best theories and models, recommending belief in both observable and unobservable aspects of the world described by the sciences" (p. 1). Kuhn's (1962/2012) *The Structure of Scientific Revolutions* was seminal in articulating that scientific theories of what he called "normal science" evolve as scientific knowledge matures; rarely, a "revolutionary science" that is disruptive emerges, and a paradigm shift ensues. Consequently, our best scientific theories must be reconfigured to accommodate this new perspective. Such revolutions are exemplified in mature disciplines such as astronomy and physics, and include the 16th-century work of Copernicus, who revealed that the Earth revolves around the sun (not the other way around, as was the belief of the Church). Followers of Copernican theory, such as Galileo, were deemed heretics, and the rationalist philosopher Giordano Bruno was burned at the stake (Leveillee, 2011). In biology, a relatively young discipline compared to astronomy and physics, a period of normal science followed after Darwin's theory of evolution was presented, and was again disrupted when Watson and Crick revealed the double-helical structure of the DNA as the blueprint of life, which became the central paradigm of molecular biology (Bussard, 2005).

Chakravartty (2017) recommends first understanding the distinction between epistemic achievements and epistemic aims before unpacking scientific realism. *Epistemic achievement* refers to the epistemic status and belief that the best scientific theories give us the knowledge of certain aspects of the world in their approximately true form. *Epistemic aims* are the intentions of scientific inquiry, which are basically to describe and understand aspects of the world in its true or approximately true form using logic and scientific methods.

To fully understand realism in the context of science, and to distinguish it from the antirealist stance, it is helpful to contrast the metaphysical, semantic, and epistemological dimensions of realism (Chakravartty, 2017). The *metaphysical* dimension views the world and objects in the world, their properties and relations, as independent of our thought, perception, and scientific inquiry. Metaphysical realism is "a doctrine of what it is for such irreducible theoretical claims to be true, specifically that the concept of truth involves a primitive non-epistemic idea—for example, 'correspondence with reality'—not entirely captured" (Horwich, 2004, p. 8). How, then, can we use reductionist scientific methods of experimentation or investigation of the world and its objects if we cannot think about them or perceive them? Science takes us up to a point of understanding or grasping an approximate truth of reality that then must be subjected to metaphysical theorizing. Metaphysical realism is important and of critical historical significance. Neo-Kantian views contest the idea that knowable reality can be mind-independent. However, examples abound in theoretical physics (e.g., black holes, dark matter) to support the view that one can know and understand the abstract that our senses do not and cannot perceive.

Semantic realism refers to the literal interpretation of scientific claims, accepting unobservable scientific objects, entities, processes, and properties at face value. It is "the anti-reductionist, anti-verificationist, anti-instrumentalist view to the effect that claims about theoretical entities should be taken at 'face value'" (Horwich, 2004, p. 8). This commitment to literal meaning of unobservable entities is similar to instrumentalism's acceptance of the unobservable as a mere means to explain or validate the observable.

Epistemological realism (Horwich, 2004) is "the commonplace claim concerning some specified class of postulated entities that [such entities] really do exist" (p. 7). Epistemological realism accepts the idea of the literal interpretations or true value of theoretical understanding of mind-independent reality as knowledge of the world. For instance, the discipline of molecular biology is built on acceptance of the proposed double-helical structure of DNA as the true representation of the genetic blueprint of each organism.

Structural realism, introduced by Worrall, is "considered by both realists and anti-realists as the most defensible form of realism" (Ladyman, 2016, p. 1). It arose as a way to reconcile the contentions concerning (1) the fact that theories change in scientific realism (so why accept current scientific theories that will most likely be proven to be incorrect in the future) and (2) belief in the ability of scientific theories to accurately describe the unobservable in the absence of empirical evidence. A powerful counterargument for accepting scientific theories, while knowing that they change, is that some *a priori* assumptions and theoretical constructs have been proven correct by the rigorous scientific process. There is evidence that empirical data has been used to show that human beings can generate theories that correctly explain certain realities. Worrall opposes the anti-realists, but he also does not accept the premise of standard scientific realism that "the nature of unobservable objects that cause the phenomenon we observe is correctly described by our best theories" (as cited in Ladyman, 2016, p. 3). His epistemic commitment is only to "the mathematical or structural content of our theories" that is retained when theories change (as cited in Ladyman, 2016, p. 3). In other words, we accept the truth of the structural content of scientific theory without necessarily accepting that these theories accurately represent the true natures of unobserved entities. It is unclear if Worrall's version of structural realism is a "metaphysical or epistemological modification of standard scientific realism" (Ladyman, 2016, p. 3).

Like structural realism, *entity realism* commits to entities that are stable and remain unchanged regardless of scientific theories and their changes over time. Entity realism is therefore a form of scientific realism which states that causal interactions between unobservable entities—e.g., molecules—is sufficient for taking the existence of such entities at face value. Eronen (2017) cites Hacking and Cartwright as the originators of entity realism, which was "based on actual scientific practices of experimental manipulation and causal explanations" (p. 2342). Entity realism differs from scientific realism primarily in its skepticism about the truth of theories that postulate the existence of the unobservable. Eronen (2017) opines that although scientific realism is the default philosophy of the life sciences, it is at times discordant with the biological sciences. He has proposed a *robustness-based* version of entity realism that he claims is better suited for the practice of science. Entity realism is based on experimentation and explanations of causality and hence its application to life sciences is obvious. Entity realism based on robustness differs from its original doctrine in its holding that an entity is most likely to be real if validated by using multiple methods to measure and describe the entity and obtaining consistent results (Eronen, 2017). What all dimensions and forms of realism described so far have in common is a commitment to the epistemic status of our best theories as yielding knowledge of certain aspects of the observable and unobservable world.

The social sciences are foundational to occupational therapy, as humans live in society and engage in occupations in context of social structures, norms, roles, and laws. Kincaid (2008) makes a case for structural realism in the social sciences with regard to social structures and structural relations that can be preserved across diverse social science theories. Social structures look at microphenomena and macrophenomena in society where structural relationships are never between individuals, but instead reside in the relationships between social status, position, or roles. According to Kincaid (2008), "social structures relates organizations, classes, groups, practices and so forth without any explicit reference to individuals" (p. 723). The practice of causal modeling in the social sciences—for example, the idea of supply and demand, and in equilibrium explanations of phenomena that depict the consistency of a set of variables—is also amenable to structural realism. In a dynamic social system, typically various components interact in a manner that gravitates toward equilibrium. For instance, a fundamental concept in evolutionary biology is the necessity for a certain male-to-female sex ratio for the survival of a species. The sex ratio influences aggression, courtship behavior, and parental care of progeny; more recently, experiments have revealed that human economic behaviors are influenced by sex ratio (Székely & Székely, 2012).

Constructive realism argues that all realities that are constructed are real and claims that considering mind-independent entities alone causes one to lose or miss important realities about human experience (Jansen, 2017; Wallner, 2016). Constructive realism opposes rationalism and its proponents, such as Plato and Augustine, who argue that reality is independent from the human mind. Many constructivists do not see their work as opposed to realism but as evidence of it (Jansen, 2017). Ethnicity, social status, groups, and roles, for example, exist as socially constructed realities. The argument that socially constructed reality is not real is thus perceived by constructivists as logically invalid.

Anderson's *situational realism* is concerned with features of reality (ontology) more than with epistemology, human inquiry, or linguistic analysis (Hibberd, 2009). As Hibberd (2009) puts it, situational realism is "one of process—the world is something continuously changing and infinitely complex, one that moves through 'cycles' or alternating phases—Heraclitus' 'ex-changes'—such as day and night, waking and sleeping, utilitarianism and classicism, conservatism and liberalism" (p. 67). *Existence* is defined as situations and occurrences in time and space; situations are historical, changing and complex, distinct but connected. Individuals are historical, contextualized, and cannot be seen as outside of society.

Situational realism is a nonreductionist alternative to disciplines that study organism–environment relations and dynamic interactions, such as ecology or psychology (Petocz & Mackay, 2013). It is a dynamic systems approach to realism that sees reality as a collection of infinite and complex situations that are historically and contextually embedded. Traditional dualisms such as mind/body, matter/spirit, free/

determined, or universal/particular are irrelevant. Although antecedent conditions give rise to situations, the process goes beyond a linear cause-and-effect relationship. Causality is tripartite, consisting of cause, causal field or conditions, and effect (Petocz & Mackay, 2013).

The British philosopher Roy Bhaskar introduced the idea that social sciences, like the physical sciences, can produce distinct and valid knowledge (Frauley & Pearce, 2007). Bhaskar's *critical realism* is an ontological realism concerned with the natural world as well as the social world, and hold that reality exists at different levels such as biological, psychological, social, and cultural levels. It is a philosophy based on the existence of real social structures and systems that are entities which operate independently of mind but are dependent on human activity to exist and transform (Wikgren, 2005). The basic tenets of critical realism are (1) that social reality exists independent of our knowledge or awareness, and systemic inequalities, though real, are always mediated through "perceptual filters"; hence, our knowledge is imperfect and will undergo revision. (2) Social objects exist in a stratified reality, and arise from complex intersections of material and discursive relations. (3) Unobservable features of social life can be understood to some extent, and must be revealed to explain existence, reproduction, and transformation of empirically captured social phenomenon. Power and privilege, for instance, affect class privilege, racial inequities, oppression, and exploitation that are social and occupational injustices. (4) All human action is situated in a context and social structure which exists prior to social action. Social structures create social institutions such as marriage, family, religion, and the like that are long-lasting or transient; they can enable or constrain actions (Frauley & Pearce, 2007).

Critical realism distinguishes between a reality independent of what we think of it (the intransitive dimension) and our thinking of it (the transitive dimension). To believe that "what we think is all what is" is, according to Bhaskar (1989), to commit the "epistemic fallacy." We will only be able to understand—and so change—the social world if we identify the structures at work that generate those events and discourses. Critical realism focuses on social reality as consisting of social structures that exist "independently of the various ways in which they can be discursively constructed and interpreted by social scientists and other social actors located in a wide range of sociohistorical situations" (Reed, 2001, p. 214). Describing Bhaskar's transformational model of social action, Harvey (2002) notes that society does not directly create humans any more than humans directly create society. An important assumption is that society can effectively socialize people *if* a multitude of social relations is already in place. Although all social phenomena are dependent on human action, action nonetheless requires structures.

THE OBJECTIVE OF REALISM

Over millennia, realism has sought to inspire a quest for truth about the existence and nature of things. Ancient philosophy saw science as part of philosophy, the one discipline that sought to understand reality and truth about our world. But as science matured, it gradually departed from philosophy and came to be viewed as a different field, particularly as logical positivism increased the need for concrete science, leading to increased rejection of metaphysical speculation (Solomon, 2008). Scientific methods were for a while perceived as the only reliable forms of inquiry into objective reality. However, the claim that reality can be revealed solely through science is now questioned, and thus a return to metaphysics is recommended in our day. Ellis (2014) expresses this concern:

> For science is limited in what it can tell us about reality. What is needed, it will be argued, is not more science, but the progressive development of higher and higher levels of explanation of the world that is revealed to us by science. For the aims of metaphysics are different from those of science, and the structures of metaphysical explanations are different from those of scientific explanations. Metaphysical explanations all proceed from the premise that truth supervenes on being. (p. 7)

IMPACT ON UNDERSTANDING OF OCCUPATION AND OCCUPATIONAL ENGAGEMENT

Are occupations and occupational performance things that exist in themselves or things that we socially or individually construct in our minds? Realism challenges us to reflect on this question. One who takes an anti-realist position describes occupation and occupational performance as subjective, nonrepeatable, and personally constructed experience (Frauley & Pearce, 2007). Yerxa et al. (1989) also takes an anti-realist (constructivist) stance in defining occupation as "specific chunks of activity within the ongoing stream of human behavior which are names in the lexicon of the culture" (p. 5). Yerxa's definition makes the reality of occupation dependent on language and culture, which thus makes it mind-dependent. But Nelson (1988) perceived occupation as something out there that structures human experience. He evokes memory of Plato's theory of forms by defining what he terms *occupational form* as the "preexisting structure that guides, or structures subsequent human experience" (p. 633). If we choose to embrace occupation as something out there (independently existing) that structures human experience, we become realists. If we choose, as is often the case, to identify occupation as a thing that is dependent on human schemes such as theory, language, and/or culture, we become anti-realists.

Realism argues that understanding humans as occupational beings using purely scientific approaches will reveal only partial truth. This is because current scientific methods reduce occupations to aspects that can be studied using scientific methods which are limited in what they can reveal about truth, whereas human experience of occupation and performance is an amalgamation of doing, feeling, and valuing that requires more than what the scientific methods, taken in total, can reveal about reality. Nevertheless, science provides essential facts which, when seen in conjunction with other known realities, can provide hints regarding even some unknown but related phenomena. Having more factual information regarding related phenomena facilitates informed metaphysical reflections which can enable *a priori* creation of theory, and theories created through metaphysical reflections can generate new hypotheses and support science.

A founding philosophy of occupational therapy was American pragmatism, originated by Charles Sanders Peirce and then popularized by William James, John Dewey, and others (Breines, 1986; Cutchin, 2004; Ikiugu & Schultz, 2006). Pragmatism developed to disprove the use of authority in justifying speculative propositions (Ikiugu, 2007); in other words, pragmatism was a repudiation of Plato's form of realism. It is not surprising, then, that a vast majority of current definitions of *occupation* reflect anti-realism. Many anti-realists, however, including constructive realists, reject this label and consider themselves realists who define realism differently. Overall, the pragmatism that grounds American occupational therapy appears incongruent with realism, as "pragmatism emphasizes usefulness as opposed to truthfulness" (Gupta, 2015, p. 64); it is skeptical about a realist view of knowledge founded on science and logic, and the belief that the "only support available for our knowledge claims is common human agreement among those who seek it" (Gill, 2013, p. 369). This has far-reaching implications for occupational therapy. For instance, the evidence-based practice pyramid ranks research methods, and a realist will contend that evidence from methods at the top of the pyramid are closer to truth. A pragmatist view "is that any one kind of knowledge, such as that offered by [the evidence pyramid], is not necessarily the most useful in responding to all clinical questions" (Gupta, 2015, p. 64). Occupational performance is usually explained as motivated by meaning and purpose: subjective concepts understood and accepted in occupational therapy as dependent on individual and cultural dispositions. This, perhaps, is the basis for the dissonance that pragmatist practitioners experience in the realist world of medicine.

Are there ways in which realism can inform occupation and occupational performance today? There are ways in which speculative propositions can sharpen our understanding and facilitate creation of theories. Such speculative theories can become the basis for scientific testing or experimentation. However, we posit that even greater insight will result not simply from subjecting speculative theory to scientific testing, but from subjecting scientific findings to metaphysical analysis to determine if scientific findings reflect the real world they seek to explain or discover. It seems clear that integrating both scientific and metaphysical methods would facilitate deeper understanding of the reality of occupation. The risk of embracing metaphysical methods is that occupational scientists may appear unscientific at a time when the discipline seeks to establish itself as a valid science. It is our stance that the integration of science and philosophy will yield the greatest advancements in authentically meeting the world's occupational needs.

KEY IMPLICATIONS FOR OCCUPATIONAL THERAPY EDUCATION, RESEARCH, AND PRACTICE

Education

- Realism considers knowable aspects of the world as the content to be learned. The focus for instruction is realities believed to be known or knowable, including the things we may not presently know but are speculating about or seeking to know using theories. These may be observable or unobservable realities. Educators in general believe that truth is acquired through logic and scientific methods. Therefore, occupational therapy education must aim to develop curiosity and build capacity for logical and scientific inquiry among students and educators.

- A realist curriculum in occupational therapy embraces and utilizes new knowledge generated through valid methods drawing from a variety of research paradigms. The content is presented using different methods that reflect the nature of knowledge being developed. For kinesiology or neuroscience, the teaching methods focus on mastery of factual knowledge and basic observational skills tested through demonstration, presentation, and performance on exams. Knowledge regarding how to interact with clients is presented through simulated or laboratory demonstration and practice using standardized patients.

- Realism holds that there is more to be discovered to better support the discipline. As future clinicians and researchers, students must demonstrate their ability to think critically, apply scientific theories, and access and critique evidence. To become producers and good consumers of research, students must learn to critique research paradigms, methods, and designs to better inform themselves about the validity of research studies on specified problems.

Research

- The occupational therapy profession's "taken for granted" attitude about occupation and its relationship to health and well-being as the fundamental premise of the profession exemplifies belief in the espoused theory in its holistic form. However, the belief in occupation as a mind-dependent or constructed reality can limit the scope and methods of inquiry into the reality of occupation. This presents barriers to understanding occupation, as it does not support speculative theories that hold potential to increase our understanding of certain realities.

- The increasing demands for accountability have required evidence-based practice and production of research evidence from the profession. Aligning with the dominant paradigms of health care that embrace the hierarchy of evidence, with randomized controlled trials as the accepted gold standard for research methodology, the profession is challenged to produce high-level research evidence. However, an increase in the number of such studies must not be assumed to be enough. Realism challenges us to go further and uncover the fuller realities revealed by scientific studies that apply a variety of study methods and designs.

- Quantitative and objective research methods that are replicable and generalizable constitute the dominant and accepted paradigm in medicine and the scientific disciplines that are foundational to occupational therapy. Developing knowledge about human occupation and its causal links to health and well-being, using a systematic and scientific approach, is in keeping with Aristotelian realism.

- Platonic realism, referred to as an ideal form of realism, would tell us that scientific methods limit our understanding of reality, and that science is just the starting point for uncovering the truth about reality. A metaphysical approach is required to understand reality in its entirety and true form. Once scientific studies are completed, metaphysical methods should be applied to gain deeper understanding of the realities being studied.

Practice

- A systematic, logical, and analytical approach to clinical reasoning exists that is based on the premise that optimal body structure and body function are prerequisites to occupational performance. Impairments to structures disrupt body functions and thus affect the ability to perform occupations. Deductive reasoning is a realist approach to clinical reasoning in which logical conclusions are drawn from a given situation. Individual occupational issues are understood from how occupations occur universally.

- Plato's theory of forms is applied by those who understand occupation as constituting a range of activities that may be predetermined; therefore, a clinician is able to do an activity analysis for a specified occupation. Playing soccer requires a different set of skills than taking a shower; a therapist will have a general idea of occupation before interacting with an individual client.

- Occupations occur in social context and are influenced by societal expectations, roles, and access to opportunities.

RECOMMENDED READINGS

Bhaskar, R. (1989). *Reclaiming reality: A critical introduction to contemporary philosophy*. Verso.

Brock, S., & Mares, E. (2014). *Realism and anti-realism*. Routledge.

Kuhn, T. S. (2012). *The structure of scientific revolutions*. University of Chicago Press. (Original work published 1962)

REFERENCES

Allison, H. E. (2004). Kant's transcendental idealism (Rev. and enlarged ed.). Yale University Press.

Bhaskar, R. (1989). *Reclaiming reality: A critical introduction to contemporary philosophy*. Verso.

Breines, E. (1986). *Origins and adaptations: A philosophy of practice*. Geri-Rehab.

Brock, S., & Mares, E. (2014). *Realism and anti-realism*. Routledge.

Bussard, A. E. (2005). A scientific revolution? *EMBO Reports, 6*(8), 691–694. https://doi.org/10.1038/sj.embor.7400497

Chakravartty, A. (2017). Scientific realism. In E. N. Zalta (Ed.), *The Stanford encyclopedia of philosophy* (June 12, 2017 ed.). https://plato.stanford.edu/archives/sum2017/entries/scientific-realism

Cutchin, M. P. (2004). Using Deweyan philosophy to rename and reframe adaptation-to environment. *American Journal of Occupational Therapy, 58*(3), 303–312. https://doi.org/10.5014/ajot.58.3.303

Devitt, M. (1991). Aberrations of the realism debate. *Philosophical Studies, 61*(1), 43–63. https://doi.org/10.1007/BF00385832

Ellis, B. D. (2014). *The metaphysics of scientific realism*. Routledge.

Eronen, M. I. (2017). Robust realism for the life sciences. *Synthese, 196*(6), 2341–2354. https://doi.org/10.1007/s11229-017-1542-5

Frauley, J., & Pearce, F. (2007). *Critical realism and the social sciences: Heterodox elaborations*. University of Toronto Press.

Gadenne, V. (2014). Why realism needs ontology. In B. Guido, J. Cumpa, & G. Jesson (Eds.), *Defending realism: Ontological and epistemological investigations*. De Gruyter Oldenbourg.

Gill, J. H. (2013). It's turtles all the way around: Realism and pragmatism, yet again. *Philosophy Today*, 57(4), 369–375. https://www.pdcnet.org/philtoday/content/philtoday_2013_0057_0004_0369_0375

Gupta, M. (2015). Why pragmatism cannot save evidence-based psychiatry. *Philosophy, Psychiatry, & Psychology*, 22(1), 63–65. https://doi.org/10.1353/ppp.2015.0008

Guyer, P., & Horstmann, R. P. (2018). Idealism. In E. N. Zalta (Ed.), *The Stanford encyclopedia of philosophy* (Winter 2018 ed.). https://plato.stanford.edu/archives/win2018/entries/idealism

Hale, B. (2017). Realism: Varieties of realism. *Encyclopedia Britannica*. https://www.britannica.com/topic/realism-philosophy

Harvey, D. L. (2002). Agency and community: A critical realist paradigm. *Journal for the Theory of Social Behaviour*, 32(2), 163–194. https://doi.org/10.1111/1468-5914.00182

Hibberd, F. J. (2009). John Anderson's development of (situational) realism and its bearing on psychology today. *History of the Human Sciences*, 22(4), 63–92. https://doi.org/10.1177/0952695109340493

Horwich, P (2004). Three forms of realism. In P. Horwich (Ed.), *From a Deflationary Point of View* (pp. 7–31). Clarendon Press.

Ikiugu, M. N. (2007). *Psychosocial conceptual practice models in occupational therapy: Building adaptive capability*. Elsevier.

Ikiugu, M. N., & Schultz, S. (2006). An argument for pragmatism as a foundational philosophy of occupational therapy. *Canadian Journal of Occupational Therapy*, 73(2), 86–97. https://doi.org/10.2182/cjot.05.0009

Jansen, L. (2017). Constructed reality. In C. Kanzian, S. Kletzl, J. Mitterer, & K. Neges (Eds.), *Realism-relativism-constructivism: Proceedings of the 38th international Wittgenstein symposium in Kirchberg*. De Gruyter Oldenbourg.

Kincaid, H. (2008). Structural realism and the social sciences. *Philosophy of Science*, 75(5), 720–731. https://doi.org/10.1086/594517

Kuhn, T. S. (2012). *The structure of scientific revolutions*. University of Chicago Press. (Original work published 1962)

Ladyman, J. (2016). Structural realism. In E. N. Zalta (Ed.), *The Stanford encyclopedia of philosophy* (Fall 2019, ed.). https://plato.stanford.edu/archives/fall2019/entries/structural-realism

Leveillee, N. P. (2011). Copernicus, Galileo, and the church: Science in a religious world. *Inquiries Journal/Student Pulse*, 3(05), 1–2. http://www.inquiriesjournal.com/a?id=1675

Miller, A. (2016). Realism. In E. N. Zalta (Ed.), *The Stanford encyclopedia of philosophy* (Winter 2016 ed.). https://plato.stanford.edu/archives/win2016/entries/realism

Miller, C. (2002). Realism, antirealism, and common sense. In W. P. Alston (Ed.), *Realism and antirealism* (pp. 13–25). Cornell University Press.

Nelson, D. (1988). Occupation: Form and performance. *American Journal of Occupational Therapy*, 42, 633–641. https://doi.org/10.5014/ajot.42.10.633

Petocz, A., & Mackay, N. (2013). Unifying psychology through situational realism. *Review of General Psychology*, 17(2), 216–223. https://doi.org/10.1037/a0032937

Psillos, S. (2018). Realism and theory change in science. In E. N. Zalta (Ed.), *The Stanford encyclopedia of philosophy* (Summer 2018 ed.). https://plato.stanford.edu/archives/sum2018/entries/realism-theory-change

Reed, M. I. (2001). Organization, trust and control: A realist analysis. *Organization Studies*, 22(2), 201–228. https://doi.org/10.1177/0170840601222002

Sgarbi, M. (2013). *The Aristotelian tradition and the rise of British empiricism: Logic and epistemology in the British Isles (1570–1689)*. Springer.

Solomon, R. C. (2008). *Introducing philosophy: A text with integrated readings* (8th ed.). Oxford University Press.

Székely, Á., & Székely, T. (2012). Human behaviour: Sex ratio and the city. *Current Biology*, 22(17), R684–R685. https://doi.org/10.1016/j.cub.2012.07.056

Tegtmeier, E. (2014). Realism and intentionality. In B. Guido, J. Cumpa, & G. Jesson (Eds.), *Defending realism: Ontological and epistemological investigations* (pp. 247–264). De Gruyter Oldenbourg.

Wallner, F. G. (2016). Constructivism without a constructor. In F. G. Wallner & G. Klünger (Eds.), *Constructive realism: Philosophy, science, and medicine* (pp. 9–26). Verlag Traugott Bautz GmbH.

Wikgren, M. (2005). Critical realism as a philosophy and social theory in information science? *Journal of Documentation, 61*(1), 11–22. https://doi.org/10.1108/00220410510577989

Williamson, T. (2005). Realism. In T. Honderich (Ed.), *The Oxford guide to philosophy*. Oxford University Press.

Yerxa, E., Clark, F. A., Frank, G., Jackson, J. M., Parham, D., Pierce, D., . . . Zemke, R. (1989). An introduction to occupational science: A foundation for occupational therapy in the 21st century. In J. Johnson & E. Yerxa (Eds.), *Occupational science: The foundation for new models of practice* (pp. 1–17). Haworth Press.

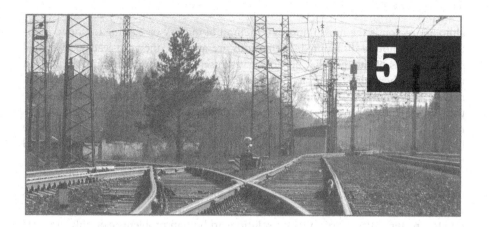

A Teleological Perspective of Occupational Engagement

Humanism Informing Occupational Therapy

Moses N. Ikiugu, PhD, OTR/L, FAOTA
Whitney Lucas-Molitor, PhD, OTD, MS, OTR/L, BCG

INTRODUCTION

As a philosophy, humanism is rooted in the constructs of social justice and human rights. It is based on the belief that opportunity should be provided to expand positive human experience in this world in a way that is consistent with diversity of human traits (American Humanist Association [AHA], 2019). It is a "human-centered" philosophy in which the goal of life is to enhance the happiness and well-being of all humanity, by meeting the material needs of all (Lamont, 1997). This philosophical school of thought originated in the European Renaissance and has been increasingly influential since the 16th century (Ikiugu, 2007; Orlov & Coleman, 1992). The philosophical foundation of humanism is that meaningful and happy living is devoted to the service of the greater good in this natural world, using the methods of science, reason, and the process of democracy. Epistemologically, humanists espouse use of reason as a way of knowing. However,

Taff, S. D. (Ed.). *Philosophy and Occupational Therapy: Informing Education, Research, and Practice* (pp. 45-52).
© 2021 Taylor & Francis Group.

although reason is the most important method of inquiry or "getting to know," emotions should not be discounted. If emotions are ignored, they can lead to irrational manifestations of thought that do not serve a useful purpose. Therefore, the human mind should be understood as a holistic entity, consisting of matter (brain) and mind, reason, and emotion. The mind and brain are thus conjoined into a holistic entity through which our consciousness arises. Ultimately, humanists argue that consciousness is not possible after death precisely because upon death, matter (in the form of the brain) ceases to exist. Therefore, there is no consciousness beyond our current material lives.

Metaphysically, reality is understood in humanism as that which is natural, consisting of matter and energy, objectively existing independent of our minds. Humanists thus do not subscribe to notions of the supernatural and myths. Rather, they are interested in material concrete reality, as solutions to human problems can only emanate from a full grasp of this reality. Human beings are part of nature and indeed evolved from nature, and therefore their actions should be firmly rooted in nature. That is why science is very important for humanists, because it is a way of dealing realistically with matters of nature.

Axiologically, humanists value action because human beings have the power and the wherewithal to determine their own destiny. Human beings do not need to rely on a supernatural being, but rather are themselves capable of using reason and science to solve problems. The goal of solving problems is, of course, to serve the greater good by creating conditions for a good existence for all people in this world. This is a utilitarian view of morality, in the fashion of John Stuart Mill (Bergson, 1911/1998). According to Bergson, it is also through action that human beings flow through time. Bergson's philosophy may be seen as closer in kinship to existentialism than to humanism, as indicated by the subjects that he covered in his writing, such as free will (Bergson, 1910/2015). However, he embraced a phenomenological perspective in his doctrine of qualitative multiplicities (the notion that our experiences are phenomenological representations in duration, which means that experiences in time are perceived holistically in the present). The notion of duration places the human being at the center of reality. That is what made his philosophy relevant to humanism, even though, as Ansell-Pearson (2018) observed, Bergson's doctrine could be seen as transcending the human condition precisely through the notion of situation in time (duration). In reflection (bringing experiences over time into the moment), human intellect emerges within a person's overall life trajectory. Such intellect is aimed at action to help humanity insert itself in the material world (Bergson, 1910/2015). In this sense, Bergson's philosophy is a form of humanism because the human being has to use intellect and act to create the desired material world.

Given this view that human beings have the power to solve problems and create desired conditions in their natural environment, they have choice about how to shape their own destiny (within limitations, of course). Given these attitudes, humanists strive to create peace and economic prosperity in the world, through scientific and democratic institutions. Ethically, the ideal goal is to serve all of humanity, working for the good of all members of the human family. In essence, the humanistic attitude can be summed up as follows:

[P]eople have but one life to lead and should make the most of it in terms of creative work and happiness; that human happiness is its own justification and requires no sanction or support from supernatural sources; that in any case the supernatural, usually conceived of in the form of heavenly gods or immortal heavens, does not exist; and that human beings, using their own intelligence and cooperating liberally with one another, can build an enduring citadel of peace and beauty upon this earth. (Lamont, 1997, p. 15)

Based on this philosophical stance, according to humanists, individuals are capable of developing their capacities so as to lead fulfilled lives (United Nations Educational, Scientific and Cultural Organization, 2015). Therefore, the major tenets of humanism as a philosophy are that human beings:

1. Arose out of nature, are continuous with, and are part of nature
2. Have the power to solve problems in their lives
3. In solving these everyday problems that arise out of their natural lives, should rely on reason and science, while also considering the value and power of emotions
4. Do not need supernatural beings or myths to help them solve problems

Based on these general principles, the goal of human life is to use rational thought and the tools of science to solve problems and create overall well-being by ensuring that basic human needs for all of humanity are met. This objective of necessity requires creation of international democratic institutions that can be used to harness human beings' creative power to solve problems for the well-being of all.

The principles just delineated were articulated by key humanistic philosophers including the Italian poet Francesco Petrarch, Dutch theologian Erasmus, and English philosophers Sir Francis Bacon and Sir Bertrand Russell, among others. Erasmus in particular is important to mention here because he came to be regarded as the originator of "Christian Humanism" (Rummel, 2017). He espoused the humanistic notion of the human capacity for self-improvement combined with a belief that education was necessary as a way of raising the human being above the status of a brute animal. In addition, Bacon (1999) introduced the line of philosophy that came to be known as British empiricism, which became the basis of today's scientific method of seeking to generalize inductively from individual instances to general principles. He challenged the *a priori* methods of ancient scholastics and Aristotelians who held that knowledge could be attained through reflection without reference to facts presented by the natural reality. In contrast, Russell is credited with the development of analytical philosophy, including logicism, which was the basis of latter-day logical positivism on which today's scientific inference is based (see his classic work, *The Problems of Philosophy*, 1912/2015).

In psychology, Abraham Maslow and Carl Rogers are the leaders in application of this school of thought. Their type of psychology is referred to as "humanistic psychology" or "Third Force Psychology" (Kirschenbaum, 2004; Maslow, 1970; Rogers, 1961). Consistent with humanistic principles, both Maslow and Rogers believed in the ability of people to make choices freely and therefore to determine their behavior and the outcomes of that behavior. Thus, they rejected the deterministic assumptions of both behaviorism and psychoanalysis (Merriam & Bierema, 2014). These two schools of psychological thought are discussed further here to illustrate their application of humanistic principles.

Abraham Maslow

Maslow proposed that the major human motivating principle is need fulfillment (Maslow, 1970). He conceptualized human needs as hierarchical in nature. Needs lower in the hierarchy have to be met before higher level needs can be addressed. For example, a person's need for food has to be met before the person can worry about self-esteem and esteem by others. Once the need for sustenance has been fulfilled, then one has to meet the need for safety. One has to know that one is safe and that one's life cannot be taken arbitrarily. Only after the need for safety has been met is one able to perceive a need for self-esteem and to be esteemed by those in one's social circle. Ultimately, the highest need for a person is to attain transcendent actualization characterized by spiritual self-expression. Maslow did not mean "spirit" in a religious sense; rather, he meant spiritual self-expression in the form of love for humanity, beauty, justice, and truth (Ikiugu, 2007). In Maslow's view, all needs must be met, beginning with the foundational psychological needs. Those who attain self-actualization have reached the pinnacle of human psychological development and present as self-confident, demonstrate open-mindedness, and feel connected to all of humanity, so they are highly empathetic.

Carl Rogers

Consistent with humanistic principles, Rogers believed that the recipient of therapy was the expert in his/her own problems, and if a therapist really listened carefully, the individual would lead in finding solutions to those problems (Rogers, 1961). In this regard, Rogers saw the therapist's role as that of a facilitator. This meant abandoning power as "an expert" and collaborating with the client person-to-person in the process of seeking answers to the client's issues. In this type of relationship, the therapist uses self as a therapeutic tool, communicating empathy, unconditional positive regard, and appreciation of the dignity of the client as a human being. Empathy comes from a therapist's willingness to enter the client's internal frame of reference so as to see the world through that individual's eyes. To enter another person's frame of reference, the therapist has to create *intersubjectivity* (a shared internal experience).

This attitude of willingness to really understand the world as the client experiences it fosters trust, and the therapeutic environment becomes a crucible in which self-exploration can occur, leading to self-understanding. As self-understanding is developed, answers to the client's issues become apparent. Rogerian principles of therapy are the basis of today's professional counseling. Both Maslow and Rogers have been very influential in the development of occupational therapy. Consistent with Erasmus's notion of the human capacity for self-improvement, Maslow (1970) conceptualized the primary human motivation as the drive toward self-actualization: a state in which one ultimately becomes all that one could be (had a sense of novelty, was confident, empathetic, nonprejudiced, and above polarities). Maslow's hierarchy of need fulfillment (which was essentially a hierarchy of self-improvement) is currently widely used in occupational therapy. Similarly, Rogers (1961) believed in the capacity for the client to guide the process of therapy by identifying issues that were a priority for that client. His therapeutic principles were central to the development of the Canadian Model of Occupational Performance and Engagement (Polatajko et al., 2013). Both Maslow and Rogers also seemed to agree with the notion of equality, not only among the genders but also between the therapist and the client, as was espoused in Lamont's (1997) rendition of humanism.

IMPACT ON UNDERSTANDING OF OCCUPATION AND OCCUPATIONAL ENGAGEMENT

Many authors in occupational therapy have associated humanism with the profession. As early as the 1990s, occupational therapy scholars were aware that many occupational therapists thought that the profession was significantly influenced by humanism, even though they were not clear about exactly how this influence manifested. Barnitt and Mayers (1993), for example, were concerned about the loose definition of *humanism* as applied to occupational therapy practice. In particular, they were concerned about therapists who espoused Christian values of "faith, self-denial, chastity, obedience, or meekness" but did "not approve of truth, responsibility, tolerance, sympathy, public spirit . . ." and yet referred to themselves as humanists (Barnitt & Mayers, 1993, p. 87). Barnitt and Mayers (1993) further argued that therapists who did not practice "client autonomy, shared decision making, and respect for the client's values" could not claim to be humanists (p. 87). Other occupational therapy authors discussed the challenges of a tension that existed in the United States between the desire to provide therapy guided by humanistic principles emphasizing respect for the individual person and the objectifying profit-seeking reimbursement environment (Burke & Cassidy, 1991).

It was, however, the Canadian occupational therapists who firmly put the philosophy of humanism at the center of the occupational therapy profession by seeking to directly apply Rogerian client-centered principles. In this endeavor, they developed the Canadian Model of Occupational Performance, which was later renamed the Canadian Model of Occupational Performance and Engagement (Canadian Association of Occupational Therapists, 1993; Townsend & Polatajko, 2013). Through this theoretical conceptual practice model, humanistic perspectives have over time become widely accepted by occupational therapy practitioners throughout the world.

In regard to occupational engagement, the principles of humanism are articulated in the notion of agency, as can be found in much of the occupational science literature (Townsend & Polatajko, 2013). This human agency is inherent in the construct of occupational justice, which signals the need to provide opportunities for individuals, groups, and populations to freely engage in meaningful occupations. However, individual agency is not considered to be isolated. Rather, individuals exercise their choices and actions in the context of broader global issues so that an individual's actions have repercussions within the larger community (Ikiugu, 2008).

KEY IMPLICATIONS FOR OCCUPATIONAL THERAPY EDUCATION, RESEARCH, AND PRACTICE

Embracing humanistic principles means that occupational therapy practitioners value the client (recipient of services) as an individual, and seek to treat the person with respect and unconditional positive regard. A therapist informed by the humanistic perspective seeks to empower and enable the client to optimize participation in personally meaningful and valued occupations. It means collaborating with clients to explore and seek solutions to barriers that prevent effective dynamic interaction with the environment through occupational participation and engagement (Polatajko et al., 2013). This view of the individual and the role of the occupational therapy practitioner has significant implications for occupational therapy education, research, and practice.

Education

Students have to be prepared to actively engage the recipient of therapeutic interventions (Mroz et al., 2015). This means that students have to learn:

- How to engage and collaborate with the recipient of services in order to get to know the person, including an understanding of occupations that are meaningful to and valued by the person, and the context within which this individual's occupational participation takes place.
- Content that fosters self-understanding and empathy for recipients of occupational therapy services, including *Therapeutic Use of Relationship*, *Cultural Humility*, and *Understanding of Population-Level Determinants of Health*.
- In a learning environment that promotes opportunities for "safe, caring, accepting, trusting, respectful, and understanding" interactions, sharing ideas and broadening their worldview through collaboration with faculty as partners (Freire, 2018; Knowles et al., 2012, p. 119).

Research

According to Mroz et al. (2015), client-centeredness should be a part of the occupational therapy research agenda. However, there are those who question whether the term *client-centered* is appropriate (Brown, 2013; Morgan & Yoder, 2012). Those who question use of that terminology argue that the term *client* denotes a transactional, businesslike relationship between an occupational therapy practitioner and the recipient of services. This would mean that the client pays, and the practitioner provides services in accordance with that fee. So, the question then becomes, What if the client is unable to pay but really needs occupational therapy services? Does the practitioner withhold necessary services? Such a course of action would be ethically untenable, not to mention inconsistent with the humanistic principle of committing one's life to improving the life circumstances of fellow human beings. This discussion suggests the need for inquiry on:

- What we, as occupational therapists, should call individuals who receive our services.

- How to define, operationalize, and investigate client-centered terminology such as collaboration, occupational participation, occupational engagement, and enablement (Mroz et al., 2015).

- Generating evidence that supports service recipient experiences in therapy as a valid outcome measure. Such research could focus on investigating how positive experiences in therapy explain variability in perceived quality of life and decreased readmission into hospitals.

Practice

As mentioned earlier, occupational therapy that is based on humanistic principles would be person-centered, collaborative, and geared toward empowerment and enablement of the recipient of services. This focus on the person implies thoughtful planning and implementation of therapeutic interventions administered in an environment that supports occupational participation and engagement. This approach to therapy would require:

- Careful interview of the recipient of occupational therapy services in order to understand the person's occupational history, priorities, and life goals (see the Occupational Profile Template by the American Occupational Therapy Association, 2017).

- Planning an individualized therapeutic protocol targeting the specific needs and priorities of the individual as identified in the occupational profile interview. This is the very definition of person-centeredness and the humanistic valuing of the individual as the author of his/her own destiny.

RECOMMENDED READINGS

Lamont, C. (1997). *The philosophy of humanism* (8th ed.). Half-Moon Foundation.

Maslow, A. H. (1970). *Motivation and personality* (2nd ed.). Harper & Row.

Rogers, C. R. (1961). *On becoming a person*. Houghton Mifflin.

REFERENCES

American Humanist Association (AHA). (2019). *Definition of humanism*. https://americanhumanist.org/what-is-humanism/definition-of-humanism

American Occupational Therapy Association (AOTA). (2017). *AOTA occupational profile template*. https://www.aota.org/~/media/Corporate/Files/Practice/Manage/Documentation/AOTA-Occupational-Profile-Template.pdf

Ansell-Pearson, K. (2018). *Bergson: Thinking beyond the human condition*. Bloomsbury.

Bacon, F. (1999). *Selected philosophical works*. Hackett.

Barnitt, R., & Mayers, C. (1993). Can occupational therapists be both humanists and Christians? A study of two conflicting frames of reference. *British Journal of Occupational Therapy, 56*(3), 84–88. https://doi.org/10.1177/030802269305600302

Bergson, H. (1998). *Creative evolution*. Dover. (Original work published 1911)

Bergson, H. (2015). *Time and free will: An essay on the immediate data of consciousness.* Martino. (Original work published 1910)

Brown, T. (2013). Person-centred occupational practice: Is it time for a change of terminology? *British Journal of Occupational Therapy, 76*(5), 207. https://doi.org/10.4276/030802213X13679275042609

Burke, J. P., & Cassidy, J. C. (1991). Disparity between reimbursement-driven practice and humanistic values in occupational therapy. *American Journal of Occupational Therapy, 45*(2), 173–176. https://doi.org/10.5014/ajot.45.2.173

Canadian Association of Occupational Therapists. (1993). *Occupational therapy guidelines for client-centered mental health practice.* Author.

Freire, P. (2018). *Pedagogy of the oppressed* (4th ed.) (M. Bergman Ramos, Trans.). Continuum.

Ikiugu, M. N. (2007). *Psychosocial conceptual practice models in occupational therapy: Building adaptive capability.* Elsevier.

Ikiugu, M. N. (2008). *Occupational science in the service of GAIA: An essay describing a possible contribution of occupational scientists to the solution of prevailing global problems.* PublishAmerica.

Kirschenbaum, H. (2004). Carl Rogers's life and work: An assessment on the 100th anniversary of his birth. *Journal of Counseling and Development, 82*(1), 116–125. https://doi.org/10.1002/j.1556-6678.2004.tb00293.x

Knowles, M. S., Holton, E. F., & Swanson, R. A. (2012). *The adult learner: The definitive classic in adult education and human resource development* (7th ed.). Routledge.

Lamont, C. (1997). *The philosophy of humanism* (8th ed.). Half-Moon.

Maslow, A. H. (1970). *Motivation and personality* (2nd ed.). Harper & Row.

Merriam, S., & Bierema, L. L. (2014). *Adult learning: Linking theory and practice.* Jossey-Bass.

Morgan, S., & Yoder, L. H. (2012). A concept analysis of person-centered care. *Journal of Holistic Nursing, 30*(1), 6–15. https://doi.org/10.1177/0898010111412189

Mroz, T. M., Pitonyak, J. S., Fogelberg, D., & Leland, N. E. (2015). Health policy perspectives—Client centeredness and health reform: Key issues for occupational therapy. *American Journal of Occupational Therapy, 69*, 6905090010p1–8. https://doi.org/10.5014/ajot.2015.695001

Orlov, A. B., & Coleman, M. (1992). Carl Rogers and contemporary humanism. *Russian Social Science Review, 33*(5), 89. https://doi.org/10.2753/RSS1061-1428330589

Polatajko, H. J., Townsend, E. A., & Craik, J. (2013). Canadian Model of Occupational Performance and Engagement (CMOPE). In E. A. Townsend & H. J. Polatajko (Eds.), *Enabling occupation II: Advancing an occupational therapy vision for health, well-being & justice through occupation* (2nd ed., pp. 27–32). CAOT.

Rogers, C. R. (1961). *On becoming a person.* Houghton Mifflin.

Rummel, E. (2017). Desiderius Erasmus. In E. N. Zalta (Ed.), *The Stanford encyclopedia of philosophy* (2017 Winter ed.). https://plato.stanford.edu/archives/win2017/entries/erasmus

Russell, B. (2015). *The problems of philosophy.* Createspace. (Original work published 1912)

Townsend, E., & Polatajko, H. (2013). *Enabling occupation II: Advancing an occupational therapy vision for health, well-being, & justice through occupations* (2nd ed.). CAOT.

United Nations Educational, Scientific and Cultural Organization. (2015). *Rethinking education.* http://www.unesco.org/new/fileadmin/MULTIMEDIA/FIELD/Cairo/images/RethinkingEducation.pdf

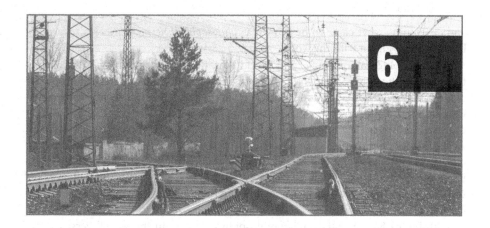

Occupation and Meaningful Living

An Existential Perspective

Aaron M. Eakman, PhD, OTR/L, FAOTA
Moses N. Ikiugu, PhD, OTR/L, FAOTA

INTRODUCTION

Existentialism is more of a literary than a philosophical phenomenon. It was associated with a cultural movement that flourished in Europe in the 1940s and 1950s (Crowell, 2017). However, its origin can be traced back to, and may appear indistinguishable from, phenomenology (Jones, 2001). Its development can be conceptualized as having occurred in three phases. Phase one consisted of the phenomenology of Franz Brentano and Carl Stumpf, which arose as a reaction to scientific positivism, which the authors of phenomenology thought was too reductionistic and, therefore, not a good representation of human experience. Edmund Husserl extended this notion of human experience as a lived phenomenon in what may be seen as phase two of the movement's development. In phase three, Martin Heidegger developed Husserl's ideas further by adding an ontological perspective

Taff, S. D. (Ed.). *Philosophy and Occupational Therapy: Informing Education, Research, and Practice* (pp. 53-60).

and developing what came to be known as *philosophical hermeneutics*—a respect for being as engagement with the world.

After the outbreak of the Second World War, these phenomenological ideas contributed significantly to the work of leading existential philosophers in Europe, including Gabriel Marcel, Simone de Beauvoir, Maurice Merleau-Ponty, and Albert Camus, among others. However, it was in the work of Jean-Paul Sartre that the ideas of existentialism as they have been applied particularly in psychotherapy crystallized. According to Jones (2001), Sartre's work consisted of a blend of Husserl's phenomenology, Heidegger's ontology, and elements of Marxism. The key constructs of existentialism, according to Sartre (1956, 2007), are thinking (reflection), freedom, choice, and responsibility. These constructs are vital to the ontology, epistemology, and ethics of existentialism.

Ontologically, existentialism is a philosophy of "being-in-the-world" versus "nothingness" (Sartre, 1956). The basic proposition is that human beings cannot rely on God or any supernatural being to provide meaning to existence. Thus, the defining characteristic of existentialism is that "existence comes before essence" (Sartre, 2007, p. 27). In other words, a human being first exists, then encounters self, and then defines the self in the world through action. The fact that human beings are free to define their existence in the world, however, is also the source of their anguish. Because they cannot attribute their essence to any supernatural being, including God, in that sense humanity is condemned to be free, and our existence as human beings is that of a continual state of becoming. This becoming is determined in part by the situations in which we find ourselves, though ultimately by the choices we make through our actions. As is detailed later in this chapter, the ontological nature of "being" found in existential philosophy also recognizes others in the world, and we time-bind together past, present, and possible future selves through day-to-day action.

Epistemologically, the fact that as human beings we are free to make ourselves what we will means that we should know ourselves. Sartre (2007) was in agreement with Descartes that "cogito, ergo sum" ("I think, therefore I am"). He saw this as the absolute truth in the sense that "it consists in one's immediate sense of oneself" (p. 52). Therefore, any objective knowledge of the world must be based on the foundation of self-knowledge. This perspective of epistemology was based on the phenomenological view of knowledge as primarily consisting of the lived experience. Importantly, this knowledge of the self requires action: that is, the creation of the self and related self-knowledge is manifested through our everydayness, our day-to-day occupations.

Ethically, because human beings are free to define their own existence through their life choices and actions, it means that they should live an authentic life (Sartre, 1956). In other words, good living is authentic living, which means living in such a way that one "acts in good faith." Acting in good faith means that one is acting for the purpose of "being-in-the-world" rather than conforming to whatever forces that bear upon one. Nevertheless, making decisions that enable one to "live in good faith" does not mean that one must be isolated. There is intersubjectivity in human action and experience. One cannot be anything unless others recognize one as such. This means that when one chooses for oneself, those choices are not just for oneself alone. Each person is choosing for all of humanity. This is the basis of existential ethics. We are responsible, not only for ourselves but also for all of humanity. So, the rightness or wrongness of whatever choices we make in life and the actions that follow is immanent in the fact that if they are right for us, they are right for everybody else. This places considerable responsibility on the individual. Every time you make a choice, it means you are choosing what is acceptable behavior for all of humanity.

IMPACT ON UNDERSTANDING OF OCCUPATION AND OCCUPATIONAL ENGAGEMENT

Existentialism has expanded Western thought regarding the nature of human existence, consciousness, and meaning (Solomon, 1993). As discussed earlier, to be fully human, one has to exercise freedom by making choices and acting in the process, creating and defining oneself. This means acting in such a way as to engage fully (passionately) with the world through occupations in which one participates. However, imagine the anxiety that can arise when your hope for the future is uncertain, and you lack the confidence and skills to perform essential tasks needed to achieve your goals. Then imagine engaging fully in the world through your masterful use of occupation, thereby shaping a meaningful and satisfying life—a life you wish to live (Eakman, 2015; Ikiugu & Pollard, 2015). Drawing from the work of Martin Heidegger (Heidegger, 1927/2010) and Jean-Paul Sartre (Sartre, 1956), we can understand occupation and occupational engagement as a way by which human beings make choices in life, a process of exercising our freedom to create ourselves and thus to live authentically.

To elaborate further on this perspective, we as fellow humans find ourselves nested in sociocultural contexts (situations), and we make moment-to-moment choices regarding why and how we engage in occupation. We often choose to engage in occupations that connect us to others, offer experiences of mastery and goal progress, and add joy to our lives (Eakman et al., 2018; Ikiugu, 2005). As we develop, we strive to manage our ever-evolving system of occupations. We create meaning in our lives, and our sense of selfhood, in this system of occupations. Yet, as my life plays out, up to its end, my occupational experiences exist as part of my "being," reflecting my past and indicating my possible future occupations (Sartre, 1956).

Central to this ontological perspective is the experiential awareness that we are thrown into a world with no inherent meaning (Solomon, 2000). The nature of "being" human centers on the fact that we are free to choose our destinies by choosing our own actions—in fact, this freedom is a day-to-day responsibility until the time of our death when we cease to "be." We choose our actions, and in doing so we define ourselves (Sartre, 1956). Furthermore, we bear full responsibility, to ourselves and others, for the actions we choose—as well as the actions we choose not to undertake. Unceasingly, on a day-to-day basis, we must face this responsibility to act—to do—and we bear ultimate responsibility for the ramifications of our choices (Catalano, 1974/1985).

Existential thought offers an avenue for optimism and hope when human beings experience anxiety about their future, according to Sartre (1957). Regardless of our circumstance or situation, we can and should create the person we wish to be. Through our acts, whether we are poorly skilled or masterful, we have a responsibility to engage with the world and to shape it into one we can understand—a world in which we aspire to live. We are compelled to act because of our freedom. Regardless of our past and seemingly dire situations, we are responsible for our acts, and for the meanings those acts engender in our lives (Solomon, 1993).

The Ontology of Being and Being with Others. Heidegger and Sartre drew upon Edmund Husserl's phenomenological method to develop their related ontologies of the human "being" (Collins & Selina, 1999). Existential phenomenology was essential to providing an ontological or descriptive study of "being" in which human consciousness and subjectivity were of central concern (Catalano, 1974/1985). Consciousness, according to Heidegger, was a practical matter: the study of consciousness must necessarily rely on our engagement in practical, everyday life as a starting point. What this would mean in practical terms is that the here-and-now experience of our daily occupations serves as a foundation of our experiences, subjectivity, and meaning. My being at this moment, for example, is contextualized in the occupation of writing; I am "the one-who-is-writing-a-chapter-on-existentialism-for-which-the-initial-deadline-has-passed" (Solomon, 1981). In other words, one can conceptualize Heidegger's idea of the ontology of being (*Dasein*) as constituting the practical aspects of daily life (which consist of a repertoire of occupations), and our related states of mind (e.g., our concerns and emotions) as being necessary constituents of our conscious experience of *being-in-the-world*. Thus, we experience the world through our day-to-day practices, and masterful use of occupation enables us to understand the nature of our world (Heidegger, 1927/2010).

Furthermore, if we are living authentically, we are choosing to participate in occupations that Sartre (1956), in his ontology, referred to as *being-for-itself*, by working toward our "life projects" that should be foremost in our conscious experiences (or subjectivity). This is the basis on which we make choices to engage in our projects and their underlying occupations, which then would help us create future selves in which meaning may be found. Occupational therapy practitioners can be seen as experts who help people learn how to "be-in-the-world" by choosing occupations that enable the fulfillment of valued life projects (Ikiugu & Pollard, 2015).

In terms of ethics, according to Sartre, meaning is an extension of our freedom, which is realized through the web of our choices related to our ongoing life projects. Our projects serve as symbols and expressions of our values: we choose our projects, and by extension, we choose our values and their related meanings (Solomon, 2000). Further, Sartre's philosophy denotes a central ethic, within which we choose to engage fully and passionately in the world through our projects. This ethic comes with the understanding that we can actively foster personal awareness of our responsibility for our acts, and their role in shaping our situations, our communities, and our world (Catalano, 1974/1985; Sartre, 1957).

Heidegger and Sartre describe the ontology of "being" as involving the "other" as a necessary and irreducible aspect of our subjectivity. According to Heidegger, we live day-to-day as participants in a world with others, such that our *being-in-the-world* is enmeshed with our *being-with-others* (Collins & Selina, 1999). The nature of our subjective, lived experience is that the "other" (individuals, their social practices, and societies) influences the experience and meaning of our day-to-day occupations—so much so that our "being," or *Dasein*, can become lost to, or dissolved in, the "other" (Heidegger, 1927/2010). Our experiences of autonomy and choice inevitably blur across the life course as we pursue our projects in our social worlds (Deci & Ryan, 2008; Little et al., 2007). However, ethically, an authentic "being," according to Heidegger, must experience autonomy and mastery in day-to-day occupations. Therefore, existential ethics require that as occupational therapy practitioners, we strive to help our clients live authentic lives, by choosing occupations that enhance their autonomy and further their life projects of "being-in-the-world" (Yerxa, 1967). However, because "being-for-itself" is bound in relation to the "other" in a perpetual conflict, according to Sartre (1956), we must encourage our clients to construct their occupations and their lives based on the awareness of the "other," and that *being-for-itself* should adopt an awareness of *being-for-others*. In practical terms, this could mean facilitating participation in occupations that are shared with family, friends, lovers, and co-workers.

Structures of Temporality. Existential philosophers have described three related temporal structures of human experience: past, present, and future. These three temporal experiences are essential concepts for describing "being" and the nature of human consciousness. Heidegger (1927/2010) proposed that the temporal nature of our past, present, and future actions was the basis of human existence, a fundamental aspect of our subjectivity. Temporality offers an ontological structure in which the conscious experience of "being" is a totality (or whole), comprised of distinct experiences of a past "occupational" self, a present "occupational" self, and a projected "occupational" self seeking future possibilities of "being." This experience of "being" is described as ecstatic or *ekstasis*, which refers to the ability to know oneself as a past self, a present self, and a projected future self, as well as the totality of these three selves (Catalano, 1974/1985). Heidegger suggests that the future should predominate in the study of the temporal structure of "being," given that the nature of *Dasein* is to will or project itself onto future possibilities in an ongoing process of self-transcendence (Heidegger, 1927/2010; Mulhall, 2005).

Sartre's (1956) perspective on ecstatic temporality is similar to Heidegger's, which is that humans are temporal beings who exist in time, and whose experience of "being" is a synthetic unity or totality of their past, present, and future selves (Palmer, 1995). We can posit that experiences from one's past occupations, one's present situation, and anticipation of one's future possibilities for occupations constitute a formative structure for "being," and therefore can inform the nature of meaning in occupation. Sartre indicates that the experience of the present should be the focus for exploring the temporal nature of "being," not the future, as suggested by Heidegger (Catalano, 1974/1985). It is in the present that we choose to act toward an unknown future and create possibilities for a future self (Sartre, 1957). Also, consider that it is in the present that we experience the personal meanings of our past occupations and possible future selves. Past occupations signify the beliefs and values that we have held and exist as facts informing our present situation—a situation in which we inevitably must choose again to act in order to create a hoped-for future self.

Engaging With the World: Occupation, Emotion, and Meaning. Both Heidegger (1927/2010) and Sartre (1956) identify how our level of awareness of our present situation influences our choices and shapes the nature of meaning in our projects and our lives. Heidegger referred to this awareness as "a moment of vision" in which one became "tuned in" to one's situation, which involved an awareness of one's moods and emotions. Awareness of emotions in the here and now offers a sign that something matters or is of concern to the individual in the present moment. Awareness of emotions (moods and desires) is therefore of critical concern because those emotions acted as signs to the individual regarding the individual's projects and underlying occupations, and in doing so, had implications for realizing future possibilities and an idealized future self. This means that when we work with clients to help them construct meaningful lives, the occupations that constitute those lives must not only contribute to their life projects but must also provide emotional valence by tapping into their wants and desires. Robert Solomon's (1993) philosophy of emotions has advanced existential thought by making explicit ties among human subjectivity, human emotion, meaning in our acts, and life. Emotions reflect our engagements with our world, and emotions reflect our judgments and appraisals of our situation, including our past acts and future possibilities. Further, we are responsible for our emotions, and by extension responsible for the occupations that give rise to our emotions. Occupational therapists can discover the meanings clients hold regarding their occupations, and their lives, by uncovering the client's narratives (Eakman, 2015). Personal and contextual barriers to masterful occupation may thwart the experience of essential meanings such as belonging, autonomy, self-esteem, continuity, pleasure, and satisfaction. A client's appraisals of such situations may lead to multiple emotions, such as loneliness, anger, loss, fear, and sadness. Occupational therapists can listen carefully to the stories of their clients, and create situations that enable masterful occupation, thereby building a bridge of health-promoting occupations from the present to a hoped-for future.

KEY IMPLICATIONS FOR OCCUPATIONAL THERAPY EDUCATION, RESEARCH, AND PRACTICE

Embracing existentialism requires that occupational therapy transform the education of future researchers and practitioners as follows.

Education

Provide students with an experiential awareness of the human condition as a way of preparing them to work with clients in the future as occupational therapy practitioners. This would mean guiding students to identify:

- Their experiences as human beings who are living in the world
- The nature and breadth of their life projects and related occupations
- The way they choose daily occupations to live authentic lives geared toward their life projects

Research

Questions that arise for investigation by occupational therapy scholars would include:

- How do people construct their life projects and underlying occupations in order to live authentic lives?
- How could occupational therapy practitioners enhance awareness of meanings in occupations, such as choice, autonomy, and mastery, for their clients?
- What are the relationships among past, present, and future occupations that enhance authentic living, meaning in life, health, and well-being?

Practice

Occupational therapy interventions that are based on existentialist principles would develop an awareness of occupational experiences (Atler et al., 2017) and emphasize the client's ability to:

- Identify the capacity of occupations to realize the individual's life projects
- Shape occupations that enhance masterful action toward those life projects and make them part of the individual's day-to-day life (e.g., routines)
- Exercise freedom, autonomy, and choice in the masterful practice of day-to-day occupations

RECOMMENDED READINGS

Heidegger, M. (2010). *Being and time* (J. Stambaugh, Trans.). State University of New York Press. (Original work published 1927)

Husserl, E. (1962). *Ideas: General introduction to pure phenomenology*. Collier.

Sartre, J. P. (1969). *Being and nothingness*. Routledge.

Solomon, R. (1993). *The passions: Emotions and the meaning of life*. Hackett.

REFERENCES

Atler, K. E., Barney, L., Moravec, A., Sample, P. L., & Fruhauf, C. A. (2017). The daily experiences of pleasure, productivity, and restoration profile: A case study. *Canadian Journal of Occupational Therapy, 84*(4–5), 262–272. https://doi.org/10.1177/0008417417723119

Catalano, J. S. (1985). *A commentary on Jean-Paul Sartre's being and nothingness*. University of Chicago Press. (Original work published 1974)

Collins, J., & Selina, H. (1999). *Introducing Heidegger*. Totem Books.

Crowell, S. (2017). Existentialism. In E. N. Zalta (Ed.), *The Stanford encyclopedia of philosophy* (Winter 2017 ed.). http://plato.stanford.edu/archives/win2017/entries/existentialism

Deci, E. L., & Ryan, R. M. (2008). Facilitating optimal motivation and psychological well-being across life domains. *Canadian Psychology, 49*, 14–23. https://doi.org/10.1037/0708-5591.49.1.14

Eakman, A. M. (2015). Meaning, sense-making and spirituality. In C. H. Christiansen, C. M. Baum, & J. Bass (Eds.), *Occupational therapy: Performance, participation, and well-being* (4th ed., pp. 313–331). SLACK Incorporated.

Eakman, A. M., Atler, K. E., Rumble, M., Gee, B. M., Romriell, B., & Hardy, N. (2018). A qualitative research synthesis of positive subjective experiences in occupation from the *Journal of Occupational Science* (1993–2010). *Journal of Occupational Science, 25*(3), 346–367. https://doi.org/10.1080/14427591.2018.1492958

Heidegger, M. (2010). *Being and time* (J. Stambaugh, Trans.). State University of New York Press. (Original work published 1927)

Ikiugu, M. N. (2005). Meaningfulness of occupations as an occupational-life-trajectory attractor. *Journal of Occupational Science, 12*, 102–109. https://doi.org/10.1080/14427591.2005.9686553

Ikiugu, M. N., & Pollard, N. (2015). *Meaningful living across the lifespan: Occupation-based intervention strategies for occupational therapists and scientists.* Whiting & Birch.

Jones, A. (2001). Absurdity and being-in-itself. The third phase of phenomenology: Jean-Paul Sartre and existential psychoanalysis. *Journal of Psychiatric and Mental Health Nursing, 8,* 367–372. https://doi.org/10.1046/j.1365-2850.2001.00405.x

Little, B. R., Salmela-Aro, K., & Phillips, S. D. (2007). *Personal projects: Goals, action, and human flourishing.* Lawrence Erlbaum.

Mulhall, S. (2005). *Routledge philosophy guidebook to Heidegger and being and time* (2nd ed.). Routledge.

Palmer, D. D. (1995). *Sartre for beginners.* Writers and Readers.

Sartre, J. P. (1956). *Being and nothingness: The principal text of modern existentialism* (H. E. Barnes, Trans.). Washington Square Press.

Sartre, J. P. (1957). *Existentialism and human emotions.* Citadel Press.

Sartre, J. P. (2007). *Existentialism and humanism.* Methuen. (Original work published 1996)

Solomon, R. (1981). *Introducing the existentialists: Imaginary interviews with Sartre, Heidegger, and Camus.* Hackett.

Solomon, R. (1993). *The passions: Emotions and the meaning of life.* Hackett.

Solomon, R. (2000). *No excuses: Existentialism and the meaning of life.* The Teaching Company.

Yerxa, E. J. (1967). 1966 Eleanor Clarke Slagle lecture. Authentic occupational therapy. *American Journal of Occupational Therapy, 21*(1), 1–9.

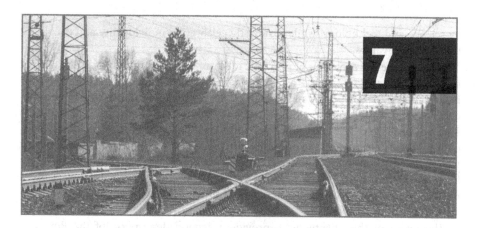

Romanticism and Transcendentalism
Ideas That Made Occupational Therapy Possible and Holistic Practice Necessary

Charles H. Christiansen, EdD, OTR, FAOTA

INTRODUCTION

Considered broadly, *romanticism* can be described as a set of transformative ideas that evolved significantly in 18th-century European philosophy and took root in the United States in the 19th century, largely through their cultural expression in literature, poetry, religion, and significant social movements. Romanticism and its cousins, aestheticism and transcendentalism, worked individually yet synergistically to provide a more complete and benevolent view of existence than what was offered by the rational scientific empiricism that was influencing (and dividing) philosophy at the time. The Romantic Movement encompassed various expressions of a widespread cultural reaction against scientific reductionism, materialism, and a rapidly evolving industrial world. The intent was to more fully and contentedly comprehend and inhabit a world that was being dramatically changed

Taff, S. D. (Ed.). *Philosophy and Occupational Therapy:*
Informing Education, Research, and Practice (pp. 61-74).
© 2021 Taylor & Francis Group.

by science and technology, while steadfastly celebrating individuality and deeply felt humanitarian values.

Here, I trace the evolution of romantic ideas as expressed in their emphasis on the subjective, difficult-to-measure aspects of being, such as feelings, intuition, and spiritual connectedness with the natural environment. I then examine how these influences were manifested in literature, music, and art, primarily in the late 18th and early 19th centuries. Finally, I show how these ideas combined with the religious traditions of the United States and its dynamically changing landscape to fuel transcendentalism, which added a bold agentic dimension that inspired dissent, activism, and social reform. The combination of these evolving ideas and movements created an ideal context for the founding of occupational therapy, and these ideas continue to manifest themselves in the 21st century.

The intent of this chapter is to provide a general description of the Romantic Movement and its uniquely American expression through transcendentalism, identifying major ideas and influences on the culture. However, it should be emphasized that, as social movements, romanticism and transcendentalism evolved by influencing attitudes and beliefs among large segments of diverse and changing societies. Hence, ideas were fluid, and views evolved over time, even as they were debated by their own adherents (Riley, 1918). One could easily get lost trying to explain nuances and complexities, so a balance of detail and generalization is needed. Thus, to use an artistic metaphor, the chapter attempts to exhibit romanticism (and its uniquely American expression through transcendentalism) through more than a caricature, but less than a finely detailed portrait.

CAN ROMANTICISM BE DEFINED? OR IS IT BEST "DESCRIBED"?

As many writers have noted, no definition of romanticism is capable of fully capturing the magnitude of its scope and influence. Perhaps an attempt at an inclusive description is a better approach: *Romanticism* can be described as set of ideas embraced by Western societies that arose in opposition to the reductionism of scientific empiricism, the emptiness of materialism, and the negative consequences of mechanization and industrialization. Romanticism contended that a full explanation of existence and experience must recognize individual emotions, sensations, imagination, and inspiration, often revealed through the creative genius evident in beauty as it appears in the arts and nature. The beauty and perfection of inspired art, unspoiled nature, and human benevolence were seen as evidence that the universe and human evolution itself were products of an intelligence that transcended the physical world.

FACETS OF ROMANTICISM: THE WHOLE IS GREATER THAN THE SUM OF ITS PARTS

Romanticism is not principally associated with any one philosopher and is anything but monolithic. It is perhaps better understood as a period in which rebellious ideas that challenged the *status quo* found expression, emerging from a time of political and social chaos in Europe coinciding with the French Revolution. These ideas challenged the dominant orthodoxies that were influencing the civilized Western world at the time. Berlin (1999) has argued that the Romantic Movement (which was at its peak from the late 18th century to the mid-19th century) resulted in such a transformative change in the world that nothing remained the same afterward. Romantic ideas challenged the dominance of classical science and the traditional thinking advanced by luminaries such as Isaac Newton, Roger and Francis Bacon, and René Descartes (among others).

The major problem was that these figures emphasized the pre-eminence of measurable phenomena in a rational, objective world that provided little accommodation for notions such as benevolence, patriotism, beauty, and inspiration. Yet, in spite of these shortcomings, the path prescribed by classical science was seen by many as providing a more traditional and familiar set of foundations for living that were directly linked with progress—and that progress was evident in the inventions that led to industrialization, mechanization, and material or practical improvements in the modern lifestyle (e.g., factory jobs, transportation, electricity, sanitation, communication).

Romantics, however, viewed these "modern" manifestations of progress as an assault on nature, authenticity, and the values that they used to define a good life. Against this backdrop and in the political chaos surrounding the French Revolution, German philosophers such as Kant, Hegel, and Fichte, among others, insisted that classical scientific explanations of the universe, including human evolution, were incomplete without accounting for the existence of the unseen (noumenal) world, or a reality beyond the ability of the individual to directly sense or apprehend it. Not unlike today's "black holes" of the universe that were once imagined and theorized in quantum physics, the idea of a noumenal world specified real but undiscovered and incomprehensible aspects of existence.

Romantic conceptions of reality featured a more complete view of the universe that acknowledged a divine intelligence (genius) in natural beauty and in humanistic societal reforms. They asserted that consciousness (being) itself and human feelings of passion, inspiration, intuition, and benevolence had to be accounted for in any complete and rational explanation of the world (Tarr, 1994). Hegel in particular, along with his contemporary Fichte, viewed social progress and its humanitarian advances as a manifestation of the rational plan of a divine intelligence (Sharp, 2004). Important threads of romanticism and transcendental thought can be seen in the work of Rousseau, particularly those related to the importance of the individual and the beauty and sanctity of nature (Robinson, 2004). Thus, romanticism (and its close cousins, transcendentalism and aestheticism) agreed with some ideas of philosophers such as Rousseau and the German idealists (e.g., Kant, Hegel, Fichte) while reacting against a longer line of philosophers who championed knowledge through science, objectivism, and rational empiricism. This "fault line" between mind and matter was delineated by Descartes (in his mind/body dualism), and continues to separate physics from metaphysics, quantitative science from qualitative science, and science and technology from the arts and humanities.

What makes some music so emotional? Or some poetry or art awe-inspiring? Why does the beauty of nature often seem to make us feel connected to the universe? Why does the history of civilization seem to describe a series of progressive struggles, with humankind gradually gaining an enlightened understanding of the world as it overcomes each challenge?

Clearly, no mathematical formulas can be used to answer these questions. The ideas of romanticism and its philosophical underpinnings addressed a human need to acknowledge the significance and reality of personal experiences that were dismissed by empiricists as "subjective." Kant challenged the idea that the mind was a passive observer of an external reality, suggesting that it was, instead, human perception that made objects possible. After Kant's forays, Hegel, Fichte, and Schiller set the stage for romanticism by further challenging science as incomplete and asserting that rather than being fixed, reality was dynamic and evolving (Robinson, 2004). Schiller (1794), in particular, extended Kantian ideas by proposing that humans had a "play" drive that emerged through artistic creativity. Through contemplating beauty, Schiller asserted, people were able to connect thought and sensation and find a place of balance between freedom and necessity. Aesthetic proponents believed that through unfettered creativity, beauty, and art, humans might find important insights into wisdom and their "true nature" (Arnold, 1994). These ideas became important cornerstones of romantic thought.

Not surprisingly, then, romanticism valued nature over civilization, individual agency over social conformity, authenticity over formality, and emotion and imagination over scientific rationality (Berlin, 1999). These sentiments evolved easily into a spiritual sentiment that was quickly inhabited by transcendentalists, who quite readily associated the power of the human spirit with the divine hand of God.

In some ways, the Romantic Movement, and its expression through transcendentalism, became a new period of "enlightenment" that cast aside classical science as inadequate for solving social inequities and moral dilemmas. Romantic ideas both acknowledged and confronted the injustices of humanity. Romantics recognized that human development (particularly in childhood) and the importance of the individual were important aspects of a world befitting the common person (Berlin, 1999). These are particularly key points, as they link directly to the ideas behind the founding and development of occupational therapy (a discussion to which this chapter turns later).

How Did the Ideas That Powered These Social Movements Gain Momentum?

Since I have observed that there was no principal spokesperson behind the philosophical social movements discussed in this chapter, it seems appropriate to briefly discuss the means through which they gained awareness and support. The social media of the 18th and early 19th century were plays, books, magazines, lectures, speeches, and concerts. Also, thoughtfully written letters, social gatherings, and salons were important. Salons, made famous in France, were highly visible organized social gatherings that often featured influential ideas and speakers and encouraged the active participation of women (Kale, 2002).

In addition to salons, speeches, and written modes of idea-sharing, the creative arts were especially prominent in the Romantic Movement, particularly to the extent that they presented opportunities to defy conventional norms or elicit strong emotions, whether through painting, architecture, or the performing arts, such as musical performances, theater, opera, and dance (particularly ballet), which in essence were the multimedia presentations of the era.

CREATIVE WORKS THAT ILLUSTRATE THE AESTHETIC, ROMANTIC, AND TRANSCENDENTAL MOVEMENTS

This section identifies a sample of authors, poets, musicians, and painters whose work illustrates the manner in which romanticism was expressed in creative work. These works variously elicit intense emotion; inspire patriotism or reverence; acclaim the beauty of nature; applaud self-reliance, originality, and nonconformity; celebrate individualism; and connect the commonplace with the divine. The order of presentation here is chronological; the reader can assume that the works of earlier authors may well have influenced those who followed. Indeed, the great musical composer Beethoven is reported to have said: "Goethe's poems exercise a great sway over me, not only by their meaning but also by their rhythm. It is a language that stimulates me to composition" (Goethe, 1808/2018, p. 7).

Johann Wolfgang von Goethe. A pre-romantic writer and poet, Goethe's hugely popular novella *The Sorrows of Young Werther: The New Melusina Novelle* (1949), written during the *sturm und drang* period, described the events leading to the suicide of a young man (Werther) who was despondent over unrequited love. So widely influential and intensely emotional was this work that multiple suicides throughout Europe followed its publication, and it has been used as an exemplar to describe the suicide copycat phenomenon in modern psychiatry (Jack, 2014). The following is a brief excerpt from the novella in which Werther, the central character, explains how his despondency (over having fallen in love with a married woman who cannot return his affections) justifies his thoughts of suicide:

> "Human nature," I continued, "has its limits. It can endure a certain degree of joy, sorrow, and pain, but collapses as soon as this is exceeded. The question, therefore, is not whether a man is strong or weak, but whether he is able to endure the measure of his suffering, moral or physical; and in my opinion it is just as absurd to call a man a coward who kills himself as to call a man a coward who dies of a malignant fever." (Goethe, 1949, p. 11)

Goethe is most famously known for his immensely popular play in two parts, titled *Faust* (1808/1867), which was published over a series of years beginning in 1790 and ending in 1832. *Faust* included both prose and poetry, and became an exalted work of German literature. These lines brilliantly express Goethe's (1808/1867) view of the importance of human agency (acting with intention), a key idea in occupational therapy philosophy:

> What you can do, or dream you can, begin it,
>
> Boldness has genius, power, and magic in it.
>
> Only engage, and then the mind grows heated,—
>
> Begin it, and the work will be completed! (p. 14)

Friedrich Schlegel. A German poet, philosopher, literary critic, and contemporary of Goethe, Schlegel wrote widely and on principles fundamental to romanticism; he is considered by some to be among the leading influences in the Romantic Movement. Following are excerpts from *Athenaeum*, a journal Schlegel published with his brother August in the German town of Jena, known as an early center of romantic thought. In the first excerpt, Schlegel (1798/2014) asserts that poetry is an ideal medium for conveying the essence of Romantic ideas.

> The Romantic form of poetry is still in the process of becoming. Indeed, that is its true essence, that it is always in the process of becoming and can never be completed. It cannot be exhausted by any theory, and only a divinatory criticism would dare to want to characterize its ideal. Romantic poetry alone is infinite, just as it alone is free and recognizes as its first law that the poetic will submits itself to no other law. The Romantic kind of poetry is the only one which is more than a kind—it is poetry itself. For, in a certain sense, all poetry is or should be Romantic. (Schlegel, 1789/2014, pp. 37–38)

> The one true fountain of beauty and the art is feeling. It is feeling which reveals to us true ideas and correct intentions, and gives that indefinable charm, never to be conveyed in words, but which the hand of the painter, guided by the poet's soul alone, can diffuse throughout all his works. (Schlegel, 1789/2014, p. 143)

Friedrich Schiller. Another important pre-romantic writer, playwright, poet, and philosopher from the aesthetic tradition, Schiller is often cited for his views that Kantian idealism was possible to achieve through emulating some of the characteristics of ancient Greek culture. He emphasized the alienation stemming from industrialization and importantly described a *human play drive* in an important collection titled *Letters on the Aesthetic Education of Man* (Schiller, 1794). Scholars generally agree that in describing play, Schiller was intending to communicate a state of creativity not influenced by preconceived forms of beauty as defined by society, but rather as enabled by the freedom of expressing oneself within an unconstrained natural universe (Sharpe, 2004). The relevance of this idea to occupational therapy is reflected in its growing literature on play as a therapeutic medium (Nestor & Moser, 2018). The following excerpt (with allowances for the patriarchal forms of writing of the time) illustrates Schiller's ideas on the importance of play and creativity in human expression:

> For, to speak out once for all, man only plays when in the full meaning of the word he is a man, and he is only completely a man when he plays. This proposition, which at this moment perhaps appears paradoxical, will receive a great and deep meaning if we have advanced far enough to apply it to the twofold seriousness of duty and of destiny. I promise you that the whole edifice of aesthetic art and the still more difficult art of life will be supported by this principle. But this

proposition is only unexpected in science; long ago it lived and worked in art and in the feeling of the Greeks, her most accomplished masters; only they removed to Olympus what ought to have been preserved on earth." (1794, p. 20)

Matthew Arnold. An important writer in the aesthetic movement, Arnold argued against critics of education who asserted that there was no practical benefit to studying literature and art at a time when science and engineering were making material improvements in the lives of people. Arnold's sentiments were shared by early occupational therapy educators and continue in contemporary philosophical statements of occupational therapy education (American Occupational Therapy Association, 2018). In his essay *Culture and Anarchy* (1994), excerpted here, Arnold famously defended the "liberal arts" using the term *sweetness and light* as his shorthand for emphasizing the importance of appreciating beauty (sweetness) and the virtues of a more enlightened and complete education (light):

> The pursuit of perfection, then, is the pursuit of sweetness and light. He who works for sweetness works in the end for light also; he who works for light works in the end for sweetness also. But he who works for sweetness and light united, works to make reason and the will of God prevail. He who works for machinery, he who works for hatred, works only for confusion. Culture looks beyond machinery, culture hates hatred; culture has but one great passion, the passion for sweetness and light. Yes, it has one yet greater!—the passion for making them prevail. (1994, p. 47)

Ralph Waldo Emerson. An American lecturer, essayist, poet, and philosopher, Emerson is considered the father of American transcendentalism. Emerson wrote beautifully about key romantic ideas such as genius, and transcendental ideas such as individual potential, self-reliance, the soul, and the dangers of conforming to a misguided social order (Emerson, 1929). Because he had such a wide audience (perhaps more than any other American writer), Emerson's published lectures, essays, and poems profoundly influenced readers of the era, most notably those of his most influential disciple, Henry David Thoreau. A short excerpt from Emerson's essay *Nature* (1849) describes the connection between the natural world and spirit and the limitations of objective definitions of reality, urging the reader to transcend the obvious and see the perfection in all things designed by the Creator. The entire essay is filled with arguments that reflect romantic ideas from aestheticism and transcendentalism. Note especially the transcendental idea that the environment (natural world) is not simply a phenomenon to be passively observed, but rather is reified (made real) through the mind, intentions, and actions of the individual.

> Know then, that the world exists for you. For you is the phenomenon perfect. What we are, that only can we see. All that Adam had, all that Caesar could, you have and can do. Adam called his house, heaven and earth; Caesar called his house, Rome; you perhaps call yours, a cobbler's trade; a hundred acres of ploughed land; or a scholar's garret. Yet line for line and point for point, your dominion is as great as theirs, though without fine names. Build, therefore, your own world. As fast as you conform your life to the pure idea in your mind, that will unfold its great proportions. (Emerson, 1849, p. 75)

Henry David Thoreau. An American poet and author and devoted disciple of Emerson, Thoreau is perhaps best known for his widely known and beautifully reflective description of solitude and self-reliance while living in the wilderness. In many ways, his book, titled *Walden* (Thoreau, 1854/1995) masterfully conveys essential romantic and transcendental ideas such as self-reliance; the beauty, truth, and authenticity of nature; and the value of solitude and self-reflection. Perhaps notions of self-reliance and rugged individualism became popular because of their perceived relevance to an age where pioneers and explorers were inhabiting the American frontier. It can be argued that this "can do" sentiment presaged a national spirit that was evident during and after World War I, where national plans for a reconstruction program to assist wounded veterans propelled the growth of occupational therapy. Ideas of independence and self-reliance continue in occupational therapy and were evident in the independent living movement. Wrote Thoreau (1854/1995):

> I went to the woods because I wished to live deliberately, to front only the essential facts of life, and see if I could not learn what it had to teach, and not, when I came to die, discover that I had not lived. I did not wish to live what was not life, living is so dear; nor did I wish to practice resignation, unless it was quite necessary. I wanted to live deep and suck out all the marrow of life, to live so sturdily and Spartan-like as to put to rout all that was not life, to cut a broad swath and shave close, to drive life into a corner, and reduce it to its lowest terms, and, if it proved to be mean, why then to get the whole and genuine meanness of it, and publish its meanness to the world; or if it were sublime, to know it by experience, and be able to give a true account of it in my next excursion. (p. 31)

Walt Whitman. Few American poets from the 19th century rival Whitman as a transmitter of romantic and transcendental ideas. Controversial in his day because of his candid and authentic written reflections on sensuality, Whitman lived the principles of transcendentalism by refusing to conform to social norms and resourcefully self-publishing his own work, collected in the volume titled *Leaves of Grass* (1855/2018), which evolved over several editions. Nearly every poem by Walt Whitman reflects some concept of romanticism, from emotional self-reflection and celebration of the individual to the wonder of nature and the divine plan of human progress. In *O Me! O Life!* (1855/2018), Whitman seems to express anguish at the misguided, material concerns of the industrial time, finding inspiration in the idea of the larger march of humankind and the opportunity to make his life matter. These are themes of spirituality, divine genius, self-reflection, agency, and self-determination.

Oh Me! Oh Life!

Oh me! Oh life! of the questions of these recurring,

Of the endless trains of the faithless, of cities fill'd with the foolish,

Of myself forever reproaching myself, (for who more foolish than I, and who more faithless?)

Of eyes that vainly crave the light, of the objects mean, of the struggle ever renew'd,

Of the poor results of all, of the plodding and sordid crowds I see around me,

Of the empty and useless years of the rest, with the rest me intertwined,

The question, O me! so sad, recurring—What good amid these, O me, O life?

Answer.
That you are here—that life exists and identity,
That the powerful play goes on, and you may contribute a verse. (p. 30)

ROMANTICISM IN MUSIC AND PAINTING

It has been mentioned that the Romantic Movement touched many areas of culture. In addition to those illustrated through plays, prose, poetry, and education, it also influenced music and painting. Although they were not compatible friends, it has been well documented that Beethoven (1770–1827) wrote compositions on some of Goethe's work (Biederman, 2009), and music historians consider Beethoven the finest composer of the romantic era. They explain how his compositions changed from the more formal baroque style typical of classical composers before him to ones more innovative, patriotic, emotional, and even philosophical in tone (Charlton, 1989). Other composers seen as representative of the romantic era include Chopin, Brahms, Wagner, and Berlioz, but this is not an exhaustive list.

In addition to music, another artistic medium that readily communicated romantic ideas was painting. Romantic art was known for its exaltation of nature as well as emotion and individualism. Romantic art also featured patriotism and glorification of the past. Though there are many 19th-century painters whose work can be seen as emblematic of the romantic period, some celebrated painters of the genre include Thomas Cole, Emmanuel Leutze, Casper Friedrich, Francisco Goya, Eugene Delacroix, and J. M. W. Turner. For a quickly accessible and well-organized collection of romantic images, readers are encouraged to consult wikiart.org, a nonprofit organization with a mission to make visual art accessible to internet users around the world.

ROMANTICISM EXPRESSED IN
TRANSCENDENTAL SOCIAL REFORMS IN AMERICA

As was observed earlier, romantic ideas were expressed in social reform movements that were natural consequences of the ideas of self-reliance, individualism, and self-determination. These movements also exhibited nonconformism with social norms such as consumerism, which greatly influenced much of society, fueled by the prosperity of American ingenuity, advances in technology, industrialization, and capitalism. Nearly all of these advances were in some way connected to the exploitation of enslaved persons, so it should hardly be surprising that many transcendentalists were proponents of the abolition of slavery. One of the more eloquent spokespersons for this cause was **Frederick Douglass**, a slave who escaped and was given refuge in a New York safe house and eventually made his way to Massachusetts, where he married and changed his name. Self-educated, Douglass became an accomplished orator and writer, advocating for the abolition of slavery and for the rights of women. Eventually, he gained widespread public recognition, both in the United States and abroad, especially after the publication of his autobiography. With his widespread notoriety, Douglass became an advisor to other social reform leaders and politicians, including Presidents Abraham Lincoln and Andrew Johnson.

Douglass became acquainted with Emerson and Thoreau and other transcendentalist leaders. Perhaps no description of Douglass better makes the case for his transcendental beliefs than this excerpt from Andrews (1996): "Frederick Douglass's basic idea of his own individuality, his own quintessential identity, lay not in his racial affiliations or his American allegiances but in his sense of himself as a person with a moral mission . . . [he] stood, not just for freedom, but for intellectual and moral integrity in the articulation and pursuit of freedom" (p. 17).

Notably, several well-known leaders in the transcendentalist movement were women. Two prominent examples are **Margaret Fuller** and **Elizabeth Palmer Peabody**. Fuller, largely self-educated, partnered with her friend Ralph Waldo Emerson to start a small journal called *The Dial* that published articles on transcendental thought. As a persuasive spokesperson for women's rights, an essay she wrote for *The Dial* later became a book, *Woman in the Nineteenth Century*, now considered a classic of feminist thought. As the precocious child of a congressman, Fuller learned Greek, Latin, German, and Italian, which proved useful when she became a foreign correspondent for the *New York Tribune* and traveled to Europe to cover the revolution taking place in Italy. While there, she married an Italian revolutionary and joined the war effort. Unfortunately, during her return voyage home in 1850 with her husband and son, the ship on which she was traveling ran aground and sank within sight of shore, drowning the entire family—and in so doing depriving women's rights activists of an articulate and powerful spokesperson. Sadly, women would not be granted the right to vote for nearly 70 years following her death.

Other transcendentalists, such as Elizabeth Palmer Peabody, a contemporary of Fuller, used their influence and writing skill to advance causes in education. Peabody advocated for the importance of early childhood education, importing the idea of kindergartens from Friedrich Froebel in Germany, who highlighted the importance of guided childhood play. Peabody advocated for kindergarten to become a universal part of public education in America, and started many schools herself in her quest to see this idea universally adopted. Consistent with transcendentalist ideals (Jones, 1992), Peabody was an avid proponent of the inclusion of art education in the kindergarten curriculum.

Although there were other social activists who embraced transcendental ideas, one can readily trace advances in women's rights (such as the right to vote) to Fuller's early leadership. Some women's rights issues, such as those related to equal pay, women's health, and freedom from sexual harassment, continue even today. The reader may well wonder about the extent to which early transcendental ideas influenced significant developments in occupational therapy, such as the Settlement House Movement advanced by Jane Addams (Greenstone, 1979) or the strong, confident personality of Eleanor Clarke Slagle, one of the founders of the occupational therapy profession (Loomis, 1992; Metaxas, 2000).

IMPACT ON UNDERSTANDING OF OCCUPATION AND OCCUPATIONAL ENGAGEMENT

Romanticism and its American expression in transcendentalism included:

- A recognition of the importance of subjective states, such as emotion, intuition, and inspiration
- The celebration of art, music, literature, and nature as counterweights to mechanization, industrialization, and materialism
- Belief in self-reliance and individualism
- Belief in a divine sense of genius that transcends the physical world and is expressed in the beauty of nature, art, music, and literature, especially poetry
- A commitment to the plight of the common man and the reform of social injustices

In this section, we examine these romantic ideas in the context of the emergence and identity of occupational therapy.

To fully comprehend the impact of romanticism and transcendentalism on occupational therapy, one must imagine America's contradictory social context at the time the profession was founded. The United States was teeming with optimism and confidence at the wealth, advancements, opportunities, and geographic expansion afforded by industrialization and technology. The transcontinental railroad, the automobile, the airplane, and the Panama Canal were recent game-changing technological realities. The sentiments behind the humanitarian reforms of the 19th century, such as the abolition of slavery and more humane treatment of persons with mental illness, continued into the 20th century. Social activism and wise leadership supported laws and regulations that were enacted to protect workers, create a national park system to preserve the country's natural beauty, and rein in industrial monopolies.

Nevertheless, segments of society were simultaneously concerned with the social consequences of these developments. The widespread exploitation of factory workers and the deplorable living conditions facing immigrants who struggled with language and discrimination were societal realities. Women continued to be denied voting rights, emancipated slaves and their offspring were still subject to cruel discrimination and exploitation, and medical practice was inconsistent, newly re-organized, and just on the cusp of becoming science-based. Many of the negative consequences of science and technology that had led to the creation of romanticism in the first place remained; efforts such as the Settlement House and Arts and Crafts Movements (Clancy, 2009) reflected romantic sentiments of reform. In short, conditions were ideal for the emergence of a profession that embodied social reform, the value of the individual, the virtues of work and creativity, and opportunities for educated women in the workforce. Ironically, and perhaps fortuitously, World War I came at the precise time when occupational therapy could gain a national opportunity to demonstrate its value.

Over the next 100 years, the history of occupational therapy would re-enact the tension between emphasis on the scientific and mechanical and emphasis on the subjective and meaningful. Indeed, the phrase "the art and science of occupational therapy" reflects the imperfect marriage of the profession's longstanding attempt to integrate the two traditions; the literature of occupational therapy also documents this history of competing paradigms (Kielhofner & Burke, 1977), which continues today. Occupational therapy emerged from traditions deeply rooted in mental health movements, and then experienced great influence from the science-driven paradigms of medical practice (Christiansen & Haertl, 2019). A return to occupation as a basis for practice gained traction, but did so just as opportunities for practice in mental health dissipated with the closure of large mental hospitals (Bonder, 1987). Large-scale employment in schools focused efforts on education-related disabilities of children (Colman, 1988). As this chapter is written, cost-containment efforts in health care within the United States emphasize evidence-based practices that generally favor medically oriented occupational therapy at the expense of highly individualized occupation-based interventions that consider romantic ideals of personal meaning, spiritual fulfillment, and purpose in life.

KEY IMPLICATIONS FOR OCCUPATIONAL THERAPY EDUCATION, RESEARCH, AND PRACTICE

What implications do these philosophies (romanticism, transcendentalism, and aestheticism) hold for occupational therapy education, research, and practice? Here key implications are summarized for each area.

Education

- Education in the profession has always emphasized a holistic approach to the patient, considering both mind and body (and more recently, spirit). This perspective honors the insistence of romantics and transcendentalists that we embrace a more complete view of the world, including subjective or unseen elements.
- Historically, occupational therapy education has valued arts and crafts and opportunities for creative expression. This reflects romantic aesthetic sensibilities advanced by transcendental reformers. Yet, occupational therapy's appreciation for the importance of a solid grounding in science requires that the profession straddle both romantic and classical traditions.

Research

- Occupational therapy research often includes qualitative or mixed-methods approaches. This directly reflects the romantic/transcendentalist view of a universe that both values the participation of the individual and recognizes the importance of spiritual dimensions of existence. It also acknowledges the broad societal mandate for scientific explanations of phenomena in science-driven health care.
- Narrative-based research, focusing on the individual stories of patients or clients, can be traced to the romantic/transcendentalist tradition of the importance of the individual and his/her perceptions and experience of the world.

Practice

- Practice is client-centered, reflecting a valuing of the individual. This includes an expectation that the client's individual goals will be considered in planning intervention and an acknowledgment that the individual is an active agent in the provision of care. Individualism and agency are definitive ideas from romanticism and transcendentalism.

- The fundamental idea behind therapy itself involves the romantic and transcendental sentiments of benevolence and goodwill in the service of helping others overcome life's challenges.

- Important romantic and transcendental ideas involve how individual humans acting in the world are an expression of the fundamental genius underlying the universe and how the arc of history expresses an evolution of progressive reform. The essence of occupational therapy practice involves understanding and harnessing the therapeutic opportunities "hidden" within human occupation or doing, as well as advocating for the rights of all individuals to access occupational opportunities, a concept termed *occupational justice*.

RECOMMENDED READINGS

Arnold, M. (1994). *Culture and anarchy.* Yale University Press. (Original work published 1869)

Berlin, I. (1999). *The roots of romanticism.* Princeton University Press.

Emerson, R. W. (1929). *Ralph Waldo Emerson: The complete writings.* William Wise.

REFERENCES

American Occupational Therapy Association (AOTA). (2018). Philosophy of occupational therapy education. *American Journal of Occupational Therapy, 72*(Suppl. 2), 7212410070p1–7212410070p2.

Andrews, W. L. (1996). *The Oxford Frederick Douglass reader.* Oxford University Press.

Arnold, M. (1994). *Culture and anarchy.* Yale University Press. (Original work published 1869)

Berlin, I. (1999). *The roots of romanticism.* Princeton University Press.

Biederman, W. (Ed.). (2009). *Goethes Briefwechsel mit Friedrich Rochlitz.* Kessinger. (Original work published 1887)

Bonder, B. (1987). Occupational therapy in mental health: Crisis or opportunity? *American Journal of Occupational Therapy, 41*(8), 495–499. https://doi.org/10.5014/ajot.41.8.495

Charlton, D. (Ed.). (1989). *ETA Hoffmann's writings on music, collected in a single volume.* Cambridge University Press.

Christiansen, C., & Haertl, K. (2019). A contextual history of occupational therapy. In B. Schell & G. Gillen (Eds.), *Willard and Spackman's occupational therapy* (13th ed., pp. 11–41). Wolters Kluwer.

Clancy, J. (2009). Elbert Hubbard, transcendentalism and the arts and crafts movement in America. *Journal of Modern Craft, 2*(2), 143–160. https://doi.org/10.2752/174967809X463088

Colman, W. (1988). The evolution of occupational therapy in the public schools: The laws mandating practice. *American Journal of Occupational Therapy, 42*(11), 701–705. https://doi.org/10.5014/ajot.42.11.701

Emerson, R. W. (1849). *Nature.* https://play.google.com/store/books/details Ralph_Waldo_Emerson_Nature_and_Other_Essays?id=j8ld3fVaoioC

Emerson, R. W. (1929). *Ralph Waldo Emerson: The complete writings.* William Wise.

Goethe, J. W. (1867). *Faust* (J. Anster, Ed.). Bernhard Tauchnitz. (Original work published 1808)

Goethe, J. W. (1949). *The sorrows of young Werther: The new melusina novella*. Holt, Rinehart, and Winston.

Goethe, J. W. (2018). *Faust*. Lerner. (Original work published 1808)

Greenstone, J. D. (1979). Dorothea Dix and Jane Addams: From transcendentalism to pragmatism in American social reform. *Social Service Review, 53*(4), 527–559. https://doi.org/10.1086/643782

Jack, B. (2014). Goethe's Werther and its effects. *The Lancet Psychiatry, 1*(1), 18–19. https://doi.org/10.1016/S2215-0366(14)70229-9

Jones, D. B. (1992). Elizabeth Palmer Peabody's transcendental manifesto. *Studies in the American Renaissance*, 195–207. http://www.jstor.org/stable/30227626

Kale, S. D. (2002). Women, the public sphere, and the persistence of salons. *French Historical Studies, 25*(1), 115–148. https://doi.org/10.1215/00161071-25-1-115

Kielhofner, G., & Burke, J. P. (1977). Occupational therapy after 60 years: An account of changing identity and knowledge. *American Journal of Occupational Therapy, 31*(10), 675–689.

Loomis, B. (1992). The Henry B. Favill school of occupations and Eleanor Clarke Slagle. *American Journal of Occupational Therapy, 46*(1), 34–37. https://doi.org/10.5014/ajot.46.1.34

Metaxas, V. A. (2000). Eleanor Clarke Slagle and Susan E. Tracy: Personal and professional identity and the development of occupational therapy in progressive era America. *Nursing History Review, 8*(1), 39–70. https://doi.org/10.1891/1062-8061.8.1.39

Nestor, O., & Moser, C. S. (2018). The importance of play. *Journal of Occupational Therapy, Schools, & Early Intervention, 11*(3), 247–262. https://doi.org/10.1080/19411243.2018.1472861

Riley, W. (1918). Two types of transcendentalism in America. *Journal of Philosophy, Psychology and Scientific Methods, 15*(11), 281–292. https://doi.org/10.2307/2940664

Robinson, D. N. (2004). *The great ideas of philosophy* (2nd ed.). The Learning Company.

Schiller, F. (1794). *Letters upon the aesthetic education of man*. https://openspaceofdemocracy.files.wordpress.com/2017/03/letters-on-the-aesthetic-education-of-man.pdf

Schlegel, F. (2014). *The aesthetic and miscellaneous works of Frederick von Schlegel* (E. J. Millington, Trans.). https://doi.org/10.1017/CBO9781107049451 (Original work published 1789)

Sharp, L. (2004). Metempsychosis and social reform: The individual and the collective in romantic socialism. *French Historical Studies, 27*(2), 349–379. https://doi.org/10.1215/00161071-27-2-349

Sharpe, L. (2004). *Friedrich Schiller: Drama, thought and politics*. Cambridge University Press. https://doi.org/10.1017/CBO9780511597749

Tarr, C. A. (1994). Romanticism: A variety of views. *The Lion and the Unicorn, 18*(2), 227–230. https://doi.org/10.1353/uni.0.0239

Thoreau, H. D. (1995). *Walden*. Dover. (Original work published 1854)

Whitman, W. (2018). *Leaves of grass: 1855*. CreateSpace Independent. (Original work published 1855)

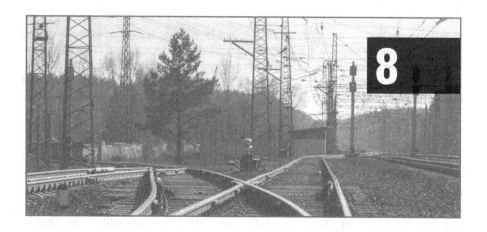

Slouching Toward Utopia

Hope, Fear, and the Pursuit of the Unattainable

Richard L. Whalley, OTD, OTR/L
Anna J. Neff, OTD, MSCI, OTR/L
Steven D. Taff, PhD, OTR/L, FNAP, FAOTA

A map of the world that does not include Utopia is not even worth glancing at.

—*Oscar Wilde*

INTRODUCTION

Utopianism is a philosophical tradition rife with dualities and contradictions. A *utopia* is essentially an imagined place where life is easy, needs are met, and society is orderly and peaceful; its counterpart, *dystopia*, suggests a bleak, often post-apocalyptic world of scarcity and inequality under an oppressive totalitarian regime. Both are part of utopianism, which dwells in hope—and in fear. It is this dualism that led Lyman Tower Sargent (2010) to the conclusion that utopianism is simultaneously "essential for the improvement of the human condition" and a grave threat to it, depending on whether it is employed from a place of hope or a place of fear (p. 9). The overarching goal of utopian philosophy is an improved

Taff, S. D. (Ed.). *Philosophy and Occupational Therapy:*
Informing Education, Research, and Practice (pp. 75-81).
© 2021 Taylor & Francis Group.

society. In practice, such improvement may best be approached not as a zero-sum goal but as a continuous, aspirational process. Here we discuss two general areas of utopian writings: utopian fiction and utopian philosophy for practical application to real life. Finally, we will reflect on the implications of utopianism as it pertains to daily life and occupational engagement.

LITERARY UTOPIA

The word *utopia* comes from the Greek *ou-* (not) and *topos* (place) and first appeared in Sir Thomas More's (1478–1535) satirical book *Utopia* (1516/2008). Over time, the word has come to signify a perfect or blissful place rather than simply a nonexistent place, due in part to More's wordplay, as he also employed the similar-sounding *eutopia* (good place). Stories of paradise existed in many cultures long before More, but his tale of an island inhabited by a highly structured, largely equitable society sparked a literary genre of utopian and dystopian fiction that remains popular to this day. Novels in this tradition typify a key facet of utopianism, which is its highly contextual nature. Whether literary or practical, realistic or surreal, utopian visions arise from an individual's sense of what is wrong with society in a given time and place and imagine a world where those problems do not exist (utopia) or where those problems, unaddressed, have led to something much worse (dystopia). Context, however, is also subject to individual perceptions and interpretations, which is why there can be no singular utopia. One person's utopian paradise could be another's dystopian nightmare. What sounded like an improved society to a 16th-century English audience may sound harsh and tyrannical to today's reader, or to a contemporaneous reader from another corner of the world.

Stories of "body utopia," at the opposite end of the utopian literature spectrum, can be found throughout recorded history. These are places known to be fictional or believed to have existed at some point in the past (such as the Garden of Eden) and characterized by surrealist levels of excess and abundance. The Land of Cockaigne is one such fable which has been identified in some form or another as far back as ancient Greece; it describes a land where no one has to work, human desire is magically fulfilled, and food and drink simply materialize and present themselves for consumption (Bonner, 1910).

Francis Bacon's (1561–1626) *New Atlantis* (1627/2008), published posthumously, shared many utopian characteristics with *Utopia*. Both the island of Utopia and *New Atlantis's* Bensalem are societies that could hypothetically exist in the real world (i.e., they contain no fantastical rivers of wine or crops that reap themselves), reflect the author's time and place, and are considered to be the author's aspiration of what his society *could* be. Bacon's Bensalem is an advanced society positively dominated by science. The proliferation of scientific endeavor in Bacon's era is reflected in the fictional institution of Solomon's House, which is similar to today's research university and ultimately guides the development of society in New Atlantis (Bacon, 1627/2008).

The early modern utopias described by More and Bacon served as a foundation for later utopian writers and philosophers. The historian J. C. Davis asserts that in practice, there is no "easy out" in utopianism. The fantastical excess of Cockaigne is clearly unattainable, but even those fictions that could hypothetically exist would be unsustainable because individuals are still subject to human nature; in no place does the entire populace exhibit unflinchingly high moral character. At every turn where hope drives societal change, fear may yet derail or redirect it. Davis argues that even in a utopia, organization and institutions are necessary to address the reality of human desire, supply and demand, transgression, and management of available resources (Davis, 1983). The imposition of rules to govern conduct is inherently limiting. One person's utopia is another's oppressive regime.

UTOPIAN PHILOSOPHY IN PRACTICE

Utopianism has influenced social and political movements since its inception, as groups and individuals have attempted to apply utopian principles to the problems they perceived in their respective societies—or in the world at large. A school of thought later dubbed "utopian socialism" arose in the early 19th century, and eventually influenced such heavyweight philosophers as Friedrich Engels and Karl Marx, whose *Communist Manifesto*, in turn, affects social and political movements even today. In France, utopian socialism was based initially on the ideas of two rival thinkers, Henri de Saint-Simon (1760–1825), a businessman and political philosophizer who participated in both the American and French Revolutions, and Charles Fourier (1772–1837), a philosopher who espoused extraordinarily progressive views on sexuality but also held hostile, anti-Semitic beliefs common among French socialists of the time (Morris, 2012).

Saint-Simon rejected the utopian label as suggestive of reactionary naïveté, but in his writings embraced the goal of the perfection of human civilization (Saint-Simon, 1817/1975). His vision of a better society involved a departure from aristocratic, religious, or monarchic rule in favor of a hierarchical, merit-based system governed by knowledgeable managers and scientists, who would place as little restriction on productivity as possible. He considered humans to be innately lazy and self-interested and valorized those who overcame their natural sloth by becoming industrious, productive members of society; this group he termed the "working class." The "idle class," in contrast, were "throngs of parasites," those who "use force to live off the work of the rest, either off what they are given or what they can take . . . they are idlers, that is, thieves" (Saint-Simon, 1817/1975, p. 158). Unlike some of his revolutionary socialist contemporaries, Saint-Simon was not opposed to utilizing existing channels of government to usher in a new kind of society (Simon, 1956).

Fourier, though similar in age to Saint-Simon, responded differently to the social-political conditions of their shared time and place. Fourier more closely resembled the traditional utopian thinker, with cooperation, equality, and communalism at the heart of his hopeful vision for society. He supported skilled education for all children, accessibility of all occupations to women (though some jobs were still reserved for women alone), and a system in which individuals would choose their work according to their skills and preferences, never keeping at a task for more than a couple of hours in order to prevent boredom (Goldstein, 1982, p. 102). The options Fourier envisioned for women represented a great liberation from the limitations many women would have lived under at the time, even wealthy women. However, in retrospect, many of the jobs he imagined significant numbers of them opting into (e.g., "bait for industrial armies"; Goldstein, 1982, p. 104) may sound less than liberating to a contemporary reader.

Harmony, Fourier's conception of utopia, would be composed of thousands of "phalanxes," or communal households that would minimize the importance of the nuclear family unit. At times, Fourier described Harmony in terms that sound too similar to the pleasure festival of Cockaigne to be realistically tenable, yet a number of communities based on his vision were established in Europe and North America.

Robert Owen (1771–1858) was Fourier's British counterpart, an early proponent of utopian socialism. Owen believed in the overwhelming influence of community and environment on one's behavior and well-being. He owned a textile mill at New Lanark, Scotland, and came to see that the conditions of his employees, in work and in life, were reflected in the functioning of his mill, much the way the condition of a mechanical machine affected its operation and performance (Owen, 1813/2013, p. 12). A social reformer, Owen advocated improved child care, free education, and better working conditions (including an 8-hour workday) and experimented with these ideas in his own mill community. The results were beneficial not only to his employees and the community at large, but also to the productivity of his mill.

A relatively common manifestation of utopian practice is the *intentional community*, a broad, generally neutral label for what might once have been called a commune or, at the dystopian end of the spectrum, a cult. Followers of Saint-Simon, Fourier, and Owen all established utopian communities based on their respective ideas, with varying degrees of success. Owen himself traveled to North America and spent several years establishing such communities and espousing the potential of socialist communities and policies to people with influence there, including the U.S. Congress and current and former presidents (Harvey, 1947, pp. 99–100).

Intentional communities are not unique to the utopian socialist movement. They have existed in one form or another for millennia; the earliest known examples were likely monasteries and other religious communities (Sargent, 2010, pp. 35–41). The kibbutzim of Israel are one of the most enduring examples, but all over the world, groups both religious and secular have established such communities of like-minded people seeking to live by a common code in hopes of creating improved societies.

IMPACT ON UNDERSTANDING OF OCCUPATION AND OCCUPATIONAL ENGAGEMENT

Evidently, one's personal vision of what constitutes a better world has immense influence on the choices made and actions taken in realizing it. A common thread in utopian thought is the firm belief in humans' capacity to effect meaningful change in society. In many cases, this assertion is coupled with a delineation of what individual people should *do*, that is, the specific roles and occupations each member should assume or engage in to manifest that change. The historical and literary proponents of utopianism discussed earlier stipulated a wide variety of occupational goals and limitations for their real or imagined community members, frequently driven by the authors' hopes and fears about the state of their own societies at the time.

Even without the deliberate application of a utopian philosophical lens, many daily occupations can be viewed as attempts to move the needle of one's life or one's community—however locally or globally—closer to one's ideal world. Though many (at times, most) of our daily activities are carried out in the service of keeping ourselves and our loved ones alive and well, once basic needs are met, we turn our attention to activities that we believe will make our societies better. Through interactions with others, we seek to learn about and influence our social environments.

Given utopianism's practical emphasis on the functioning of societies over individual lives, it is easy to see how it may be applied at the community level. Many occupations of communities are innately associated with efforts to improve those communities and could easily accommodate a utopian perspective. The collective activities of health promotion, organization and distribution of resources, advocacy, and civic engagement all are typically intended to sustain the community and increase the comfort and security of its members. For communities across the socioeconomic spectrum, collective engagement in occupation furthers the ultimate goal of a better future. As with individuals, communities engaging in occupations in the pursuit of change may do so in hopes of betterment or out of fear of degradation. At this level, intentional application of a utopian approach can unite a community under a common goal.

Engaging in occupations that offer an appropriate level of challenge may be a defining characteristic that differentiates fantastical utopias of fiction from the real-life efforts of everyday people to improve their societies. The self-efficacy built from trying, learning, and achieving goals through occupation contributes to overall well-being, increasing the competence and confidence of groups and individuals in pursuit of their ideals. When societal problems impose greater challenges, the occupations in which a community engages may determine if collective self-efficacy is built (potentially increasing hope) or lost (potentially increasing fear). Regardless, the actions a community takes to address a problem may affect the perspectives of its members and influence how utopian thought is employed.

The perspectives from which we engage with daily life can affect our motivations and goals for societal improvement. In utopianism, as we have seen, such goals may be pursued primarily out of hope or fear. While the latter may seem to carry a higher risk of resulting in a dystopia, both may also be employed simultaneously toward the same goal. An optimist may view actions inspired by hope for continual betterment to be moving society *toward* the utopian end of the spectrum, regardless of the starting point. A more fearful or pessimistic person might seek the same improvements through application of the same occupations, focused not on pursuing utopia, but simply on moving *away* from dystopia. In either case, the intention to better society is the same.

A major cause of instability in utopian experiments may be the difficulty of maintaining a common vision of the future. The greater the number of people involved, the more complex and nuanced the structure and regulation required to keep order and manage resources. More people also often means greater variance of opinion, which makes attaining consensus more difficult. It is when the envisioned *results* of our activities differ that utopianism's greatest challenges arise.

Perhaps the greatest Achilles' heel of utopianism is subjective morality. Discord between differing beliefs or perceptions of what makes an ideal world can lead to conflict. If one entity's utopian vision involves increasing the concentration of power and control over resources, their engagement in occupations that further that goal to their benefit can contribute to scarcity of resources for others. History is rife with examples of this occurring on every scale, from opposing factions within a single neighborhood to the enduring and devastating effects of colonialism on indigenous societies the world over. On a less dramatic level, even differences of opinion on the future directions of a family, a department, or an organization may exemplify this type of conflict. By the same token, communication and cooperation at any of these levels can ignite new utopian visions among oppressed or disadvantaged parties, fostering their participation in activities to manifest their own occupational justice. Critical evaluation of how our occupations affect others near and far may reduce the potential for negative (dystopian) impact of our own utopian efforts.

Whatever a person's perspective or underlying motivation may be, engagement in meaningful occupation is the catalyst for substantive, positive change for individuals, for communities, and for the world. Like occupation in occupational therapy, utopianism may be considered both the process and the product. Striving to attain a utopian ideal—a state or a place better than the one we have—does not mean failure if that goal is not fully realized. The process alone is a worthy pursuit when it inches us away from dystopia and toward a more just, accessible, and equitable world.

KEY IMPLICATIONS FOR OCCUPATIONAL THERAPY EDUCATION, RESEARCH, AND PRACTICE

Education

- Occupational therapy curricula can be designed to provide students the tools, confidence, and inspiration to improve society through occupational engagement.
- Educators in occupational therapy programs and fieldwork supervision can demonstrate and foster an interest in the role and utility of utopian thought in our professional origins as well as the trails we are blazing today.

Research

- Posing research questions with the overarching aim to improve society is a worthy goal whether or not we achieve our ideal outcomes.
- In the design and execution of research, it is vital to elicit and respect the perspectives of participants and avoid projecting our own utopian ideals onto their lives.

Practice

- We prioritize client-centered care because we recognize the importance of honoring the client's personal "utopian vision" and working toward it.

- Through an occupational therapy lens, we are uniquely equipped to facilitate the establishment of intentional interprofessional communities, with our neighbor at the next desk to our colleagues on a national and global scale. This approach can improve the efficiency, efficacy, and small- and large-scale impact of health services everywhere.

RECOMMENDED READINGS

Owen, R. (2013). *A new view of society: Essays on the principle of the formation of the human character, and the application of the principle to practice.* Prism Key Press. (Original work published 1813)

Reece, E. (2016). *Utopia drive: A road trip through America's most radical idea.* Farrar, Straus and Giroux.

Sargent, L. T. (2010). *Utopianism: A very short introduction.* Oxford University Press.

REFERENCES

Bacon, F. (2008). New Atlantis. In S. Bruce (Ed.), *Three early modern utopias: Utopia, New Atlantis, and the Isle of Pines* (pp. 152–186). Oxford University Press. (Original work published 1627)

Bonner, C. (1910). Dionysiac magic and the Greek land of Cockaigne. *Transactions and Proceedings of the American Philological Association, 41,* 175–185. https://doi.org/10.2307/282723

Davis, J. C. (1983). *Utopia and the ideal society: A study of English utopian writing 1516–1700.* Cambridge University Press.

Goldstein, L. F. (1982). Early feminist themes in French utopian socialism: The St.-Simonians and Fourier. *Journal of the History of Ideas, 43*(1), 91–108. https://doi.org/10.2307/2709162

Harvey, R. H. (1947). *Robert Owen: Social idealist.* University of California Press.

More, T. (2008). Utopia (R. Robinson, Trans.). In S. Bruce (Ed.), *Three early modern utopias: Utopia, New Atlantis, and the Isle of Pines* (pp. 1–129). Oxford University Press. (Original work published 1516)

Morris, P. (2012). Judaism and capitalism. In R. H. Roberts (Ed.), *Religions and the transformations of capitalism: Comparative approaches* (pp. 88–120). Routledge.

Owen, R. (2013). *A new view of society: Essays on the principle of the formation of the human character, and the application of the principle to practice.* Prism Key Press. (Original work published 1813)

Saint-Simon, H. (1975). Declaration of principles. In K. Taylor (Ed. & Trans.), *Henri Saint-Simon (1760–1825): Selected writings on science, industry and social organization* (pp. 158–161). Holmes and Meier. (Original work published 1817)

Sargent, L. T. (2010). *Utopianism: A very short introduction.* Oxford University Press.

Simon, W. M. (1956). History for utopia: Saint-Simon and the idea of progress. *Journal of the History of Ideas, 17*(3), 311–331. https://doi.org/10.2307/2707547

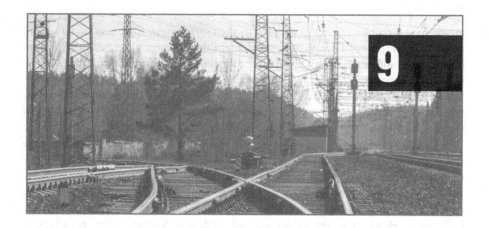

Pragmatic Foundations
Instrumentalism and Transactionalism in Occupational Therapy

Moses N. Ikiugu, PhD, OTR/L, FAOTA
Ranelle M. Nissen, PhD, OTR/L

INTRODUCTION

Pragmatism is a conspicuously American philosophy underlying the ethos of action rather than abstract discourse in U.S. culture. It was founded by Charles Sanders Peirce in the late 19th century (Buchler, 1955). Peirce was particularly concerned about what he saw as a speculative tradition in philosophy and wanted to make it more aligned with scientific methods, or to create what he referred to as "laboratory-philosophy" (Muelder et al., 1960, p. 363). He asserted that all reasoning should be aimed at deducing the unknown from the known, and that "reasoning is good if it be such as to lead to true conclusions from true premises and not otherwise" (Fisch, 1996, p. 57). Peirce further asserted that it was not enough merely to believe, but that belief must drive action in order for the belief to be meaningful (Ikiugu, 2007; White, 1973). This is what he referred to as "belief as a rule for action." He also viewed action originating from belief as a critical

Taff, S. D. (Ed.). *Philosophy and Occupational Therapy:*
Informing Education, Research, and Practice (pp. 83-90).
© 2021 Taylor & Francis Group.

means by which human beings adapted to their environment. He was in agreement with Darwin's theory of adaptation and thought that Darwin was one of the greatest intellectual giants of his time who had freed the human mind from the dogma of fixed species by demonstrating that biological organisms could evolve from nature without a need to be created as a fixed genera (Buchler, 1955). One can therefore see, as will be discussed later, how the notion of adaptation came to be central to occupational therapy discourse and practice through the influence of pragmatism.

According to Peirce, the only way to verify the truth of a belief was to examine the consequences of acting on that belief. If the consequences of action based on a belief were as expected or desired, then the belief had been verified. In other words, if belief was not supported by the results of acting on it, then that belief was not grounded in fact and, therefore, was not real. Failure to verify belief in that manner created doubt in the mind. However, doubt was an uncomfortable state for human beings and therefore people tended to act in order to re-establish belief. This meant either changing the belief or doing further experimentation to test the current belief. The goal was to expel doubt and re-establish belief so as to attain balance of the mind. Furthermore, when the consequences of acting on a belief were as expected, the belief persisted in the mind and consequent action was repeated, leading to formation of habits of the mind (Ikiugu, 2007).

Although Peirce was an astute logician and effectively created pragmatism, he was not an effective communicator, and therefore his philosophical doctrine was not widely shared—that is, until it was popularized by William James (McDermott, 1977). James was a close friend and greatly influenced by Peirce. He held strictly to Peirce's original philosophical thought that if evidence from action does not support belief, we should move to re-examine that belief or to identify a new belief that would result in action supported by the evidence (what Peirce called *verifiability* in his doctrine of belief as a rule for action). However, James further expanded his view of verifiability to include religious beliefs (James, 1981), which was a huge departure from Peirce, and a stance with which Peirce disagreed strongly (Ikiugu, 2007). This new extension included testing the truth of a person's moral and religious beliefs based on the satisfaction a person had due to holding those beliefs (White, 1973). In this expanded view of belief as a rule for action, James viewed humans as co-creators of nature in collaboration with God. Thus, "through doing, one was creative, and in being creative, one existed" (Ikiugu, 2007, p. 20).

In addition, James elaborated on Peirce's notion of habit formation as a result of acting on beliefs (McDermott, 1977). His view of habit formation was largely based on his training as a psychologist. James belonged to the functionalist school of psychology (the same school of psychology in which Ivan Pavlov, the creator of classical conditioning theory, was educated), which emphasized examination of behavior as a way of understanding the mind (Ikiugu, 2007). Thus, according to James, habits were created by repetition of actions that were meaningful. Also, habits were seen as critical to the functioning of human beings. By creating a habit, one was able to do things without investing too much thought into them, which reduced the cognitive load and allowed one to focus on more important, intellectually demanding tasks. The reduced demand on cognitive energy was possible because of brain plasticity that allowed the mind to streamline movements with minimal conscious thought (Andersen & Reed, 2017). James's work was very influential in occupational therapy, as indicated by the importance of assisting clients to develop desired habits, as will be made clear in the following discussion.

The third major personality in the philosophy of pragmatism whose work significantly influenced the development of occupational therapy was John Dewey. Like Peirce, Dewey saw himself as an experimentalist (Murphy, 1990). His most significant contribution was to apply pragmatism to education. He was highly influenced by the work of Francis Bacon, who saw knowledge as measurable only by its consequences (Dewey, 1957). In this regard, learning abstract, fantastic theories that did not produce a difference in the real world was not useful. Therefore, learning had to occur by doing (experimentation and exploration of nature). This was the thinking on which Dewey's Laboratory School in Chicago was founded. Students developed their own learning objectives and learned by doing and exploring their environment (Knoll, 2016; McDermott, 1981). For example, to learn about the social structure during the Stone Age, students would actually fashion stone tools and try to use them in a variety of applied tasks.

Dewey was close to James and ultimately was highly influenced by James's philosophical views. In addition, he drew from the philosophy of Georg Wilhelm Friedrich Hegel, a German philosopher (McDermott, 1981). He adopted the Hegelian dialectic, in which human institutions and even human beings were perceived to develop through a conflict between tradition or status quo (thesis), change or the principle challenging the status quo (antithesis), leading to a synthesis (hybrid) consisting of a melding of the old and the new, thereby creating a better institution or human being. By adopting this philosophical approach to analysis, he concluded that the role of intellectual inquiry was to facilitate that dialectic process, thereby improving social institutions and simultaneously improving the lot of humanity. In this sense, the focus of Dewey's philosophy was meliorism, and the whole purpose of education, according to him, was to improve democratic institutions and society.

Furthermore, Dewey viewed historical examination of a situation as the best possible means to deconstruct what is, in order to understand how it came to be (White, 1973). In his view, one used the mind to analyze and come to understand history (the grounding of thesis), identify challenges to those historical traditions, and then to facilitate a useful synthesis. Dewey named this process of applying one's mind to solve personal or social problems *instrumentalism* (Ikiugu, 2007), which referred to instrumental use of the mind to create preferred circumstances, make the environment suitable to human existence, and thus adapt, survive, and thrive. In other words, the mind was seen as a tool like any other, that human beings used to their advantage in the process of adaptation. This instrumental view of the mind was a way of operationalizing Darwin's theory of evolution in a way that was applicable to human beings in their current circumstances as they strived to survive in their natural environments (Ikiugu, 2007). The philosophical propositions of James and Dewey were very influential on Adolf Meyer, who articulated the oft-cited "philosophy of occupation therapy" (Meyer, 1922), in which he discussed the need for human beings to remain in balance and in harmony with the environment through occupation in order to survive and thrive as biological organisms.

IMPACT ON UNDERSTANDING OF OCCUPATION AND OCCUPATIONAL ENGAGEMENT

The philosophy of pragmatism was very influential to the development of occupational therapy during the formative years of the profession. Two of the three leading pragmatists were well acquainted with Eleanor Clark Slagle, who has been widely accepted as the mother of occupational therapy, through their mutual activities at the Hull House in Chicago and the Chicago School of Civics and Philanthropy (Breines, 1986; Loomis, 1992). The Chicago School of Civics and Philanthropy was founded in 1908 to offer instruction in occupations as a therapeutic modality to help poor immigrants from Europe adapt to their new country. Important figures at the school were also key figures in the Mental Hygiene Movement. Mental hygienists such as Jane Addams, Emil G. Hirsch, Julia Lathrop, Adolf Meyer, and Eleanor Clark Slagle were all highly influenced by pragmatism and the Arts and Crafts Movement. Pragmatism and the Arts and Crafts Movement, along with the Moral Treatment Movement, were all pivotal in the formal founding of occupational therapy as a profession (Breines, 1987; Ikiugu, 2007).

This influence of pragmatism in the profession can be seen today in the valuing of the environment and the importance of habits as key foci in occupational therapy, and the adoption of terminology such as *adaptation*, which filtered into the profession from Darwin through pragmatism. The American Occupational Therapy Association (AOTA, 2017) statement of the philosophical base of occupational therapy and the World Federation of Occupational Therapists (WFOT, 2010) statement on occupational therapy both emphasize the importance of adaptation of the person to the environment through experience. John Dewey's notion of "learning by doing" is also clearly apparent in occupational therapy practice. Because of these pragmatic influences, occupational therapy practice was founded in, and continues to be centered on, occupation and occupational engagement through a person-centered lens (AOTA, 2014).

Furthermore, the pragmatic concept that experience is individual, and a person must be viewed holistically in context, was the foundational principle supporting the use of occupation to create change in mind and body. Also, consistent with pragmatism, occupational therapy practitioners view knowledge as based in experience. As such, this knowledge is always changing (is in flux), because human response to the environment is different in different situations and this response changes our understanding of and thus our knowledge of something (Hooper & Wood, 2002). This changing experience of our environment occurs as we interact with it through occupations, a fact that underlies the importance of occupations to the human ability to interact with and thus adapt to the environment.

To illustrate this point, imagine someone whose productive occupation is construction. Let's say this person is engaged in a project to construct a new building in an area that was hitherto wild. The initial experience for the person is that of interacting with the natural untamed environment. Part of the project involves clearing vegetation, leveling the ground, and digging the foundation and using the materials to create the desired structure. As the building goes up, the environment is tamed and becomes more and more comfortable for individuals sheltered by the structure, including the construction worker who did and continues to do the work. In creating the building, the construction worker has expended energy, and the effort has helped develop that person's muscle fibers, and he/she has learned a few things about constructing a building (developing experience in the trade). Therefore, in the process, the worker has changed the environment by installing a human-made structure where previously there was wilderness, and this interaction with the environment has in turn resulted in better-developed muscles, some learning and experience, and therefore change in the brain structure and function. The two entities have mutually changed each other. In other words, engagement in occupations is an active experience of understanding our world and changing it as we desire, while in the process understanding who we are as occupational beings (Andersen & Reed, 2017; AOTA, 2014; Muelder et al., 1960; WFOT, 2010). The premise of humans as occupational beings who can adapt to and effect change in the environment to improve their context is the core of occupational therapy (Andersen & Reed, 2017; AOTA, 2014).

This centrality of occupation to human adaptation is the reason that an occupational therapy practitioner can use occupation to reach the person's mind to enhance the individual's overall well-being (Ikiugu, 2014). As McDermott (1977) asserted, the process of active learning leads to development of the mind's ability to interpret, process, and understand one's experience. This understanding is what leads to knowledge of the world and informs how we act in the future (Muelder et al., 1960; White; 1973). James's (and Dewey's) principle of active learning maps perfectly into occupation-based interventions in occupational therapy. Through occupations, we are actively engaged with the context in which we are performing, and this engagement provides us with the experience that changes us as we change the context through what we are doing. As we engage in occupations, we interpret and re-examine our performance so that we can adapt as our understanding of performance shifts due to changes in ourselves, the environment, and/or the occupation (AOTA, 2014; WFOT, 2010).

Furthermore, through a pragmatic lens, we can understand occupational engagement as the process through which we gain knowledge of occupations experientially. Knowledge of occupations cannot occur prior to engagement in the experience itself (Muelder et al., 1960; White, 1973). The experience in the natural context is the means by which we experiment, in the process gaining new knowledge and modifying our existing conceptual understanding of the world in which we exist (Andersen & Reed, 2017). Experiencing occupation in context thus changes our sense of the meaning and value of that occupation within the environmental context in which we are acting. As our knowledge increases based on multiple experiences, we increasingly understand the occupation and develop a sense for what to expect in engagement in that occupation in the future.

KEY IMPLICATIONS FOR OCCUPATIONAL THERAPY EDUCATION, RESEARCH, AND PRACTICE

Education

Based on Dewey's notion of "learning by doing," it is clear that an occupational therapy student should be educated in a collaborative, experiential environment. The student should be encouraged to experiment with constructs, examining how they may be applicable in clinical settings. Real-life experiences should be used to design learning activities and the social function of learning should be emphasized. Such education would emphasize:

- The student's life experiences as the foundation for learning clinical skills
- Exploration of the ethics and social role of occupational therapy
- Exposure to real-life situations where the student can solve problems as he/she would solve them in clinical settings (learning by doing)

Research

Application of pragmatic principles in occupational therapy practice has been proposed in the literature (Cutchin, 2004; Hooper & Wood, 2002; Ikiugu & Schultz, 2006; Morrison, 2016). Ikiugu (2007) operationalized Dewey's construct of instrumentalism to formulate the theoretical conceptual practice model called Instrumentalism in Occupational Therapy and a later version, Modified Instrumentalism in Occupational Therapy (Ikiugu & Pollard, 2015). In a number of studies, the theoretical guidelines of the model were tested (Ikiugu, 2007, 2012, 2014; Ikiugu & McCollister, 2011; Ikiugu & Pollard, 2015). However, more extensive research should be conducted to test a number of constructs adopted from pragmatism by the profession. Following are a few possible research questions:

- What are the best interventions to help a client develop the most adaptive habits through occupations?
- What are the relationships among habits, occupational participation, and health?
- To what extent does social consciousness motivate participation in healing occupations?

Practice

Constructs based on pragmatism have been used in occupational therapy since the early days of its formal founding. Slagle, for example, developed habit training programs based on James's ideas about the importance of sound habits to good health (Loomis, 1992; Serrett, 1985). Constructs such as adaptation to the environment through participation in occupations, and the importance of good habits for optimal occupational participation, continue to be emphasized in current theoretical conceptual practice models such as the Model of Human Occupation, the Person-Environment-Occupation model, and the Instrumentalism in Occupational Therapy model. More specifically, therapy founded on pragmatic principles focuses on:

- Occupation as the vehicle through which people experience life
- The subjective experience of occupational participation as the person, environment, and occupation dynamically interact to foster adaptation
- Learning through doing as the gold standard of occupational therapy intervention

RECOMMENDED READINGS

Breines, E. (1986). *Origins and adaptations: A philosophy of practice*. Geri-Rehab.

Buchler, J. (1955). *Philosophical writings of Peirce*. Dover.

McDermott, J. J. (1977). *The writings of William James*. University of Chicago Press.

McDermott, J. J. (1981). *The philosophy of John Dewey*. University of Chicago Press.

REFERENCES

American Occupational Therapy Association (AOTA). (2014). Occupational therapy practice framework: Domain and process (3rd ed.). *American Journal of Occupational Therapy, 68*(Suppl. 1), S1–S48. https://doi.org/10.5014/ajot.2014.682006

American Occupational Therapy Association (AOTA). (2017). Philosophical base of occupational therapy. *American Journal of Occupational Therapy, 71*(Suppl. 2), 7112410045p1. https://doi.org/10.5014/ajot.2017.716S06

Andersen, L., & Reed, K. (2017). *The history of occupational therapy: The first century*. SLACK Incorporated.

Breines, E. (1986). *Origins and adaptations: A philosophy of practice*. Geri-Rehab.

Breines, E. (1987). Pragmatism as a foundation for occupational therapy curricula. *American Journal of Occupational Therapy, 41*(8), 522–525. https://doi.org/10.5014/ajot.41.8.522

Buchler, J. (1955). *Philosophical writings of Peirce*. Dover.

Cutchin, M. P. (2004). Using Deweyan philosophy to rename and reframe adaptation-to-environment. *American Journal of Occupational Therapy, 58*, 303–312. https://doi.org/10.5014/ajot.58.3.303

Dewey, J. (1957). *Reconstruction in philosophy*. Beacon Press.

Fisch, M. (1996). *Classic American philosophers*. Fordham University Press.

Hooper, B., & Wood, W. (2002). Pragmatism and structuralism in occupational therapy: The long conversation. *American Journal of Occupational Therapy, 56*(1), 40–50. https://doi.org/10.5014/ajot.56.1.40

Ikiugu, M. N. (2007). *Psychosocial conceptual practice models in occupational therapy: Building adaptive capability*. Mosby Elsevier.

Ikiugu, M. N. (2012). The test-retest reliability and predictive validity of a battery of newly developed occupational performance assessments. *Occupational Therapy in Mental Health, 28*(1), 51–71. https://doi.org/10.1080/0164212X.2012.650985

Ikiugu, M. N. (2014). Convergent validity of a newly developed occupational performance assessment: A pilot study. *International Journal of Therapy and Rehabilitation, 21*(5), 219–226. https://doi.org/10.12968/ijtr.2014.21.5.219

Ikiugu, M. N., & McCollister, L. (2011). An occupation-based framework for changing human occupational behavior to address critical global issues. *International Journal of Professional Practice, 2*(4), 402–417.

Ikiugu, M. N., & Pollard, N. (2015). *Meaningful living across the lifespan: Occupation-based intervention strategies for occupational therapists and scientists*. Whiting & Birch.

Ikiugu, M. N., & Schultz, S. (2006). An argument for pragmatism as a foundational philosophy of occupational therapy. *Canadian Journal of Occupational Therapy, 73*(2), 86–97. https://doi.org/10.2182/cjot.05.0009

James, W. (1981). *Pragmatism*. Hackett.

Knoll, M. (2016, August 17–20). *John Dewey's laboratory school: Theory versus practice*. [Paper presentation]. International Standing Conference for the History of Education 38th Annual Conference, Chicago, IL, United States.

Loomis, B. (1992). The Henry B. Favill School of Occupations and Eleanor Clarke Slagle. *American Journal of Occupational Therapy, 46*(1), 34–37. https://doi.org/10.5014/ajot.46.1.34

McDermott, J. J. (1977). *The writings of William James*. University of Chicago Press.

McDermott, J. J. (1981). *The philosophy of John Dewey*. University of Chicago Press.

Meyer, A. (1922). The philosophy of occupation therapy. *Archives of Occupational Therapy, 1*, 1–10.

Morrison, R. (2016). Pragmatist epistemology and Jane Addams: Fundamental concepts for the social paradigm of occupational therapy. *Occupational Therapy International, 23*, 295–304. https://doi.org/10.1002/oti.1430

Muelder, W. G., Sears, L., & Schlabach, A. V. (1960). *The development of American philosophy: A book of readings*. Houghton Mifflin.

Murphy, J. P. (1990). *Pragmatism from Peirce to Davidson*. Westview Press.

Serrett, K. D. (1985). *Philosophical and historical roots of occupational therapy*. Haworth Press.

White, M. (1973). *Pragmatism and the American mind: Essays and reviews in philosophy and intellectual history*. Oxford University Press.

World Federation of Occupational Therapists (WFOT). (2010). *Statement on occupational therapy*. https://wfot.org/resources/statement-on-occupational-therapy

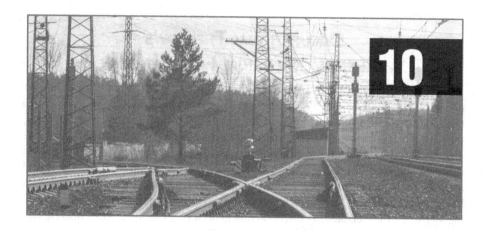

Phenomenology
Returning to the Things Themselves
With Wonder and Curiosity

Valerie A. Wright-St Clair, PhD, MPH, DipProfEthics, DipBusStud, DipOT
Elizabeth Anne Kinsella, PhD, MAdEd, BSc(OT)

INTRODUCTION

This chapter's purpose is to make phenomenology accessible to and useful for occupational therapy educators, researchers, and practitioners. We begin by taking the reader through a phenomenological perspective of occupational therapy's philosophical foundations. Then we define phenomenology and describe the philosophy's major facets and central characteristics. Finally, we introduce some of the main philosophers and consider what their distinctive ways of thinking bring to phenomenology, all with an eye toward phenomenological thinking regarding occupational therapy.

Taff, S. D. (Ed.). *Philosophy and Occupational Therapy:*
Informing Education, Research, and Practice (pp. 91-100).
© 2021 Taylor & Francis Group.

Occupational Therapy's Phenomenological Foundations

Occupational therapy can be viewed as having deep roots in philosophical phenomenology. Meyer's (1922/1977) republished work on a philosophy of occupational therapy elaborated on a "philosophy of reality, of work and time . . . [with respect for] the simple and yet most valuable experiences of real life" (p. 640). The philosophy he offered the profession early in its evolution was founded in thinking of the human entity as "an organism that maintains and balances itself in the world of reality and actuality by being in active life and active use" (Meyer, 1922/1977, p. 641). Though Meyer does not claim his philosophy to be phenomenological in nature, his thinking aligns with understanding phenomenology as a philosophy of "the concrete and ordinary things of everyday life" (van Manen, 2014, p. 118) in moments as they are lived. In further alignment between occupational therapy and phenomenology, Meyer proposed the occupation worker's beacon-lights of "awakening to a full meaning of time as the biggest wonder and asset of our lives and the valuation of opportunity and performance as the greatest *measure* of time" (Meyer, 1922/1977, p. 642). It is easy to hear Heidegger's (1927/1962) phenomenological philosophy of being and time, and his focus on *lived time*, in Meyer's words and way of thinking. Recently, Reed (2017) contended that "time and the organization of occupations within time are important concepts in Meyer's philosophy" (p. 116). Although her writing was critical of Meyer's scholarship, it is interesting that his ideas are in the spotlight again, almost a hundred years after they were first published.

Turpin (2007) challenged the occupational therapy profession to retrieve its phenomenological knowledge foundations. Turpin draws on Kielhofner's (1997) conception of occupational therapy's existence at the nexus of scientific and artful practice and Mattingly's (1994) "two-body" theory to explain practitioners' thoughtful engagement with the physical biomedical and lived phenomenological bodies to make the case for retrieving the profession's phenomenological knowledge. Although, if it was always already there—for instance, in the foundational work of Meyer—then perhaps it is a case of *illuminating* occupational therapy's philosophical phenomenological way of thinking, knowing, and doing rather than *retrieving* it.

Defining Phenomenology

In its most general sense, *phenomenology* is the study of phenomena (Zahavi, 2019b), yet all fields of study could be defined as the study of phenomena of one form or another. Specifically, phenomenology lets a phenomenon be seen for what it is and how it appears (Inwood, 1999). Therefore, phenomenology can be defined as the study of the "forms in which something appears or manifests itself" (King, 2001, p. 109). A generally familiar definition of phenomenology is that of a research approach that explores a phenomenon "from the perspective of those who have experienced it" (Neubauer et al., 2019, p. 91). However, there are various twists on the definition depending on whose phenomenological tradition is considered. In the world of descriptive phenomenology, it can be defined as the "systematic study of the *essential* content of our experiences" of phenomena (Kaufer & Chemero, 2015, p. 27) as they appear in human consciousness. In comparison, in the world of interpretive phenomenology, it can be defined as the "study of phenomena as they manifest in our experience . . . and of the meaning phenomena have" (Neubauer et al., 2019, p. 92) in that experience. In both approaches, phenomenology involves an attempt to "return to the things themselves" before they have been laden with the meanings inherent in a culture (Crotty, 2015). Descriptive phenomenology aims to bracket out the pre-understandings of the interpreter, whereas interpretive or hermeneutic phenomenology questions whether it is ever possible to achieve such bracketing. Thus, phenomenology is the study of phenomena, with the aim to return to the things themselves, freshly and pre-reflectively. In accord, descriptive Husserlian approaches aim to uncouple (bracket out) the pre-understandings of the interpreter, and to hold assumptions and interpretations of the phenomena in abeyance; in contrast interpretive, hermeneutic, and Heideggerian schools question whether it is ever possible to bracket out our pre-understandings and instead point to the need to recognize the situated nature of all human interpretation (Crotty, 2015; Dowling, 2007; Lala & Kinsella, 2011c).

The Major Facets and Goals of Phenomenology

Phenomenology can be approached as both a philosophy and a method of inquiry, as well as a human science (Qutoshi, 2018; van Manen, 2019). From a philosophical perspective, it offers a way of looking at the world: a phenomenological gaze, so to speak. From a practical perspective, it offers tools for inquiring into a phenomenon through the existential and embodied lifeworld of people.

The general goals of phenomenology may vary and overlap depending upon the context in which it is being applied. One of the overarching aims is to apprehend phenomena through wonder and curiosity by returning to the *lifeworld* (lived time, lived space, lived body, lived relations), as a means of perception and coming to "the things themselves" with fresh eyes.

Major Philosophical Concepts

Three major philosophical concepts within phenomenology are phenomenon, lifeworld, and a call to "return to the things themselves." Understanding what *phenomenon* means in the context of phenomenology is an important starting point. Looking at its Greek origins, the "word *phainomenon* means the manifest, the self-showing" (King, 2001, p. 110). Thus, in the world of phenomenology, a phenomenon is an event or thing that manifests in some way in "the lived world of human beings" (Qutoshi, 2018, p. 215). Taking this way of thinking a step further, a phenomenon in phenomenology is not about what appears at first glance (Zahavi, 2019b) or a thing that is self-evident. It is a thing that is hidden or concealed in some way and not readily seen. Inwood's (1999) explanation is useful for making sense of Heidegger's (1927/1962) classic definition of a phenomenon as that which "shows itself from itself" (p. 58) and not simply from something it seems to be.

The idea that phenomenology is the study of lived experience, or that phenomena can be apprehended through the lifeworld of people, is widely understood. *Lifeworld* in phenomenology refers to the "prereflective or prepredicative life of human existence" (van Manen, 2007, p. 26). In other words, it is the raw, before-thinking-about-it experiences in particular moments or events in life. As Husserl (1907/1990) describes it, "I find myself at all times, and without my ever being able to change this, set in relation to a world . . . it is continually 'present' for me, and I myself am a member of it . . . this world is not there for me as a mere world of facts and affairs, but, with the same immediacy, as a world of values, of goods, a practical world" (p. 103).

One of the calls of phenomenological thinkers is to "return to the things themselves" as a means to apprehend the phenomenal world through our lived experience of it. For Zahavi (2019b), phenomenology recognizes that we are "first and foremost beings constituted by our relationship to the very world that we inhabit" (p. 73).

Phenomenology: Its Thinkers and the Concepts They Originated

Three influential thinkers in phenomenology are Husserl, Heidegger, and Merleau-Ponty. While there are family resemblances across the work of these different philosophers, they also exhibit distinct styles and foci.

Husserl's (1859–1938) transcendental or descriptive phenomenology (Husserl, 1913/1962). Husserl is considered by many to be the founding father of phenomenology (Kaufer & Chemero, 2015) because of his work in formalizing and making the philosophy popular. Husserl posited the development of an objective science of phenomenology, in which the perceiver could "bracket out" his/her pre-understandings and return through what he called the "transcendental reduction" to the things themselves. In such an approach, the perceiver "seeks to elicit clarity and dispel the darkness of preconceived assumptions" (Lala & Kinsella, 2011c, p. 198) in order to approach phenomena from a fresh perspective. He posited his approach as an alternative to what he described as "an unphilosophical study of mere facts" (Spiegelberg cited in Okoro, 2005, p. 131), which he argued had lost its significance for understanding life as a whole.

Heidegger's (1889–1976) existential phenomenology (Heidegger, 1927/1962). Heidegger was a German phenomenologist. His interests in Husserl's phenomenology were sparked when he studied philosophy at the University of Freiburg, where he later taught (Dahlstrom, 2012). He reformed "phenomenology in ways that significantly depart[ed] from Husserlian phenomenology" (Dahlstrom, 2012, p. 51). Heidegger thought deeply about the ontology of human existence and understanding of the ordinary everyday of human existence, or "being-in-the-world" (Inwood, 1999). He brought his fascination with language and the hermeneutic method, which requires interpretation of texts, into his understanding of being human and the meaning of being (Dreyfus, 1991). Hence, Heideggerian phenomenology is often termed *hermeneutic* or *interpretive phenomenology*. *Being and Time* (Heidegger, 1927/1962) is commonly regarded as his most important work (Dahlstrom, 2012). In this, he used the term *Dasein* to designate "the particular being with an understanding of being" (Dahlstrom, 2012, p. 53) in the manner of human existence.

Merleau-Ponty's (1908–1961) phenomenology of perception and the lived body (Merleau-Ponty, 1945/2012). Merleau-Ponty was a French phenomenologist influenced, to a great extent, by Husserl and Heidegger, and was also a contemporary of Sartre (Macann, 1993). He is most widely known for his phenomenological attention to the body as a means of perception (Merleau-Ponty, 1945/2012). For Merleau-Ponty (1945/2012), our active engagement with the world—our performance as opposed to our thoughts—is what brings existence to light. In this view, "day to day experiences cannot be fully encompassed through a conception of human beings as thinking things"; rather, "the body is the absolute source . . . human beings are not spectators, but are rather involved, interwoven, and living in the world as embodied beings" (Lala & Kinsella, 2011a, p. 78). Merleau-Ponty's (1945/2012) work brings the lived body into a place of prominence, recognizing it as a path of direct access, beyond thinking, to the phenomenal world.

IMPACT ON UNDERSTANDING OF OCCUPATION AND OCCUPATIONAL ENGAGEMENT

Phenomenology for Educators

Educators might use people's evocative stories of doing occupations as a way to throw light on how occupations may be lived and experienced by various people and populations. Focusing on phenomenological existentials, such as lived time, lived space, lived bodies, and lived relationships, can broaden students' (and practitioners') understandings of what it might mean to live with and through occupational disruptions or transitions. Phenomenological insights about occupation can be instructive for students and therapists. For instance, findings from a study about phenomenological perspectives on occupation in the latter stages of terminal illness illuminate older adults' insights into existential dimensions (Lala & Kinsella, 2011b). Education about the phenomenology of occupations in different contexts—for instance, toward end of life—might consider unique aspects, such as the ways in which living with the knowledge of impending death changes occupations, how everyday occupations are reworked in light of illness, how occupations are guided by the will of the body, how relationships may become prioritized over productivity, how attending to "the small things" can become a priority, and how engaging existential reflections shapes everyday occupations (Lala & Kinsella, 2011b). Phenomenological perspectives as discussed by those living with terminal illness may help students and practitioners respond in more meaningful ways in their own future practices.

Conversely, educators might use phenomenology as a means to reveal hidden, real-world aspects of being a learner or student practitioner. For example, understandings of how medical learners experienced shame from sentinel events in practice might now inform medical educators' recognition of students' feelings of shame and approaches to intervening in a meaningful way (Bynum et al., 2019). Further, phenomenological perspectives can inform the practices of educators and the design of educational initiatives. A phenomenological study into arts-based approaches to ethics education in an occupational therapy curriculum is a case in point (Kinsella & Bidinosti, 2016).

Students variously described how they became aware of values, (re)discovered creativity, came to value reflection, deepened self-awareness, and developed capacities to imagine future practices through engagement with the arts. These phenomenological insights revealed unique ways in which arts-informed approaches could contribute to occupational therapy curricula, and the possibility of arts to activate imaginative engagement, foster interpretive capacities, inspire transformative understandings, engage new ways of knowing, deepen reflection and awareness, and enrich the inner lives of students.

Phenomenology for Researchers

For phenomenological researchers of people's engagement in occupations, the goal is to describe lived experiences of a phenomenon and/or to interpret the meaning of these experiences "both in terms of what was experienced and how it was experienced" (Neubauer et al., 2019, p. 91). The goal is to do phenomenological research in a way that makes it phenomenology and not any other approach to qualitative research (Wright-St Clair, 2015, 2018). This means that the concern, the research question, the methodology and research methods are congruent in the way they endeavor to understand something of people's lifeworld experiences of phenomena. Because "contemporary phenomenology is based on many intellectual strands and traditions that are developed in response to current and earlier thoughts" (van Manen, 2007, p. 21), van Manen encourages researchers to gain inspiration for their methodological attitudes and insights by engaging with the primary writings of leading philosophers. Zahavi (2019a) suggests that doing so prevents trivializing philosophical phenomenology as merely a research method.

Further, phenomenological research offers a unique approach to advancing knowledge and improving understanding of the lived worlds of human occupation in various contexts and domains. The existential phenomenological frameworks of lived time, lived space, lived relationships, and lived body have the potential to offer unique insights into investigations into occupation (Lala & Kinsella, 2011b). Phenomenological research has the potential to draw attention to the phenomenology of "being," "becoming," "belonging," and "doing" in everyday occupation (Lala & Kinsella, 2011c). Further, it can help us think through what engagement in occupation may reveal and conceal, as demonstrated in a study into occupation and aging by Wright-St Clair et al. (2011), which showed that "the ordinary ways of 'being in the everyday,' such as having a routine and a familiar purposefulness" may *conceal* being aged; whereas "'experiencing the unaccustomed,' such as suddenly noticing an unaccustomed weakness or oldness, in the midst of doing deeply familiar occupations" (Wright-St Clair et al., 2011, p. 88) may *announce* or *reveal* being aged. Phenomenological perspectives may also advance understanding of the lived embodied experiences of occupation while living with disability, illness, or periods of transition. For instance, a 2018 phenomenological investigation of the body with multiple sclerosis revealed dimensions of living with multiple sclerosis—bodily uncertainty, having a precious body, being a different body, and the mindful body—that clearly have implications for occupational engagement (van der Meide et al., 2018).

In considering the critical possibilities of phenomenological investigation, Doyle (2001) notes that phenomenological research can offer critiques of master or dominant cultural narratives and destabilize fixed or oppressive perspectives. Doyle's (2001) study, which examined the everyday lifeworld of political prisoners, showed how prisoners re-inscribed meanings, even while living in severely restricted environments. Her work and that of an emerging group of feminist and transformational phenomenologists opens possibilities for more explicit attention to critical perspectives in phenomenology: perspectives that attend to power, politics, discourse, agency, and culture.

Phenomenology for Practitioners

For occupational therapy practitioners, a phenomenological gaze fuels a wonderment for things and attunement to the lifeworld of everyday occupation in the world; it is an approach that may be used to inquire into the artistry of life as it relates to occupation. A phenomenological lens brings attention to how knowledge develops through our being-in-the-world, through "doing" and lived experiences of that which occupies us, and to our embodied being in the world. In thinking about a phenomenological relation to the world, Heidegger writes:

> The less we just stare at the thing called hammer, the more actively we use it, the more original our relation to it becomes and the more undisguisedly it is encountered as what it is, as a useful thing. The act of hammering itself discovers the specific "handiness" of the hammer. (cited in Zahavi 2019b, p. 74)

Reed, Hocking, and Smythe (2011) view the promise of phenomenology for occupation as implicated in discernment of the meaning of the call to particular occupations, recognition of the ways in which occupations allow us to "be with" others, and the possibilities that occupations open up with respect to who we are and who we are becoming.

Practitioners may inquire into the phenomenology of occupation by asking questions such as "What was that like for you?," "What were your feelings?," "What resonated for you?," "What did you feel in your body?," "What is this activity like for you?," "What were your sensations?," "Was time fleeting or slow?," "What relations are implicated?," "What possibilities are opened?," and more. This spirit of inquiry into the phenomenal world of those with whom we work has the potential to broaden the scope of attention that practitioners, and important others, bring to everyday occupations.

From the practice horizon, "phenomenology can be practiced as a human science (*Geisteswissenschaften*) that remains grounded in its original philosophic sources" (van Manen, 2019, p. 912). Its goal for occupational therapy practitioners is, therefore, practice in the phenomenological mode. Phenomenological practice privileges "thinking and an attitude of reflective attentiveness to the primordialities of human existence" (van Manen, 2019, p. 911).

Phenomenological practitioners might also come to practice with a deeper "listening attitude" (Fiumara, 1990, p. 145). A *listening attitude* is a way of listening to those whom practitioners serve in the direction of what may lie hidden, of asking open questions about experiencing lived moments and of listening deeply (Wright-St Clair et al., 2011). A listening attitude plays out as both inviting richly descriptive accounts of occupations and showing that people's stories are heard. In summary, phenomenology can help practitioners learn from others' experiences (Neubauer et al., 2019). It can also help practitioners to remain open to new interpretations of experience, and the potential to re-imagine occupation and occupational engagement with fresh eyes and in creative ways.

KEY IMPLICATIONS FOR OCCUPATIONAL THERAPY EDUCATION, RESEARCH, AND PRACTICE

Education

- Assist students to understand how occupations may be lived and experienced by various populations served.
- Use the phenomenological existentials of lived time, lived space, lived bodies, and lived relationship to broaden students' understandings of living through occupational disruptions or transitions.

Research

- Be congruent in applying a named phenomenological tradition to the research question, the methodology for, and the methods of researching people's lifeworld experiences of phenomena.
- Gain inspiration for one's own methodological attitudes and insights by engaging with the primary writings of leading philosophers.

Practice

- Bring a phenomenological gaze to practice, with a wonderment for things and attunement to the lifeworld of everyday occupations.
- Come to practice with a listening attitude, as a way of listening in the direction of what may lie hidden and of asking open questions about lived moments.

RECOMMENDED READINGS

Luft, S., & Overgaard, S. (2012). *The Routledge companion to phenomenology*. Routledge.

Moran, D., & Mooney, T. (2002). *The phenomenology reader*. Routledge.

van Manen, M. (2014). *Phenomenology of practice: Meaning-giving methods in phenomenological research and writing*. Left Coast Press.

REFERENCES

Bynum, W. E., Artino, A. R., Uijtdehaage, S., Webb, A. M. B., & Varpio, L. (2019). Sentinel emotional events: The nature, triggers, and effects of shame experiences in medical residents. *Academic Medicine, 94*(1), 85–93. https://doi.org/10.1097/ACM.0000000000002479

Crotty, M. (2015). *The foundations of social research: Meaning and perspective in the research process.* SAGE. (Original work published 1998)

Dahlstrom, D. (2012). Martin Heidegger. In S. Luft & S. Overgaard (Eds.), *The Routledge companion to phenomenology* (pp. 50–61). Routledge.

Dowling, M. (2007). From Husserl to van Manen: A review of different phenomenological approaches. *International Journal of Nursing Studies, 44*(1), 131–142. https://doi.org/10.1016/j.ijnurstu.2005.11.026

Doyle, L. (2001). Bodies inside/out: A phenomenology of the terrorized body in prison. In L. Doyle (Ed.), *Bodies of resistance: New phenomenologies of politics, agency and culture* (pp. 78–99). Northwestern University.

Dreyfus, H. L. (1991). *Being-in-the-world: A commentary on Heidegger's being and time, division I.* MIT Press.

Fiumara, G. C. (1990). *The other side of language: A philosophy of listening* (C. Lambert, Trans.). Routledge.

Heidegger, M. (1962). *Being and time* (7th ed.) (J. Macquarrie & E. Robinson, Trans.). Blackwell. (Original work published 1927)

Husserl, E. (1962). *Ideas: General introduction to pure phenomenology* (W. R. B. Gibson, Trans.). Collier Books. (Original work published 1913)

Husserl, E. (1990). *The idea of phenomenology* (W. P. Alston & G. Nakhnikian, Trans.). Kluwer Academic. (Original work published 1907)

Inwood, M. (1999). *A Heidegger dictionary.* Blackwell.

Kaufer, S., & Chemero, A. (2015). *Phenomenology: An introduction.* Polity Press.

Kielhofner, G. (1997). *Conceptual foundations of occupational therapy.* F. A. Davis.

King, M. (2001). *A guide to Heidegger's* Being and Time. State University of New York Press.

Kinsella, E. A., & Bidinosti, S. (2016). 'I now have a visual image in my mind and it is something I will never forget': An analysis of an arts-informed approach to health professions ethics education. *Advances in Health Sciences Education, 21,* 303–322. https://doi.org/10.1007/s10459-015-9628-7

Lala, A. P., & Kinsella, E. A. (2011a). Embodiment in research practices: The body in qualitative research. In J. Higgs, J. Titchen, D. Horsfall, & D. Bridges (Eds.), *Creative spaces for qualitative researching: Living research* (pp. 77–86). Sense Publishers. https://doi.org/10.1007/978-94-6091-761-5_009

Lala, A. P., & Kinsella, E. A. (2011b). A phenomenological inquiry into the embodied nature of occupation at end of life. *Canadian Journal of Occupational Therapy, 78,* 246–254. https://doi.org/10.2182/cjot.2011.78.4.6

Lala, A. P., & Kinsella, E. A. (2011c). Phenomenology and the study of human occupation. *Journal of Occupational Science, 18*(3), 195–209. https://doi.org/10.1080/14427591.2011.581629

Macann, C. (1993). *Four phenomenological philosophers: Husserl, Heidegger, Sartre and Merleau-Ponty.* Routledge.

Mattingly, C. (1994). Occupational therapy as two-body practice: The lived body. In C. Mattingly & M. H. Fleming (Eds.), *Clinical reasoning: Forms of inquiry in a therapeutic practice* (pp. 64–93). F. A. Davis.

Merleau-Ponty, M. (2012). *Phenomenology of perception.* Routledge. (Original work published 1945)

Meyer, A. (1977). The philosophy of occupational therapy. *American Journal of Occupational Therapy, 31,* 639–642. (Original work published 1922)

Neubauer, B. E., Witkop, C. T., & Varpio, L. (2019). How phenomenology can help us learn from the experiences of others. *Perspectives on Medical Education, 8,* 90–97. https://doi.org/10.1007/s40037-019-0509-2

Okoro, C. (2005). A critique of the polarity in Edmund Husserl's intersubjectivity theory. In A. T. Tymieniecka (Ed.), *Phenomenology of life: Meeting the challenges of the present-day world. Analecta Husserliana* (The Yearbook of Phenomenological Research), *84* (pp. 129–144). Springer. https://doi.org/10.1007/1-4020-3065-7_10

Qutoshi, S. B. (2018). Phenomenology: A philosophy and method of inquiry. *Journal of Education and Educational Development, 5*(1), 215–222.

Reed, K. D., Hocking, C. S., & Smythe, L. A. (2011). Exploring the meaning of occupation: The case for phenomenology. *Canadian Journal of Occupational Therapy, 78*, 303–310. https://doi.org/10.2182/cjot.2011.78.5.5

Reed, K. L. (2017). Identification of the people and critique of the ideas in Meyer's philosophy of occupational therapy. *Occupational Therapy in Mental Health, 33*(2), 107–128. https://doi.org/10.1080/0164212X.2017.1280445

Turpin, M. (2007). Recovery of our phenomenological knowledge. *American Journal of Occupational Therapy, 61*, 469–473. https://doi.org/10.5014/ajot.61.4.469

van der Meide, H., Teunissen, T., Collard, P., Visse, M., & Visser, L. H. (2018). The mindful body: A phenomenology of the body with multiple sclerosis. *Qualitative Health Research, 28*(4), 2239–2249. https://doi.org/10.1177/1049732318796831

van Manen, M. (2014). *Phenomenology of practice: Meaning-giving methods is phenomenological research and writing.* Left Coast Press.

van Manen, M. (2019). Rebuttal: Doing phenomenology on the things. *Qualitative Health Research, 29*(6), 908–925. https://doi.org/10.1177/1049732319827293

Wright-St Clair, V. A. (2015). Doing (interpretive) phenomenology. In S. Nayar & M. Stanley (Eds.), *Qualitative research methodologies for occupational science and therapy* (pp. 53–69). Routledge.

Wright-St Clair, V. A. (2018). Doing interpretive phenomenological research in primary care research. In F. Goodyear-Smith & B. B. Mash (Eds.), *How to do primary care research* (pp. 219–225). CRC Press.

Wright-St Clair, V. A., Kerse, N., & Smythe, L. (2011). Doing everyday occupations both conceals and reveals the phenomenon of being aged. *Australian Occupational Therapy Journal, 58*(2), 88–94. https://doi.org/10.1111/j.1440-1630.2010.00885.x

Zahavi, D. (2019a). Getting it quite wrong: van Manen and Smith on phenomenology. *Qualitative Health Research, 29*(6), 900–907. https://doi.org/10.1177/1049732318817547

Zahavi, D. (2019b). *Phenomenology: The basics.* Routledge.

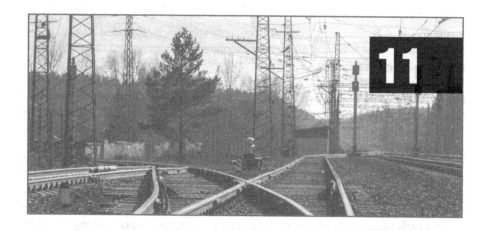

Tools, Thoughts, and Signs
Sociocultural Perspectives on Mind and Occupation

Arun Selvaratnam, MS, OTR/L
Steven D. Taff, PhD, OTR/L, FNAP, FAOTA

INTRODUCTION

In 1926, Lev Semyonovich Vygotsky, a young Soviet psychologist, completed *The Historical Meaning of the Crisis in Psychology: A Methodological Investigation.* At the time, there were a number of schools of thought in psychology, such as Pavlovian reflexology, Gestalt psychology, Freudian psychoanalysis, personalism, and more. Vygotsky analyzed these different schools and found that not only were they incompatible methodologically and theoretically, but also that they differed on what constituted the basic facts of psychology. The question of what unites psychological phenomena as disparate as a mathematician's computations or a person enjoying a tragic play would be answered differently by these different schools (Vygotsky, 1986a). To psychoanalysts, the uniting factor is the unconscious mind; to reflexologists, it would be conditioned responses to stimuli. Within a certain limit, each of these core concepts provide explanatory value. However, to gain

Taff, S. D. (Ed.). *Philosophy and Occupational Therapy:*
Informing Education, Research, and Practice (pp. 101-109).
© 2021 Taylor & Francis Group.

methodological hegemony, those core concepts were each expanded to explain all human thought and behavior, and reached a point where they failed to hold up their ideological weight (Vygotsky, 1986b).

Vygotsky originated his own concept that mental functioning in an individual could only be analyzed by exploring the social and cultural processes from which that functioning derives (Wertsch & Tulviste, 1992). This drew from a general philosophy of the Marxian and Hegelian mode, which claimed that any phenomenon could only be understood via analysis of its origin and history (Kozulin, 1984, p. 105). Vygotsky felt it essential to analyze how "lower" mental functions, such as reflexes, were organized into "higher"-end human goals. That transformation is accomplished via tools, both physical and psychological. These tools hold the history of social and cultural processes within them and define the scope of any individual's mental functioning during the use of those tools (Kozulin, 1984, p. 106). He believed that the process of learning and gaining new skills came from individuals reacting to and internalizing the context provided to them by the people and society around them. Vygotsky was concerned with the use of semiotics, or signs, as tools to mediate thoughts. Of particular interest was language, the shared signs that underscored human social interaction. He stated that humans use inner speech to plan and regulate their actions. This derives from external speech between humans and is evidenced by a period of egocentric speech in children, who are just learning to differentiate between external and inner speech (Vygotsky, 1986b).

Simultaneously, M. M. Bakhtin, a Soviet linguist, was publishing his own thoughts on language. His foundation was the *utterance*, the real unit of communication through speech, belonging to a particular speaking subject and expressing a meaning (Bakhtin, 1986). To have meaning, an utterance must be addressed to and received by a speaker (addressability). It must also be answerable and able to generate a response (Bakhtin, 1986). To understand an utterance, the listener must place it into and respond with his/her own words. Furthermore, every utterance is primarily a response to prior utterances: everything that has ever given the word in that utterance meaning as the listener receives it. This can extend voice beyond the immediate speech situation and is an exemplar of dialogism (Bakhtin, 1981).

Vygotsky's thoughts were expanded upon by thinkers who came after him. Leontiev situated his analysis of social and cultural contexts around *activities*, which he understood as meaningful, goal-driven, and socially determined interactions between human beings and their environments (Cole, 1985). He came up with a framework known as activity theory, which is explored in detail later in this chapter.

Major Concepts and Themes of a Sociocultural Philosophy of Mind

The core assumptions of a sociocultural philosophy of mind are as follows. First, all action takes place between a subject (the doer) and an object (what is being done). Objects exist in an objective reality that can be measured and analyzed. The subjects can also be analyzed via analysis of the objects. This focus on objective reality comes from the philosophy's grounding in Marxian and Hegelian origins. Second, actions/

thoughts are mediated by psychological and physical tools that define the scope of the actions. These tools are transformed over time by both the subjects and the objects between which they mediate, and therefore contain the history of the context of the action they mediate within them. In this way, the psychological tool of language contains the history of contexts for interactions between the thoughts of the individual and society. Third, transformations between the subject and the object are the mechanism through which learning occurs. Development (genetic analysis) is both described and measured within a sociocultural framework.

Zone of Proximal Development

In relation to a specific concept or action, an individual has both a level of potential development and a level of actual development. Actual development can be measured by individual problem-solving. Potential development is measured by problem-solving under the guidance of a more knowledgeable other, or expert (Vygotsky, 1978, p. 86). The zone of proximal development is the space between these two levels. During a goal-directed activity, the more knowledgeable other provides direct and indirect guidance to the learner about the actions and behaviors necessary to gain independence in and master the activity (Cole, 1985). This is done via scaffolding—providing the level of support and organization necessary to ensure the success of the learner, and then gradually removing that support as the learner becomes more adept.

The zone of proximal development measures a learner's potential. Vygotsky argued that education should focus on testing that reveals the potential for development, and less on measuring the current level of development (Vygotsky, 1978). This supports dynamic assessments, which measure the level of mediation from the more knowledgeable other during a specific activity. The assessor actively participates in the completion of the activity and provides the minimum level of mediation required for success (Lantolf & Thorne, 2007, p. 208). The zone of proximal development therefore is simultaneously a conceptual understanding of learning and an assessment framework.

Activity Theory

Figure 11-1 depicts the hierarchical structure of activity. At the top are *activities*, goal-driven actions that Leontiev framed as larger projects driven by some motive (Kaptelinin, 2013). For example, a student of finance may undertake the activity of learning to use Excel spreadsheets, with the motive of effectively completing financial analyses. *Actions* are the consciously completed components of an activity, such as entering a formula into a cell or selecting the correct range of cells. *Operations* are the unconscious components that comprise actions, such as moving a mouse pointer or typing a number. As the learner gains expertise, activities may reach the level of actions as they increase in automaticity (Hasan & Kazlauskas, 2014).

Also depicted here is activity theory's focus on object-orientedness. The subjects (activity, action, and operations) are always oriented toward some purpose that must be met (motive, goal, and task). This orientation between subject and object defines every action that a human can take. Furthermore, because the object exists in an objective reality, the subject can be objectively analyzed by examination of the object itself

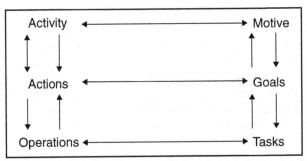

Figure 11-1. Leontiev's framework for sociocultural analysis of activity. (Reprinted with permission from Hasan, H., & Kazlauskas, A. [2014]. Activity theory: Who is doing what, why and how. In H. Hasan [Ed.], *Being practical with theory: A window into business research* [pp. 13–20]. THEORI.)

(Kaptelinin et al., 1995). This ties in with Vygotsky's ideas about understanding mental processes via analysis of the external environment (society and culture) with which they interact. Tools, thoughts, and signs all serve as mediators for activity and behavior.

Within the activity theory framework are the ideas of internalization and externalization. *Externalization* is the transformation of internal components of the activity into external ones (e.g., sketching out a concept for new adaptive equipment). *Internalization* is the transformation of external components of the activity into internal ones, such as moving from computing addition on paper to doing so in your head (Kaptelinin, 2013). The process of internalization and externalization parallels developmental exchanges between the individual and society.

Dialogism

M. M. Bakhtin formalized the concept of dialogism, which arises from the idea of literature holding a dialogue with the other literature that came both before and afterward. The previous work both informs and is informed by a piece of literature (Bakhtin, 1981). This is perhaps most readily evident in philosophical texts, which can carry on dialogues over centuries. For example, John Locke's *Second Treatise of Government* responds to and recontextualizes Thomas Hobbes's *Leviathan* on the topic of how human beings create society and government.

Bakhtin believed that all speech was dialogic. The basic unit of speech is the *utterance*. The utterance is the most straightforward unit of speech and is something that is expressed by and reflects an individual. For example, when one receives a gift, "thank you very much" is the responding utterance. All utterances are addressed at a particular object of the speaker's choosing. Here we see the subject-object relationship that defines action in the tradition of activity theory. It is in the relationship between the subject and the object, expressed by an utterance, that meaning is created (Bakhtin, 1981). Even if the object does not verbally respond, understanding of the subject's utterance is in itself a response.

Furthermore, language is itself a form of semiotics. The signs of language are the individual words and phrases that a speaker uses to communicate. In choosing a word, the speaker interacts with all past uses of that word, provides a new context for those uses, and will interact with all future uses of that word. In the same way that a psychological or physical tool holds the history of action within it, a word or phrase holds the history of communication around that word or phrase within it. In turn, this means that speech is polyphonic and holds not just one individual's voice but the intentions and voice of myriad others (Bakhtin, 1984).

IMPACT ON UNDERSTANDING OF OCCUPATION AND OCCUPATIONAL ENGAGEMENT

Leontiev's definition of activity as goal-oriented, meaningful action that occurs between a subject and an object aligns closely with popular definitions of occupation in contemporary occupational therapy. Occupations are daily activities that people find meaningful and purposeful. Within the context of a sociocultural philosophy of mind, occupations are tools (American Occupational Therapy Association, 2017), processes that people perform in order to reach some objective. They exist within a social and historical context; they transform and are transformed by the people who perform them. They are learned and mastered via interaction with others. Even seemingly solo occupations interact with the social and cultural context in a variety of ways. Through the performance of an occupation, social and cultural artifacts are created and transformed. A planted flower, the trowel used to plant it, the knowledge of what soil that flower thrives in—all of these are exchanges between the individual and the world at large.

From a sociocultural viewpoint, occupations are never truly individual. Like utterances in Bakhtin's formulation of semiotics, an occupation holds the history of the contexts for that occupation within itself. In performing an occupation, the subject interacts with the object being addressed, and with all performances of that occupation in the past and future. Even though individuals find unique meaning for themselves within their occupations, they are inextricably linked to the meanings that others have provided for that occupation. When exploring or engaging in occupation, one must address that meaning. This understanding provides an opportunity to work with that meaning, not just from the individual perspective, but also by recontextualizing it for that individual via the meanings provided by others. Individuals transform occupations through recontextualizing them, but their unique context, meanings, and goals add another aspect to what is actually a communal experience.

Activity theory shows that occupations move across levels of automaticity as the circumstances and the individual's mastery of that occupation changes. An experienced cook may focus on the overall design and theme of a dinner, whereas a novice may work on trying not to burn any food. The same occupations are performed, but the level of automaticity and engagement with the tool(s) is different. Changes in the individual's circumstances may move that occupation up or down a level of automaticity. For example, for an experienced cook a decrease in organizational ability due to changes in mental or emotional status may take cooking mashed potatoes from an unconscious action to a conscious activity.

A core belief of occupational therapy is that engagement in occupations is fundamentally valuable. Promoting and improving occupational engagement is a core mechanism through which occupational therapists treat their clients. In a sociocultural philosophy of mind, occupations are how all individuals are shaped by, and in turn themselves shape, society and culture. Through doing, one finds and affirms one's place among other people. Performing occupations is essential to creating connections with other individuals and humanity as a whole.

KEY IMPLICATIONS FOR OCCUPATIONAL THERAPY EDUCATION, RESEARCH, AND PRACTICE

Education

- Through the process of internalization, individuals receive and integrate knowledge from teachers and more knowledgeable others around them. They externalize their own understanding, thereby changing the context, and collaborating with groups to produce the desired outcome, as is often the case as a member of the allied health environment. Case-based learning groups provide a chance for occupational therapy students to practice, learn, and create knowledge via internalization and externalization in small groups, led by an expert, to prepare them for real-world practice.

- A sociocultural perspective supports educational curriculums that consistently educate students to take context, and the relationship between the client and the client's context, into consideration when adapting assessments and interventions. Learning interventions in apolitical, contextless settings is essentially meaningless because it is the subject-object relationship of the client and the intervention that will ultimately determine the usefulness of that intervention. Rather than a repertoire of intervention skills that may be applied broadly, education should focus on creativity and adaptation with a focus on the functional occupation.

Research

- Vygotsky held that potential developmental level was more important for analyzing future success than current developmental level, and designed studies comparing IQ testing to dynamic assessments as a predictor of future success. He found that dynamic assessments, which do more to measure potential to learn and were more adaptive to the specific contexts of the clients, were the better predictor (Scott & Palincsar, 2013). Health care research on a large scale can come into conflict with the innate variability of human beings when using static assessments to simplify human interaction with an occupation over large sets of data. The use of dynamic assessments can present more of a challenge in terms of methodological design, as they require ensuring and maintaining inter-rater reliability. However, they are more sensitive to the contexts of each individual within a study and ultimately provide a broader view and more points of analysis for the study as a whole.

- At times, the sociocultural theory of mind has funneled into viewing context as merely a container for an individual to interact with (Niewolny & Wilson, 2009). Although the subject-object relationship is important, that relationship is affected by and directly affects the context within which it exists. Social and cultural forces also shape this context. Sometimes those forces can be large barriers to occupational engagement for certain individuals or groups. It is important to view social criticism as a vital part of research in the sociocultural tradition, to confront and analyze those forces. Acknowledgment of the social forces that shape and change someone's context, and how that may affect results, is vital in any research study involving humans.

Practice

- All occupation takes place with the doer of the occupation, both affecting and being affected by the social and historical context behind that occupation. This means that a real understanding of what occupational engagement means for a client requires moving away from noncontextual and apolitical interpretations of occupation. People are unevenly affected by existing power structures that, in turn, define how they perceive themselves (Niewolny & Wilson, 2009). To become a more sensitive and capable practitioner, one must be open to learning about power structures and recognize that they have a vastly different effect depending on who you are. Building trust with clients to have them truly feel comfortable enough to communicate about their understanding and their needs without fear of judgment is also paramount.

- Leontiev's hierarchical structure of activity aligns well with activity analysis. At the top level is the overall activity that the client is trying to accomplish. Below are the conscious actions, then the unconscious operations, each of them oriented toward their own purpose. Transformation of activity into action or action into operation is accomplished via mastery of the skills taught in occupational therapy. Occupational therapists often have to work with clients who have had their hierarchical structure of activity uprooted. Formerly unconscious actions such as moving a hand may require conscious effort. This, in turn, disrupts higher-order conscious actions, such as putting on a shirt and elevates them to the status of conscious actions required to perform an activity. Mapping out the hierarchical structure of activity allows for a way to both analyze and map the progress of a client toward occupational goals.

- The process of continuous learning via the zone of proximal development strongly supports the use of dynamic assessments in measuring the potential for increased occupational engagement. Assessments like the Executive Function Performance Test or the Performance Assessment of Self-Care Skills have clients engage in meaningful occupation, with the therapist, who is the more knowledgeable other, participating by offering the minimum level of support needed to complete the task successfully. This establishes the level of scaffolding needed to complete the occupation, setting a baseline as well as a road map for how that support can be graded in the future.

RECOMMENDED READINGS

Bakhtin, M. M. (1981). *The dialogic imagination: Four essays* (C. Emerson & M. Holquist, Trans.). University of Texas Press.

Vygotsky, L. S. (1978). *Mind in society: The development of higher psychological processes* (M. Cole, V. John-Steiner, S. Scribner, & E. Souberman, Eds.). Harvard University Press.

Wertsch, J. V. (1991). *Voices of the mind: A sociocultural approach to mediated action.* Harvard University Press.

REFERENCES

American Occupational Therapy Association (AOTA). (2017). Occupational therapy practice framework: Domain and process (3rd ed.). *American Journal of Occupational Therapy, 68*(Suppl. 1), S1–S48. https://doi.org/10.5014/ajot.2014.682006

Bakhtin, M. M. (1981). *The dialogic imagination: Four essays* (C. Emerson and M. Holquist, Trans.). University of Texas Press.

Bakhtin, M. M. (1984). *Problems of Dostoevsky's poetics* (C. Emerson, Trans.). University of Minnesota Press.

Bakhtin, M. M. (1986). *Speech genres and other late essays* (C. Emerson and M. Holquist, Trans.). University of Texas Press.

Cole, M. (1985). The zone of proximal development: Where culture and cognition create each other. In J. V. Wertsch (Ed.), *Culture, communication, and cognition: Vygotskian perspectives* (pp. 146–161). Cambridge University Press.

Hasan, H., & Kazlauskas, A. (2014). Activity theory: Who is doing what, why and how. In H. Hasan (Ed.), *Being practical with theory: A window into business research* (pp. 13–20). THEORI.

Kaptelinin, V. (2013). Activity theory. In M. Soegaard & R. F. Dams (Eds.), *The encyclopedia of human-computer interaction* (2nd ed.). https://www.interaction-design.org/literature/book/the-encyclopedia-of-human-computer-interaction-2nd-ed/activity-theory

Kaptelinin, V., Kuutti, K., & Bannon, L. (1995). Activity theory: Basic concepts and applications. In B. Blumenthal, J. Gornostaev, & C. Unger (Eds.), *Human-computer interaction* (pp. 189–201). Springer.

Kozulin, A. (1984). *Psychology in utopia: Toward a social history of soviet psychology.* MIT Press.

Lantolf, J., & Thorne, S. L. (2007). Sociocultural theory and second language learning. In B. van Patten & J. Williams (Eds.), *Theories in second language acquisition* (pp. 201–224). Lawrence Erlbaum.

Niewolny, K. L., & Wilson, A. L. (2009). What happened to the promise? A critical (re)orientation of two sociocultural learning traditions. *Adult Education Quarterly, 60*(1), 26–45. https://doi.org/10.1177/0741713609333086

Scott, S. N., & Palincsar, A. S. (2013). *The historical roots of sociocultural theory.* https://pdfs.semanticscholar.org/37fe/8cf044514b7dbe734f2e4dad2f30c22e9doc.pdf?_ga=2.43295789.966399254.1596678130-52161774.1596678130

Vygotsky, L. S. (1978). *Mind in society: The development of higher psychological processes* (M. Cole, V. John-Steiner, S. Scribner, & E. Souberman, Eds.). Harvard University Press.

Vygotsky, L. S. (1986a). *The historical meaning of the crisis in psychology: A methodological investigation.* https://www.marxists.org/archive/vygotsky/works/crisis/index.htm (Original work published 1926)

Vygotsky, L. S. (1986b). *Thought and language.* MIT Press.

Wertsch, J. V., & Tulviste, P. (1992). L. S. Vygotsky and contemporary developmental psychology. *Developmental Psychology, 28*(4), 548–557.

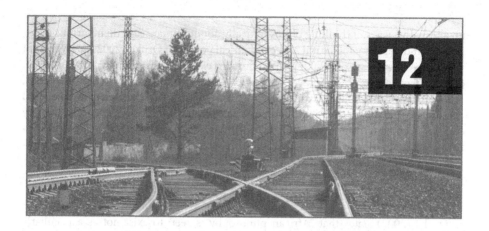

An African Philosophy of Personhood in Southern Occupational Therapy

Thuli Mthembu, BSc OT, MPH, PhD
Madeleine Duncan, DipOT, BOT, BAHons(Psych), MSc OT, DPhil(Psych)

INTRODUCTION

The philosophy of occupational therapy is based on human and social sciences that were developed during a period of imperialism in the global North. Influenced by Cartesian dualism and Kantian rationalism, the liberalist values of individualism were disseminated unidirectionally as a universal body of concepts and methods from the metropole to the peripheral majority world, most notably post-colonial Africa, Latin America, and India (Connell, 2007; Said, 1993). Capturing the thought of scholars and practitioners in formerly colonized and peripheral societies (including displaced and First Nation peoples), Southern occupational therapy seeks the advancement of multidirectional epistemologies that substantiate the philosophy of the profession in a globalizing world (Dsouza et al., 2017; Ramugondo et al., 2015). Decoloniality shifts the Euro-American and Western-centric geography and biography of knowledge, and in so doing opens

Taff, S. D. (Ed.). *Philosophy and Occupational Therapy:*
Informing Education, Research, and Practice (pp. 111-125).
© 2021 Taylor & Francis Group.

up alternative ways of thinking philosophically about humans and their various occupations in diverse sociocultural and geopolitical contexts. Oruka (2002) suggests that uniquely African ways of thinking about humans exist that are distinctly un-European, contrasting the two philosophical traditions as follows: European thought is logical, rational, and individualistic, whereas African thought is intuitive, metaphysical, and communitarian. These thought differences have implications for occupational therapy education, research, and practice in different regions of the world. The Southern positionality of this chapter draws attention to African ethno-philosophical understandings of *person* and *personhood*.

AFRICAN PHILOSOPHY

Oruka (2002) states that "African philosophy is seen to exist not as a peculiarly African phenomenon (for most philosophical problems transcend cultural and racial confines) but only as a corpus of thoughts arising from the discussion and appropriation of authentic philosophical ideas by Africans in the African context" (p. 120). There are currently 54 sovereign states and 10 nonsovereign territories in Africa, representing more than 3,000 ethnic groups and approximately 2,100 different languages and cultures. Acknowledging the diverse histories, peoples, and regions of Africa, Oruka (2002) proposes four trends in African philosophy: ethno-philosophy, philosophic sagacity, nationalist-ideological philosophy, and professional philosophy. Applying the work of African anthropologists and theologians, *ethno-philosophy* elucidates the worldview and thought systems of particular indigenous African communities with reference to, among other things, their folklore, customs, taboos, songs, dances, and other cultural artifacts (Hountondji, 1991). *Philosophic sagacity* analyzes the critical indigenous thought of African sages: men and women who may be illiterate yet whose sagacious oral wisdom reflects a dialectical frame of mind (Oruka, 1983). *Nationalist-ideological philosophy* is located in the philosophical literature of African politicians and statesmen that elucidate Pan-African, national, and individual freedoms in the context of colonization, African communalism, and development (Nabudere, 2011). *Professional philosophy* documents the academic debates of philosophers of African descent who are professionally trained across the spectrum of Greek, Egyptian, European, and Occidental philosophical traditions to teach and practice philosophy in Africa.

Given the scope of African philosophy and ethno-philosophy in particular, the ideas about person and personhood presented are by necessity broad and, therefore, potentially essentializing of the African experience: something that occupational therapists should avoid because essentialism reduces people to a fixed, predetermined, and immutable essence. Although these ideas are not representative of all Africans, they are substantiated by the writings of seminal African philosophers: hence the use of outdated references. We do not address the contemporary critique of original African thought on personhood as being gendered, ableist, and anti-queer (Manzini, 2018), nor do we cover current philosophical debates among African philosophers on individual human rights and Afro-communitarianism (Molefe, 2017). Consideration of this critique would, however, be essential for occupational therapy scholars concerned with the further articulation of Southern professional theory and practice.

FACETS OF AFRICAN ETHNO-PHILOSOPHY

In this section, we briefly describe the metaphysics of African ethno-philosophy, highlighting the worldview and existential reality of indigenous Africans within which their personhood develops. *Metaphysics* is a "branch of philosophy concerned with our conceptions of reality, position in the universe, and our relation to others and the environment—our grappling with time, space, causality and existence" (Mkhize, 2004, p. 35). *Worldview* is defined as a "set of basic assumptions that a group of people develops in order to explain reality and their place and purpose in the world" (Mkhize, 2004, p. 35). Although African philosophers are not in agreement about the existence of a unifying African worldview, three general perspectives about reality are identified. First, there is an intricate union between the object and the subject, between the observer and the observed, between God and the world and the knower and known. In other words, all reality is dialogical and relational. Second, the person is an open, engaging, and vulnerable organism within the world. Third, an African worldview believes in a personal universe that ascribes meaning and purpose in communitarianism (Foster as cited in Klassen, 2017). Figure 12-1 depicts the existential reality of African ontology: that is, how some indigenous African people conceptualize the metaphysical nature of reality.

African metaphysics emphasizes a world in which everything and everyone is connected in a communal hierarchy of beings, all of which are endowed with and energized by a creative life force (vitality, power, energy, spirit) that is extended in varying degrees directly from God (Mkhize, 2004). Every entity in Figure 12-1 is perpetually in motion, influencing and being influenced by something or someone else. Earth, nature, plants, and inanimate objects inhabit the lowest level of life force, followed by animals on the next plane of animated existence. Human beings inhabit the intermediate level of reality between the living and the living-dead (ancestors). Appeased by the homily of the living, recently deceased relatives eventually progress to the community of integrated ancestors who are capable of communicating directly with God, the highest source of life, on behalf of their living relatives. Human beings are guided throughout life by maintaining a link with their recently deceased ancestors via dreams, rituals, sacrifices, and acts of libation. The individual is subordinate first to the nuclear family community and then to the cultural community (Menkiti, 1984). In Africa, the notion of family is not nuclear as it is in Western thought. Instead, family includes and involves tightly knit and extended living and deceased relatives who are hierarchically organized in status and authority. Some humans are called by the ancestors through dreams and paranormal events to become *shamans,* traditional healers capable of mediating between the living and the living-dead. Answering the call requires the selected human to engage in a protracted training process involving mystical rituals that are monitored by an elder shaman or traditional healer. It is accepted as a natural occurrence in the intermediate reality that spirit as life force can occupy space through shapeshifting yet remain a spirit. Unlike inanimate material entities, the spirit can change into forms that can be encountered by humans in the natural intermediate realm and during dreams and trances. Both animals and humans can, therefore, be animated by varying degrees of benevolent or malevolent life force at the behest of the living-dead.

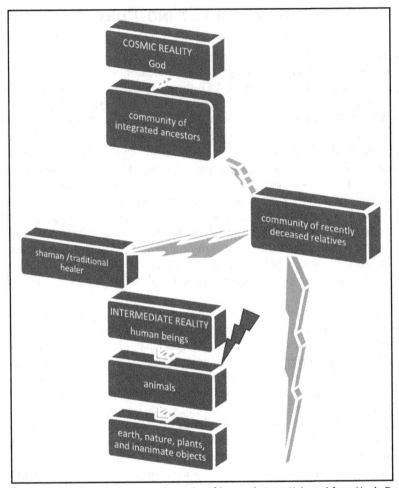

Figure 12-1. African metaphysics: hierarchy of human beings. (Adapted from Hook, D. [2004]. *Critical psychology*. Juta.)

Occult themes in African metaphysics, such as divination, sorcery, and witchcraft that affect humans, will not be addressed here. Suffice it to point out that these themes are used as causal teleological explanations for occupational choice and for understanding life events, including accidents, illness, and disability: "Why did this happen to me/at this stage/in this way?" (Teffo & Roux, 2003, p. 202). Pertinent to the creativity of African people in describing the subjectivities of African ontology to which these questions point is the use of metaphorical imagery from nature, stories, drumming, dance, and song. For example, mental distress or epilepsy may be attributed to communication by the ancestors and described as a roaring stomach filled with poisonous ants that have fed on the graves of the deceased (Keikelame & Swartz, 2015; Kpanake, 2018). Encounters with ancestors, mediated by a shaman or traditional healer, provide humans with the guidance and protection they need to participate in life through gendered and age-specific roles, responsibilities, and occupations, all of which serve to promote or disrupt the cohesion and prosperity of the family and community (Menkiti, 1984). Additionally, the relational well-being of the individual and the collective can be swayed by curses (Hachalinga, 2017).

Explaining *Ubuntu*: A Goal of African Ethno-Philosophy

A general goal of African ethno-philosophy is to explain *ubuntu*, loosely translated as "humanness" or "whole-ness of be-ing" (Ramose, 2002, p. 236). Ramose inserts hyphens to portray the "incessant continual concrete manifestation" of human "one-ness" (Ramose, 2002, p. 236). Inseparable from their social dimension, individuals in Africa appear composite in space, multiple in time, extending and carrying within and with themselves their progenitors (ancestral beings), their present selves, and their ascendants (selves yet to be born). The person cannot be conceived or function independently of social relations. Archbishop Desmond Tutu (as cited in Mulernfo, 2000) describes *ubuntu* as "I am because you are," stating that:

> it embraces hospitality, caring for others, being willing to go the extra mile for the sake of others. We believe a person is a person through another person, that my humanity is caught up, bound up and inextricable in yours. When I dehumanize you, I inexorably dehumanize myself. The solitary human being is a contradiction in terms and therefore you seek to work for the common good because your humanity comes into its own community, in belonging. (pp. 57–58)

Community in *ubuntu* is more than an association of individual persons whose interests and ends are contingently congruent. It is a group of persons linked by interdependent and interpersonal bonds, biological and/or nonbiological, who consider themselves primarily as members of that group and who have common interests, goals, and values. Communitarianism, defined as "an ongoing association of men and women who have a special commitment to one another and a distinct sense of their common life" (Coetzee, 2003, p. 322), does not deny self-determination, nor does it diminish the freedom or capability of the person to choose or question. Instead, it stresses the bidirectional benefits of interdependence: the person is part of the collective that he/ she creates, which in turn creates the more holistic personhood that he/she can attain through participation in personal and collective activities, all of which follow socially sanctioned scripts and practices. In short, *ubuntu* is a process of becoming fully human through an interdependent "community of selves" that includes metaphysical relations with the surrounding natural environment and cosmos at large.

Concepts in African Ethno-Philosophy

In this section, we describe the concepts of "person" and "personhood" in African ethno-philosophy. Although the two concepts are connected, they differ concerning the role of communitarianism in their expression.

Person

What is a person? Descartes's *cogito* ("I think, therefore I am") proposes a dualistic understanding of the person as a combination of two radically different substances: matter (body), which occupies space, and mind (thought), which does not occupy space. Kant's categorical imperative states that man—in general, every rational being—exists as an end in himself. That is, a person is an atomistic, individual, autonomous entity. Kant grounds his rational analysis of a person in the human capacity for moral and rational freedom. Thus, the person ought to be treated as an end in himself, which accounts for liberal individualism in Eurocentric thought (Serequeberhan, 2002).

In contrast, African notions of person are always relational, summed up by Mbiti (1969) as "I am because we are, and since we are, therefore I am" (p. 214). African philosophers debate the metaphysical question: Is a person a self-sufficient atomic individual who does not depend on his/her relationships with others for the realization of his/her ends and who has an ontological priority over community, or is a person by nature a communitarian being, having natural and essential relationships with others? (Matolino, 2014). The debate generally concurs that the starting point for defining a person is that "the 'I' belongs to the 'I-You-correspondence' as a stream of lived experience without which it ('I') could not be thought and would not exist" (Kurkertz as cited in Teffo & Roux, 2003, p. 204). "I" in African thought is just a "we" from another perspective. The self is, therefore, dialogical: it is always in relationship with others in a particular social context.

Against the backdrop of Figure 12-1, the person in the traditional African worldview should, therefore, "be visualized as a centrifugal force capable of emanating other complex selves that can interpermeate each other as well as other selves generated from other persona-communal centers. This centrifugality of the person reaches into all directions and touches all events that contribute to the full person—the mythical past, the generational past, the ever present nature, and the self in the process of being born" (Ogbonnaya, 1994, p. 79). Ogbonnaya's description of a "full person" situates the individual in the teleologically communal context of *ubuntu*. A person is a community of selves, a pluralistic rather than individualistic being. The African concept of a person thus differs from Western philosophy in which a decontextualized, atomized person consists of body, mind, and soul, with the soul usually, as in Descartes, identified with the mind. Writing about person and community in African thought, Gyekye (2002) also describes a person as consisting of different parts. These parts are always dialogically integrated through participation in a community of other human beings, both animate and spiritual. A person has a body, an animating force (which Gyekye metaphorically refers to as "shadow"), a principle of intelligence, and finally the heart, which is not thought of as an organic pump but as the seat of will and emotion. For Africans, mind is more than rationality, the locus of thinking; rather, it is the animating force behind the person's capacity to engage body and heart in various activities, including perceiving, reasoning, feeling, talking, and performing human occupations such as dancing, learning, playing, and working. The normative conception of the African person's will is always moral. A person is someone with the mental capacity to take responsibility for her/his actions and decisions. Children only attain the status of a person when they reach the requisite maturity in moral thinking and social action, raising philosophical questions about the social position of persons with disabilities in African cosmology (Manzini, 2018). Children are socialized into morally accountable personhood through a communitarian framework that holds the ethic of responsibility in high esteem. The individual is brought up, from the beginning, with a sense of belonging and solidarity with an extensive circle of kith and kin. The basis of this solidarity is a system of reciprocity in which each individual has obligations to a large set of other individuals, both living and living-dead. Rights match these owed to him/ her by the same individuals, all committed to interdependent moral reciprocity with the primary role of the community "as a catalyst and as prescriber of norms" (Menkiti, 1984, p. 172).

Personhood

Personhood is "not given simply because one is born of human seed"; instead, it is a state of being that one attains "through a long process of social and ritual transformation until it (*person*) attains the full complement of excellences seen as truly definitive of man" (Menkiti, 1984, p. 172). As a developmental outcome over time, personhood is a "communitarian valuation of community as ontologically, morally and epistemological[ly] before the individual" (Oyowe, 2013, p. 204). The relational dimensions of personhood highlight how the person in an African context may not be separated and completed without the involvement of others (Molefe, 2019). Because personhood is "socially acquired . . . it is something that can be had in concert with others" (Oyowe, 2013, p. 204). It is acquired in "direct proportion as one participates in communal life through the discharge of the various obligations defined by one's stations" (Menkiti, 1984, p. 176). The status of full personhood is only acquired with old age when the person takes on an ancestral quality.

Attaining personhood in the eyes of the community requires the person's participation in different rites of incorporation, notably initiation into adulthood at puberty. The attainment of personhood is a vital element of a person's existence throughout life because it is something the person has to work for *and* something at which the person can fail. Persons fail to achieve personhood when they behave contrary to the moral expectations of humanness, for example, placing curses or being cursed. There are degrees of personhood, with its lower gradations shading off into nonexistence in the life of an individual who fails in basic social decency such as not being "generous, hospitable, caring and compassionate" (Tutu, 1999). These moral standards form the crux of *ubuntu* through "a concrete enactment and realisation of the knowledge that the possession of the qualities of personhood is reflected in one's relationship with others" (Mkhize, 2004, p. 50). In short, person and personhood are two sides of the same coin in African ethno-philosophy. Understanding the dialogical interface between these two concepts creates interesting alternatives when thinking about person-environment-occupation (PEO) dynamics, occupation, and occupational engagement.

AFRICAN ETHNO-PHILOSOPHY: THINKING ABOUT OCCUPATION AND OCCUPATIONAL ENGAGEMENT

In this section, we illustrate how clarity about the African ethno-philosophical tradition regarding person and personhood may extend understanding of occupation and occupational engagement using seminal occupational therapy literature about the PEO triad as a point of reference (Law et al., 1991). Eurocentric occupational therapy literature stresses the importance of health, well-being, and quality of life through the transactional relationship among the person, environment, and occupation. The components of PEO tend to be assessed and addressed using a reductionist, individualistic lens. For example, the person is made up of mind, body, and spiritual qualities; the environment highlights cultural, socioeconomic, institutional, physical, and social considerations; and occupation looks at groups of self-directed, functional tasks and activities in which a person engages over the lifespan (Law et al., 1991). The Cartesian self exists prior to and distinct from society; it proclaims only one centralized thinker and actor. It draws sharp distinctions between the inside self and the outside non-self (Mkhize, 2004).

Although recent Eurocentric occupational therapy literature argues that the qualities of the person affect and are affected by environmental influences, the emphasis is on a paradigm shift "from performance to participation in daily life, with evidence supporting the link between participation and a person's health status" (Pizzi & Richards, 2017). The person remains atomistic, although his/her individual health status hinges on participation in daily life through engagement in personal occupations. While this dynamic between person and environment holds true in general, an African ethno-philosophical stance is more communitarian, more pluralistic. The African version of the PEO dynamic includes "the networks of participation and correspondence that bind the subject to the group and to the cosmos . . . to the important role assigned to milieu, and the inevitable reference to the sacred" (Mkhize, 2004, p. 80). An individual's health and well-being—the individual's humanity—is inextricably linked to the health and well-being of the community of selves, the collective (Kronenberg, 2019; Ramugondo, 2017). Occupations and occupational engagement are always relational (i.e., individual tasks and activities are simultaneously personal and communitarian) (Van Niekerk, 2011). The P is inextricably linked to personhood because "the community produces the individual through rites and rituals and the individual and community's growth is interrelated" (Matolino, 2009, p. 162). The E is shaped by the social power within a community, by a "struggle for power and the need for cultural reaffirmation" (Oyowe, 2013, p. 213). The O is "part of the community, population and citizens . . . [because] they share communal life, traditions, culture, morals and values" (Mthembu, 2018, p. 53). In short, in African ethno-philosophy, the PEO dynamic is always contextually determined and requires a circle around it that depicts the community, including the metaphysical realm.

In the next section, we use Figure 12-2 to illustrate an African ethno-philosophical understanding of the PEO dynamic. It depicts the ontological, interdependent

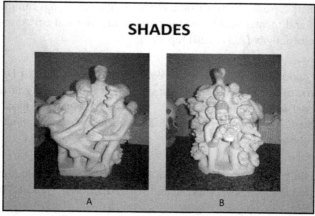

Figure 12-2. Relational interdependence between the living and the shades (living-dead). (Photograph taken by Dr. Madeleine Duncan.)

relationship between the living and the living-dead in a hand-crafted clay sculpture. Used here with informed consent from the sculptor, the photograph was taken by the second author in a rural village in the Eastern Cape Province of South Africa that is populated by isiXhosa-speaking people from the Baça tribe. The sculptor, a 40-year-old man with cerebral palsy who uses a wheelchair, generated an income through selling his sculptures at a tourist shop in a local town. Picture A, a front view, depicts a vulnerable person (either ill, has a disability, in distress, or dying) receiving assistance from living relatives and community members. Picture B, a back view, depicts ancestors surrounding the living, intimately engaged with the life events unfolding in intermediate reality.

The sculptor is an occupational therapy client. Using the American Occupational Therapy Association (AOTA, 2011) philosophical base of occupational therapy as a point of reference, we briefly clarify how an African ethno-philosophical understanding of African metaphysics, personhood, and communitarianism may assist the occupational therapist in reasoning about the occupations and occupational engagement of the sculptor and his community of selves.

- Man is an active being whose development is influenced by the use of purposeful activity (AOTA, 2011, p. S65).

The sculptor's development is influenced by his personhood as much as by engagement in purposeful activities (occupations) such as sculpting. As in the Platonic tradition, reality for the sculptor is dualistic, and he experiences both the invisible and the visible universe. However, unlike Plato's theory that invisible reality is merely a shadow of visible reality, the sculptor's ontology holds that phenomena in the invisible world are real. His development is bolstered through community interdependence as well as the purposeful activity of sculpting.

- Using their capacity for intrinsic motivation, human beings can influence their physical and mental health and their social and physical environment through purposeful activity (AOTA, 2011, p. S65).

Unlike the naturalistic metaphysics of Western philosophers such as Dewey and Castel, which situate the relationship between the self and reality entirely in the natural, materialistic realm (Okolo, 2002, p. 213), the sculptor's capacity for intrinsic motivation to influence his health and the environment is simultaneously personal and communal.

- Human life includes a process of continuous adaptation. Adaptation is a change in function that promotes survival and self-actualization (AOTA, 2011, p. S65).

The sculptor's adaptation as a person with a disability in a communitarian society depends on how the community supports his personhood (as opposed to his self-actualization as an atomistic individual person). His survival is embedded in humane relationships that enhance his potential for human growth and development (Musana, 2018). The universality of his humanness among members of his tribe, including the living-dead who constantly accompany him while he engages in the occupation of sculpting, is affirmed as he seeks the good of others above self-interest.

- Biological, psychological, and environmental factors may interrupt the adaptation process at any time throughout the life cycle. Dysfunction may occur when adaptation is impaired (AOTA, 2011, p. S65).

Figure 12-2B hints at the role that metaphysical factors may play in interrupting the sculptor's adaptation into personhood as a person with physical impairments. Contrary to the Eurocentric perspective, an African ethno-philosophy accentuates that "various types of misfortune, illness, death, and failure arise from activities of unseen forces, unknown and unseen infuriated spiritual agencies, and revengeful ancestors" (Nwoye, 2017, p. 46). There are four possible sources of dysfunction in the sculptor's life cycle: biological, psychological, social, and spiritual (Nwoye, 2015).

- Purposeful activity facilitates the adaptive process. Occupational therapy is based on the belief that purposeful activity (occupation), including its interpersonal and environmental components, may be used to prevent and mediate dysfunction and to elicit maximum adaptation. Activity, as used by the therapist, includes both an intrinsic and a therapeutic purpose (AOTA, 2011, p. S65).

Figure 12-2A illustrates ubuntu, *the humanness of the living in caring for the ailing. An* ubuntu *perspective of collective occupations highlights the value of intentionality that drives human occupations and social practice (Ramugondo & Kronenberg, 2015). The sculptor occupies his world intending to use his time and resources firstly to secure an income through the occupation of sculpting and secondly to capture, in clay form and vivid imagery, the innate need to participate in the satisfyingly ordinary and extraordinary collective human occupation of care-giving.*

Impact on Understanding of Occupation and Occupational Engagement

African ethno-philosophy accentuates the dialogical interaction among the objective, the subjective, and the metaphysical. It foregrounds the distinctions and overlaps between person and personhood as parts of the relational nature of human interconnectedness and interdependence. In contrast to the individualism of the Western worldview, African ethno-philosophy supports a communitarian approach to the PEO interaction. It envisages an understanding of occupation and occupational engagement that will promote *ubuntu* whereby "the individual and the community are in a constant shared process of becoming." An African worldview will guide a communitarian perspective on human adaptation as emerging not primarily through individual occupation but through occupational engagement with others. It foregrounds the relational values, morals, and ethics of African ethno-philosophy, and in so doing promotes the humanness of occupational therapy.

Key Implications for Occupational Therapy Education, Research, and Practice

In this section, we suggest key implications for occupational therapy education, research, and practice arising from the ideas shared in the chapter. We argue that Southern occupational therapy foregrounds the importance of interdependence and communitarianism as valued goals of persons who subscribe to an African worldview (Mthembu, 2018; Ramugondo & Kronenberg, 2015; Sherry, 2010).

Education

- Occupational therapy epistemology will benefit from decolonial scholarship (Ramugondo, 2018). Indigenous people are positioned to interpret and articulate the profession's biography so that it is fit for its purpose in particular geospatial and sociocultural contexts. Decolonial scholarship will be attuned to the hegemony of Eurocentrism in core professional constructs such as "person." It will promote actions that address the social determinants of healthy families and communities (World Health Organization [WHO], 2016).

- Education is always political. Students would benefit from a living curriculum, one that helps them understand how their personal–professional personhood unfolds through communitarian learning and authentic partnerships (Richards & Galvaan, 2018).
- Consequently, an African ethno-philosophy would socialize students around the values of the community's needs related to the social determinants of health that promote community empowerment and participation in intentional occupations (WHO, 2016).

Research

- Decolonial participatory research will pave the way for describing and theorizing Southern practice-based evidence in collaboration with historically marginalized people (Ramugondo, 2018; Smith, 2012).
- Ethno-philosophical investigation focusing on core occupational therapy concepts, beliefs, and methods will require transdisciplinary research partnerships (Frank et al., 2008).

Practice

- Occupational therapy practice will flourish if it gets "back to the basics of life, life lived and experienced in the community" (Musana, 2018, p. 31). Communicentric practice would enable occupational therapists to contribute to the United Nations Agenda 2030 and Sustainable Developmental Goals (United Nations Developmental Programme [UNDP], 2019; WHO, 2016). More importantly, it will position the profession as a change agent for mitigating the social determinants of health with the focus on occupational justice that is sensitized to local worldviews (Hocking & Townsend, 2015; WHO, 2016).
- The practice of occupational therapy should promote "the kind of life that recognises existence beyond the self as an individual, affirming the view that our individual identities are a construct of the community, and our being depends on how we relate with the immediate milieu" (Musana, 2018, p. 31).
- An African ethno-philosophy in occupational therapy practice will foreground the personhood of occupational therapists as well as the personhood of the individuals, groups, families, and communities with whom they work. A communitarian approach to practice enhances humanity on the globe. It stands for the good, desirable qualities in human beings: being good, humane, thoughtful, considerate, kind, wise, and godly (religious), generous, polite, mature, and virtuous; "the manifestation of positive and life-giving actions" (Musana, 2018, p. 32). Such a practice orientation by occupational therapists would strengthen their contribution to Sustainable Developmental Goal 17 (i.e., partnerships for the attainment of all goals; UNDP, 2019).

RECOMMENDED READINGS

Alers, V., & Crouch, R. (2010). *Occupational therapy: An African perspective.* Sarah Shorten.

Dsouza, S. A., Galvaan, R., & Ramugondo, E. L. (2017). *Concepts in occupational therapy: Understanding Southern perspectives.* Manipal University Press.

Musana, P. (2018). The African concept of personhood and its relevance to respect for human life and dignity in Africa and the global context. *Africa Study Monographs, 56,* 21–32. https://doi.org/10.14989/230172

REFERENCES

American Occupational Therapy Association (AOTA). (2011). The philosophical base of occupational therapy. *American Journal of Occupational Therapy, 65,* S65. https://doi.org/10.5014/ajot.2011.65S65

Coetzee, P. (2003). Morality in African thought. In P. Coetzee & A. P. J. Roux (Eds.), *The African Philosophy Reader* (2nd ed., pp. 321–401). Oxford University Press of Southern Africa.

Connell, R. (2007). *Southern theory: The global dynamics of knowledge in social science.* Allen & Unwin Academic.

Dsouza, S., Galvaan, R., & Ramugondo, E. (2017). *Concepts in occupational therapy: Understanding Southern perspectives.* Manipal University Press.

Frank, G., Block, P., & Zemke, R. (2008). Introduction to special theme issue anthropology, occupational therapy and disability studies: Collaborations and prospects. *Practicing Anthropology, 30*(3), 2–5. https://doi.org/10.17730/praa.30.3.w11l362702q45003

Gyekye, K. (2002). Person and community in African thought. In P. Coetzee & A. Roux (Eds.), *Philosophy from Africa: A text with readings* (2nd ed., pp. 279–311). Oxford University Press.

Hachalinga, P. (2017). How curses impact people and biblical responses. *Journal of Adventist Mission Studies, 13*(1), 1–9. https://digitalcommons.andrews.edu/jams/vol13/iss1/7

Hocking, C., & Townsend, E. (2015). Driving social change: Occupational therapists' contributions to occupational justice. *World Federation of Occupational Therapy Bulletin, 71*(2), 68–71. https://doi.org/10.1179/2056607715Y.0000000002

Hook, D. (2004). *Critical psychology.* Juta.

Hountondji, P. (1991). African philosophy: Myth and reality. In T. Serequeberhan (Ed.), *African philosophy: The essential readings* (pp. 111–131). Paragon House.

Keikelame, M., & Swartz, L. (2015). "A thing full of stories": Traditional healers' explanations of epilepsy and perspectives on collaboration with biomedical health care in Cape Town. *Transcultural Psychiatry, 52*(5), 659–680. https://doi.org/10.1177/1363461515571626

Klassen, J. (2017). The role of personhood in development: An African perspective on development in South Africa. *Missionalia, 45*(1), 29–44. http://dx.doi.org/10.7834/45-1-154

Kpanake, L. (2018). Cultural concepts of person and mental health in Africa. *Transcultural Psychiatry, 55*(2), 198–218. https://doi.org/10.1177/1363461517749435

Kronenberg, F. (2019). *Everyday enactments of human affirmations in 1994 post-apartheid South Africa: A phronetic case study of being human as occupation and health* (Doctoral dissertation). http://hdl.handle.net/11427/29441

Law, M., Cooper, B., Strong, S., Stewart, D., Rigby, P., & Letts, L. (1991). The person-environment-occupation model: A transactive approach to occupational performance. *Canadian Journal of Occupational Therapy, 63*(1), 9–23. https://doi.org/10.1177/000841749606300103

Manzini, N. (2018). Menkiti's normative communitarian conception of personhood as gendered, ableist and anti-queer. *South African Journal of Philosophy, 37*(1), 18–33. https://doi.org/10.1080/02580136.2017.1405510

Matolino, B. (2009). Radicals versus moderates: A critique of Gyekye's moderate communitarianism. *South African Journal of Philosophy, 28*(2), 160–170. https://doi.org/10.4314/sajpem.v28i2.46674

Matolino, B. (2014). *Personhood in African philosophy.* Cluster Publications.

Mbiti, J. (1969). *African religious and philosophy.* Heineman.

Menkiti, I. (1984). Person and community in African traditional thought. In R. Wright (Ed.), *African philosophy: An introduction* (pp. 171–181). University Press of America.

Mkhize, N. (2004). Psychology: An African perspective. In D. Hook (Ed.), *Critical psychology* (pp. 24–52). UCT Press.

Mkhize, N. (2004). Sociocultural approaches to psychology: Dialogism and African conceptions of the self. In D. Hook (Ed.), *Critical psychology* (pp. 53–83). UCT Press.

Molefe, M. (2017). Personhood and rights in an African tradition. *Politokon, 45*(2), 1–16. https://doi.org/10.1080/02589346.2017.1339176

Molefe, M. (2019). Solving the conundrum of African philosophy through personhood: The individual or community. *Journal of Value Inquiry, 54*(1) 1–17. https://doi.org/10.1007/s10790-019-09683-8

Mthembu, T. G. (2018). Ethics in occupational therapy—African perspectives. In N. Nortje, W. A. Hoffmann, & J. De Jongh (Eds.), *African perspectives on ethics for healthcare professionals* (pp. 49–60). https://doi.org/10.1007/978-3-319-93230-9_4

Mulernfo, M. (2000). *Thabo Mbeki and the African renaissance.* Actna Press.

Musana, P. (2018). The African concept of personhood and its relevance to respect for human life and dignity in Africa and global context. *African Study Monographs, 56,* 21–32. https://doi.org/10.1489/2301172

Nabudere, D. (2011). *Afrokology, philosophy and wholeness: An epistemology.* Institute of South Africa.

Nwoye, A. (2015). African psychology and the Africentric paradigm to clinical diagnosis and treatment. *South African Journal of Psychology, 45*(3), 305–317. https://doi.org/10.1177/0081246315570960

Nwoye, A. (2017). An African theory of human personhood. *Psychology in Society, 54,* 42–66. https://doi.org/10.17159/2309-8708/2017/n54a4

Ogbonnaya, A. (1994). Person as community: An African understanding of the person as an intrapsychic community. *Journal of Black Psychology, 20,* 75–87. https://doi.org/10.1177/00957984940201007

Okolo, C. (2002). Self as a problem in African philosophy. In P. Coetzee & A. Roux (Eds.), *Philosophy from Africa: A text with readings* (2nd ed., pp. 209–215). Oxford University Press.

Oruka, H. (1983). Sagacity in African philosophy. *International Philosophical Quarterly, 23*(4), 383–393. https://doi.org/10.5840/ipq198323448

Oruka, H. (2002). Four trends in African philosophy. In P. Coetzee & A. Roux (Eds.), *Philosophy from Africa: A text with readings* (2nd ed., pp. 120–124). Oxford University Press.

Oyowe, O. (2013). Personhood and social power in African thought. *Alternation, 20*(1), 203–228.

Pizzi, M., & Richards, L. G. (2017). Promoting health, well-being, and quality of life in occupational therapy: A commitment to a paradigm shift for the next year 100 years. *American Journal of Occupational Therapy, 71,* 298–301. https://doi.org/10.5014/ajot.2017.028456

Ramose, M. (2002). The philosophy of ubuntu and ubuntu philosophy. In P. Coetzee & A. Roux (Eds.), *Philosophy from Africa: A text with readings* (2nd ed., pp. 230–237). Oxford University Press.

Ramugondo, E. (2017). Human occupation and health. In S. Dsouza, R. Galvaan, & E. L. Ramugondo (Eds.), *Concepts in occupational therapy: Understanding Southern perspective* (pp. 32–48). Manipal University Press.

Ramugondo, E. (2018). Healing work: Intersections for decoloniality. *World Federation of Occupational Therapy, 74*(2), 83–91. https://doi.org/10.1080/14473828.2018.1523981

Ramugondo, E., Galvaan, R., & Duncan, E. (2015). Theorising about human occupation. *South African Journal of Occupational Therapy, 45*(1), 1–2. https://doi.org/10.17159/2310-3833/2015/v45no1a1

Ramugondo, E., & Kronenberg, F. (2015). Explaining collective occupations from a human relations perspective: Bridging the individual-collective dichotomy. *Journal of Occupational Science, 22*(1), 3–16. https://doi.org/10.1080/14427591.2013.781920

Richards, L., & Galvaan, R. (2018). Developing a social transformative focus in occupational therapy. Insights from South African practice. *South African Journal of Occupational Therapy, 48*(1), 3–8. https://doi.org/10.17159/2310-3833/2017/vol48n1a2

Said, E. (1993). *Culture and imperialism.* Vintage.

Serequeberhan, T. (2002). A critique of Eurocentrism and the practice of African philosophy. In P. Coetzee & A. Roux (Eds.), *Philosophy from Africa: A text with readings* (2nd ed., pp. 64–78). Oxford University Press.

Sherry, K. (2010). Culture and cultural competence for occupational therapists in Africa. In V. Alers & R. Crouch (Eds.), *Occupational therapy: An African perspective* (pp. 60–70). Sarah Shorten Publishers.

Smith, L. (2012). *Decolonizing methodologies: Research and indigenous peoples* (2nd ed.). Zed Books Limited.

Teffo, L., & Roux, A. P. (2003). Metaphysical thinking in Africa: Themes in African metaphysical. In P. Coetzee & A. Roux (Eds.), *Philosophy from Africa: A text with readings* (2nd ed., pp. 192–258). Oxford University Press.

Tutu, D. (1999). *No future without forgiveness.* Rider Random House.

United Nations Developmental Programme (UNDP). (n.d.). *Sustainable developmental goals.* https://www.undp.org/content/undp/en/home/sustainable-development-goals.html

Van Niekerk, M. (2011). Review of the book: *Occupational therapy: An African perspective,* by V. Alers & R. Crouch. *South African Journal of Occupational Therapy, 44*(1), 45–46.

World Health Organization (WHO). (2016). *Social determinants of health: It's time: Transforming health workforce education for sustainable developmental goals.* WHO Press.

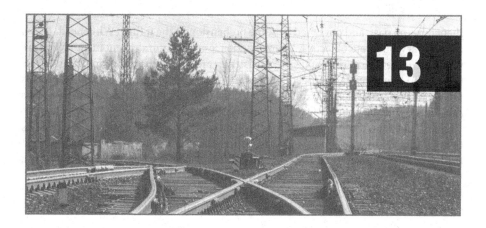

Fundamental Impermanence
Process Philosophy and
Occupational Potential

Lauren Putnam, BS
Steven D. Taff, PhD, OTR/L, FNAP, FAOTA

INTRODUCTION

Process philosophy at its core is concerned with the progressive and ever-changing nature of existence. It aims to define reality by exploring how things come to be, their existence in real time, how they come to pass, and how this results in the emergence of the ever-new. Process philosophy offers a unique perspective compared to other philosophies typically emphasized in Western philosophical development, such as philosophies of substance (Rescher, 1996). Where substance metaphysics considers the world, at its most basic parts, to be made of stable, concrete *substances* (things), process philosophy offers the opposite perspective, wherein dynamic *processes* are the most basic features of reality (Rescher, 1996; Seibt, 2017). This means that what appear to be material substances can actually be broken down into smaller subunits, these subunits being processes or "actual occasions" (Whitehead, 1929). These actual occasions are constantly evolving,

Taff, S. D. (Ed.). *Philosophy and Occupational Therapy:*
Informing Education, Research, and Practice (pp. 127-133).
© 2021 Taylor & Francis Group.

shaped by the past, and governed by some prehension of the future (Whitehead, 1929). In summary, concrete objects, human experiences, and natural phenomena which are perceived to endure in time and space (existents) are actually a collection of unit events (processes) that when taken together give the appearance of an absolute whole. Process philosophy does not deny the existence of substance in everyday life; it simply breaks substance down further to fit in the context of basic metaphysical truths (Rescher, 1996). It takes the face value of a thing and measures it against ontological questions of how, why, and what it means to exist. Upon deeper examination, it concludes that the answer lies one step further in this idea of ever-evolving and interrelated processes, without which our conception of reality would be not only disjointed, but also shallow. From a process perspective, then, the reality we see before us is actually a product of dynamic activity that only gives the appearance of enduring substance.

MAJOR FACETS AND GOALS

Although process philosophy takes a more fluid outlook than most, the role ascribed to process in defining reality is generally illustrated in one of two ways by major scholars within the tradition (Rescher, 1996). From an abstract perspective, process is considered a psychological model through which to understand a complex reality (Rescher, 1996). In this sense, process is a means to an end, rather than the actual manifestation of reality. Alternatively, among other scholars (such as Whitehead, for example), process is considered the most basic and fundamental aspect of reality. From this perspective, process is taken to be the actual ontological source of reality instead of a convenient approximation of it (Hustwit, n.d.; Rescher, 1996). Whereas one perspective presents process as a helpful concept for examining reality *in theory*, the other considers process to be at the very heart of reality. Whichever view is taken, the foundational argument remains the same: process is key in forming a comprehensive understanding of reality as it truly is.

In reconciling experience with reality, the goal of process philosophy is to bridge the gap between science, religion, philosophy, and human intuition. By attempting to synthesize these sometimes contradictory lenses into one cohesive whole, this philosophy serves as a more holistic common ground from which to make sense of the world and even accommodate what seem to be insurmountable differences of opinion (Rescher, 1996). Combining multiple disciplines into one fluid and cohesive explanation is an inevitable consequence of a philosophy based in theories of interdependency and the dynamic nature of reality. The fluidity with which this philosophy evolves also naturally promotes the continuous pursuit of knowledge (Whitehead, 1933). As far as process philosophy is concerned, there is always more to learn and new truths to contend with. In a dynamic system where truth and reality are assumed to be constantly evolving, process philosophy offers a methodical, speculative, and cohesive approach to reconcile these realities as they come to be.

Major Concepts/Themes

The foundational premise of process philosophy lies in a few basic concepts. The most fundamental is that of events' (activities') primacy over substance, as described earlier. Another equally foundational principle posits that the key to understanding reality as it truly is lies in the process (the journey) rather than the product (final outcome; Rescher, 1996; Whitehead, 1929). Consider any tangible object. Simply looking at it or labeling it does not reveal much about what it actually is. The object itself cannot be understood in any meaningful way without being put in terms of what it does, the source from which it came, or comparison to another object and its use. In addition, the object at present will inevitably change with time, whether it is discarded, redesigned to serve a new purpose, or ultimately withers away. No matter the outcome, the only real way to understand the object's existence (being) is through its entire journey or process of being (becoming). From the pre-existent conditions making its existence possible, to what it did or was used for, to its relationship with other existents, and how it continued to evolve over time, these events are what constitute that object's existence. It is the summation of all these moments and potential moments to come that give meaning to that existence. To understand reality, then, an existent cannot be taken at face value. A deeper look must be taken, revealing the inextricable relationship between an existent thing's current being and its process of becoming.

A third and integral aspect of process philosophy is that of change being the only real constant; stability and absolute duration are illusions, possible only when considering existence from a specific point in time (Bergson, 1998a; Whitehead, 1933). Time, as it exists in reality, however, cannot be taken out of context this way. Time is continuous, or it would be meaningless. If studied long enough, what appears to be unchanging will eventually become something different than it was before. In fact, many process philosophers would argue that change is not only an inevitable fact of existence, but also an almost constant one (Bergson, 1946; Seibt, 2017). If the passage of time is inevitable, so too is change. Instead of an object, now consider a human being, for example. The experiences people have in one day alone bring new knowledge, new feelings, or new perceptions that make them inherently different than they were the day before. With each new moment, then, we are somehow changing our being, simply as a result of existing in time and space. To exist in real time means to engage in this process of inevitable growth (becoming).

With this idea of change and evolutionary progress also comes that of creativity, the alternative being a reality characterized by stagnancy and theological determinism. As an example more relevant to the human experience, process philosophers such as Whitehead (1933) point to the repeated downfall of great societies throughout history. Where there was stagnancy of technology or ideas, there was failure and discontentment. It was progress and the creation of new technology or ways of thinking that led to a society's continued success. In order for this novelty to be made possible, however—to create something out of nothing—on some level there must be the possibility for creative agency (Hartshorne, 1970; Whitehead, 1933). Here process philosophy starts to scratch the surface of free will, born out of an internal drive to create our own realities. This internal drive is not unique to human beings. It is an essential component of all existents (actual occasions), serving as the driving mechanism through which change and progress are made possible. Process philosophy not only acknowledges the novel in everyday life, but also decidedly affirms its role as a fundamental feature of reality.

MAJOR THINKERS AND THEIR IDEAS

Given the open-ended and speculative nature of the process philosophical tradition, most of its major thinkers overlap in their basic explanations of reality, process, and change. Where they tend to differ is the aspect of reality upon which they chose to expand. Prior to process philosophy's development as a philosophical tradition in its own right, many sources point to Heraclitus, a 6th-century philosopher, as being the first to explore the possibility of a dynamic and ever-changing reality (Seibt, 2017). It is worthy of note, however, that many of process philosophy's ideas relating to change and impermanency were first reflected in Buddhism. This is a connection that Hartshorne (1998) was quick to make in his writings, though he acknowledged that Buddhist teachings are more abstract in nature while traditional process philosophy is grounded in scientific, logical reasoning and developed quite separately. Alfred North Whitehead is primarily credited with developing a comprehensive line of reasoning for the philosophy (Hustwit, n.d.; Rescher, 1996; Seibt, 2017). In addition to his basic explanation of the superiority of process over substance, he also outlined, in no uncertain terms, the self-creative nature of all things (Whitehead, 1929). He did so, however, without denying that a superior divine being exists. According to philosophers like Whitehead and Hartshorne, there is no predeterminism, but rather a God that also experiences the becoming of new knowledge. The divinity of this being lies in God's ability to harmonize with this new knowledge indefinitely, where lesser, imperfect forms of being cannot (Hartshorne, 1970). William James, John Dewey, and Henri Bergson also contributed to the development of this idea of self-creationism: that all entities have the ability to shape what they become. James developed his ideas from a psychological perspective, while Dewey developed his argument along more pragmatist lines of reasoning (Hartshorne, 1998; Rescher, 1996). Although Whitehead is credited with developing the most logically comprehensive argument within the philosophy, Henri Bergson contributed greatly to the idea of process relevant to evolution. Bergson took all life to be creative, in a sense, always developing, often framing this development in the context of what it means to exist in time and space (Bergson, 1998a, 1998b; Hartshorne, 1998). This preoccupation with time and space also resulted in Bergson's exploration of memory, and how psychological conceptions of the past can be possible without contradicting the fundamental impermanence that process philosophy ascribes to all existence (Bergson, 1946). This duality of past existing in the present touches on Whitehead's theory of prehension: the interrelated nature of all actual occasions and the potential for each, past and present, to shape one another (Whitehead, 1929). Where Whitehead outlined the physics supporting process philosophy's legitimacy, Bergson took a more intuitive approach. Examining the various contributions of process philosophers here, one common trend emerges: definitions of reality based upon interrelated modes of change.

IMPACT ON UNDERSTANDING OF OCCUPATION AND OCCUPATIONAL ENGAGEMENT

Process philosophy is primarily concerned with three major questions: how and why things come to be, how they exist in real time, and how the past shapes the future. In response, process philosophy offers interdependent processes, driven by activity, change, and self-creation. Taking these concepts and applying them to our understanding of occupation and occupational engagement, a strong compatibility emerges. One's occupational choices and level of engagement are the result of more than one's current situation; they are, in fact, a culmination of one's past experiences, future goals, and current contexts. Occupational scientists such as Wilcock (1999) have already made similar connections, ascribing occupation's role in the human experience to "all the things people do, the relationship of what they do with who they are as human beings and that through occupation they are in a constant state of becoming different" (p. 2). Here, occupation or activity is directly tied to who we are (being), while emphasizing the importance of the path we took to get there (becoming), and the continuity between our past, present, and future aspirations. It is our ability to engage in this process of becoming throughout our lives, by exercising different capacities in response to new needs and desires—our "occupational potential"—that is vital in shaping who we want to be and ultimately who we become (Wicks, 2005, p. 134). Without the opportunity to engage, we are denied an essential component of what it means to live: namely, the ability to shape our own destinies. Process philosophy serves to reinforce the complex and vital role occupation (doing) plays in shaping the human experience.

Process philosophy also considers each person to embody a macro process of sorts, made up of an infinite number of smaller processes, all interrelated, but also internally driven by their own agendas for self-actualization. Many models of occupational performance (Person-Environment-Occupation-Performance, Model of Human Occupation) already feature this idea of an internal drive toward self-development in the form of volition or agency, also modulated by the impact of environmental and personal factors (Baum et al., 2015; Kielhofner & Burke, 1980). From a process perspective, this internal drive is essential to our understanding of a meaningful existence. In terms of occupational engagement, then, it would seem that more emphasis should be placed on this internal drive to shape one's own reality while engaging in the therapeutic process. Rather than deciding what is most important to address for clients or relying on typical standbys within a specific practice setting, clinicians should invite clients to determine their own therapeutic goals. By doing so, clients will feel a stronger sense of ownership, purpose, and (it is hoped) a desire to engage in the therapeutic process more actively. If existence is predicated on the idea of continual progress and self-actualization as not just a goal but a fundamental aspect of nature, occupational engagement would seem an important place to start in shaping the well-being of people.

Perhaps the most progressive way process philosophy enriches our understanding of occupation, however, is through its emphasis on creativity and novelty. Through occupation, through activity, through the use of their bodies, people are fulfilling a basic inherent need to create (Reilly, 1962). Occupational therapists believe in the power of doing, in the power of rehabilitation, to enhance well-being, but also in the power of creating new solutions and approaches (novelty). Where there is no single predetermined path, there is room for occupational exploration and fulfillment by finding new and creative ways to circumvent environmental or personal barriers. From a process perspective, engaging in occupation does not have to take a traditional form to be worthwhile; if anything, it is more worthwhile if done in a new and creative way.

KEY IMPLICATIONS FOR OCCUPATIONAL THERAPY EDUCATION, RESEARCH, AND PRACTICE

Education

- Integrate the idea of ever-changing knowledge into curriculum (e.g., evidence-based practice and updating curricula as research within the profession advances).
- Understand the role the past plays in shaping current realities, so that our roots as a profession and our history should have a role in shaping our future; we should provide this foundational knowledge early on in educational programming.

Research

- Invest in the idea of creativity and novelty; push the boundaries of what we know now to find new, progressive solutions and support them with evidence.
- Because reality (and thus evidence) is subjective and constantly changing, we must challenge widely accepted therapeutic practices and test them for effective and reliable outcomes.
- Accept that some aspects of human experience are dynamic and complex, and that we thus require more comprehensive ways to measure those experiences (e.g., mixed methods).

Practice

- Embrace the idea of nature's constant evolution and natural inclination toward progress in therapeutic process; having no predestined outcome should lead clinicians to push the boundaries of what's possible and help motivate clients.
- Take advantage of intrinsic needs to shape one's own realities in motivating clients and incorporating them more into the therapeutic planning process (more client-centered).

RECOMMENDED READINGS

Browning, D., & Myers, W. T. (1998). *Philosophers of process.* Fordham University Press.

Hartshorne, C. (1970). *Creative synthesis & philosophic method.* Open Court.

Rescher, N. (1996). *Process metaphysics: An introduction to process philosophy.* State University of New York Press.

REFERENCES

Baum, C. M., Christiansen, C. H., & Bass, J. D. (2015). The person-environment-occupation-performance (PEOP) model. In C. H. Christiansen, C. M. Baum, & J. D. Bass (Eds.), *Occupational therapy: Performance, participation, and well-being* (4th ed., pp. 47–55). SLACK Incorporated.

Bergson, H. (1946). *The creative mind: An introduction to metaphysics* (M. L. Andison, Trans.). Dover.

Bergson, H. (1998a). The idea of duration. In D. Browning & W. T. Myers (Eds.), *Philosophers of process* (pp. 140–174). Fordham University Press.

Bergson, H. (1998b). The possible and the real. In D. Browning & W. T. Myers (Eds.), *Philosophers of process* (pp. 175–186). Fordham University Press.

Hartshorne, C. (1970). *Creative synthesis & philosophic method.* Open Court.

Hartshorne, C. (1998). The development of process philosophy. In D. Browning & W. T. Myers (Eds.), *Philosophers of process* (pp. 392–407). Fordham University Press.

Hustwit, J. R. (n.d.). *Process philosophy.* https://www.iep.utm.edu/processp

Kielhofner, G., & Burke, J. P. (1980). A model of human occupation, part 1. Conceptual framework and content. *American Journal of Occupational Therapy, 34*, 572–581. https://doi.org/10.5014/ajot.34.9.572

Reilly, M. (1962). Occupational therapy can be one of the great ideas of 20th century medicine. *American Journal of Occupational Therapy, 16*, 1–9. https://doi.org/10.1177/000841746303000102

Rescher, N. (1996). *Process metaphysics: An introduction to process philosophy.* State University of New York Press.

Seibt, J. (2017). Process philosophy. In E. N. Zalta (Ed.), *The Stanford encyclopedia of philosophy* (Winter 2018 ed.). https://plato.stanford.edu/entries/process-philosophy

Whitehead, A. N. (1929). *Process and reality.* Macmillan.

Whitehead, A. N. (1933). *Adventure of ideas.* Macmillan.

Wicks, A. (2005). Understanding occupational potential. *Journal of Occupational Science, 12*(3), 130–139. https://doi.org/10.1080/14427591.2005.9686556

Wilcock, A. A. (1999). Reflections on doing, being and becoming. *Australian Occupational Therapy Journal, 46*, 1–11. https://doi.org/10.1046/j.1440-1630.1999.00174.x

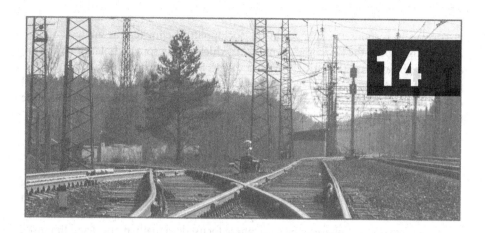

Analytic Philosophy
Guiding Method and Adding Precision
to Occupational Therapy

Marna Ghiglieri, OTD, MA, OTR/L
Ronald R. Drummond, BA
Rose McAndrew, OTD, OTR/L, CHT
Steven D. Taff, PhD, OTR/L, FNAP, FAOTA

INTRODUCTION

Definition of Analytic Philosophy

Analytic philosophy (AP) is a method-driven philosophy that uses mathematics, language, and symbolic logic as analytic tools to gain knowledge through *analysis* of problems, concepts, issues, and arguments (Schwartz, 2012). The search for truth underpins all philosophical traditions; however, it is *the approach* to seeking knowledge that sets AP apart from other branches of philosophy (Koetting & Malisa, 2004). AP is based upon the idea that absolute truth can be achieved using a logical process that requires key concepts to be reduced to their most basic elements. Many well-known thinkers have contributed to the AP tradition (Schwartz, 2012), leading to its evolution throughout the 20th century as new information is

Taff, S. D. (Ed.). *Philosophy and Occupational Therapy:*
Informing Education, Research, and Practice (pp. 135-143).
© 2021 Taylor & Francis Group.

discovered in response to changes in the sociopolitical climate. The analysis of concepts using logic is the key component of AP, which is why some scholars describe AP as "doing philosophy" (Koetting & Malisa, 2004). Students who have taken an undergraduate philosophy course in logic may be familiar with the conceptual framework of AP. AP has also been described as a philosophical perspective, delineating it from the normative and descriptive perspectives of philosophy (Koetting & Malisa, 2004).

Major Facets of Analytic Philosophy

The main facet of AP is its concern with using a logical process to define certain truths to better understand the world's problems. This logical process starts by defining a method and then clarifying concepts. Although this logical process is the foundation of AP, the range of fields where AP is applied has evolved and expanded. AP developed over two distinct phases. The early phase focused on mathematical and linguistic analysis, based upon scientific principles. AP later expanded to include other fields, such as ethics and religion, which initially were not considered open to scientific analysis. Thus, it is helpful to think of AP with respect to an early period and a contemporary period.

EARLY PHASE OF ANALYTIC PHILOSOPHY

In the early period, the application of AP was strictly scientific. Prior to the early 1900s, philosophers from varying groups believed the path toward truth depended upon the persuasive skills of the philosopher using the Socratic method (Schwartz, 2012). In other words, most thinkers viewed philosophy as a critical thinking exercise which involved asking and answering endless questions on topics such as religion or morality, where answers to these questions were speculative at best (Schwartz, 2012). Consequently, philosophy prior to the 20th century was separate and distinct from fields that applied the scientific method. In order to legitimize philosophy, a concerted effort was made to apply a logical method, which involved reducing philosophical concepts to their most basic elements to seek truth. Reductionism became a core element of many different branches of science, such as biology, chemistry, and physics, and formed the basis of the practice model for clinicians, including occupational therapists, during the 1930s and into the 1970s (Johnson & Dickie, 2019).

Students of early AP needed considerable knowledge of mathematics, which limited the number of people who could appreciate its value. Recognizing this limitation, the English philosopher Bertrand Russell applied AP's methods to language as well as mathematical operations, increasing understanding of AP beyond mathematicians. Early AP also rejected metaphysics, a branch of philosophy that presupposes the speculative nature of the universe. Thus, anything that could not be explained via logical or scientific analysis was deemed nonsense or subjective expressions of emotion. The rejection of metaphysics led to the development of logical positivism, the idea that only cognitively meaningful statements are worthy of scientific exploration. For instance, a metaphysical question such as "does God exist?", which had stymied philosophers in endless debate prior to the AP movement, was deemed unsuitable for logical analysis because it could not be analyzed scientifically.

Early AP also addressed ethics. In an attempt to put some distance between ethical issues that could not be approached with scientific inquiry, philosophers of the early AP tradition limited their students to metaethics. Metaethics is a subset of the field of ethics that explores questions in terms of their truth value (e.g., Are ethical claims objective? If so, how are these claims verified?). AP philosophers defined which ethical questions were appropriate for scientific inquiry and which were not. However, in the contemporary phase of AP, philosophers discarded the notion that AP is useful only in fields open to scientific inquiry. Leading thinkers in contemporary AP embraced multicontextual, humanistic perspectives.

RECENT DEVELOPMENTS IN ANALYTIC PHILOSOPHY

The contemporary period of AP can be considered the "art phase" of this philosophical tradition. Whereas the early period of AP embraced science, the contemporary period of AP moved to include issues previously deemed pseudoscientific and not appropriate for logical analysis. Philosophers wanted to look beyond metaethics and understand ethical behavior. Elizabeth Anscombe, a student of the leading AP philosopher, Ludwig Wittgenstein, proposed the concept of consequentialism. Consequentialism affirms that one's actions guide behavior. Contemporary AP also renewed an interest in metaphysics. Leading thinkers of the early AP tradition rejected metaphysical questions because they could not be explained through logical or scientific analysis. Recent AP thinkers have come to value metaphysics, recognizing that there are multiple ways to analyze natural phenomena. Metaphysics emphasizes that knowledge is often relative and situated in context; thus, multiple perspectives are needed to clearly acknowledge what is known and what remains unknown.

GENERAL GOALS OR INTENDED OUTCOMES OF THE PHILOSOPHY

AP proposes to increase the rigor and status of philosophy by merging it with science in a way that empirical philosophers such as Locke, Berkeley, and Hume were unable to do. In pursuit of this goal, AP has developed techniques that include use of symbolic logic and the analysis of language, concepts, or theories (Koetting & Malisa, 2004). Leading thinkers of the AP tradition believed that key concepts in scientific, moral, or religious discourse are often vague and philosophically misleading. Prominent AP thinkers clarified these concepts using science, math, or linguistics to reveal knowledge. Thus, the pursuit of knowledge is not *a priori* (rationalist's view), nor is it *a posteriori* (empiricist's view); rather, it is *analytic* (Koetting & Malisa, 2004; Schwartz, 2012). Another, more recently developed, goal of AP is to use a logical process of analysis to determine what remains unknown in order to identify the limits on our current body of knowledge or to reveal multiple perspectives on truth based on evidence and critical analysis (Schwartz, 2012). This shift in contemporary AP suggests a goal to increase interdisciplinary coordination to improve scientific results.

LEADING THINKERS OF ANALYTIC PHILOSOPHY

Gottlob Frege (1848–1925) is considered the pioneer and first thinker of AP. His work on the foundation of mathematics was adopted by Russell and built upon in *Principia Mathematica*. Also, Russell brought Frege's clarification of the issues of language to British philosophers.

Ludwig Wittgenstein (1889–1951) is considered the founding father of AP. His famous manuscript, *Tractatus,* is used for teaching symbolic logic at colleges throughout the United States today. He would have languished in obscurity if not for the famous AP philosopher Bertrand Russell.

Bertrand Russell (1872–1970) acted as the ambassador of AP during the course of his long career. He translated Wittgenstein's *Tractatus* from German into English, simplified it, added a foreword, and promoted the book. Russell was a prolific writer until his death at the age of 98. He co-wrote *Principia Mathematica* with another philosopher in the years 1910 to 1913. *Principia Mathematica* was seen as a possible guide to repairing the flaws in thinking of the classical British Empiricists, thus legitimizing certain aspects of empiricism. Russell described himself as a logical atomist, holding that knowledge could be broken down into small indivisible bits. Using this method of reduction, people would have a better understanding of the world. During the last 20 years of his life, Russell was a major proponent of metaphysical beliefs, as he popularized the idea that AP helps establish what logical thinkers know and what they still do not know (Schwartz, 2012).

The **Vienna Circle** was formed in the 1920s by Moritz Schlick, who led its biweekly meetings in Vienna with other visionary thinkers. Brilliant intellectuals from other fields (such as Otto Neurah, an economist; Kurt Gödel, a mathematician; and Albert Einstein, who was a Nobel Prize winner and leading scientist by the time the group was in its heyday) also were noted as attending meetings of inner Vienna Circle members. The founding premise of the Vienna Circle was to demystify philosophy via logical analysis of the propositions of science and common sense (Palmer, 2016). The ideas born of this first circle spread, and new circles developed in Berlin and England as philosophers met to discuss arguments against German metaphysics. Other prominent members of the Vienna Circle included Rudolph Carnap, Karl Popper, Herbert Feigl, and Felix Kaufmann (Ozmon & Craver, 2011). A. J. Ayer was a frequent visitor to the Vienna Circle and brought these ideas to thinkers in England. Similarly, many people consider Wittgenstein part of the Vienna Circle, although he was not an official member thereof. However, Wittgenstein's major work, *Tractatus,* was frequently read, discussed, and debated by circle members.

A. J. Ayer (1910–1989) was a prominent guest of and visitor to the Vienna Circle who interpreted logical positivism to the English-speaking world through teaching and writing along with radio and television (Ozmon & Craver, 2011). His most famous work, *Language, Truth, and Logic* (1936), promoted logical positivism and the Principle of Verification, both used by the Vienna Circle to discredit religious and metaphysical propositions (Ayer, 2002).

Gilbert Ryle (1900–1976) is best known for *The Concept of Mind* (1949/2009), in which he challenged the idea of mind–body dualism and emphasized the importance of splitting the concepts into separate realms, stating that the body is in the realm of matter and is studied objectively whereas the mind is in a secret realm, hidden from view, and must be studied subjectively (Ozmon & Craver, 2011). Ryle also identified that educators assume their job is primarily to teach content: what he refers to as "knowing that." However, Ryle emphasized that educators need to provide the "knowing how" as well through learning by doing after information is taught (Ozmon & Craver, 2011).

Elizabeth Anscombe (1919–2001) was a pupil of Wittgenstein. Her work *Intention* (2000), which was first published in 1957, provides an understanding of what motivates people toward their intended actions. Anscombe is credited with coining the term *consequentialism* in her article "Modern Moral Philosophy" (1958), which posits the belief that the consequences of an action are the basis for any judgment of right or wrong.

IMPACT ON UNDERSTANDING OF OCCUPATION AND OCCUPATIONAL ENGAGEMENT

The application of AP concepts can improve our knowledge by holistically framing scientific inquiries and using clearly defined methods. The analytical process can improve our understanding of occupation and occupational engagement to clarify our profession's concepts, beliefs, arguments, and assumptions. For instance, Anscombe's *Intention* (2000) can be summarized to help students develop a deeper understanding of the therapeutic value of occupational engagement. She emphasizes the importance of studying a person's *intention* to uncover motivation for occupational engagement. Anscombe writes that when people are observed, their intentions might be inferred based on their actions (e.g., someone reading would likely have intended to read). What we infer may not be true, as they may only pretend to read; therefore, how can occupational therapy practitioners understand clients' intentional actions when they are unable to engage in meaningful occupations? To answer, consider Wittgenstein's belief that using specific explanations rather than using generalized assumptions is important to avoid finding false answers after gathering information and thinking critically. These principles can be used to investigate why people are unable to engage in meaningful occupations, rather than assuming their intentions. Anscombe (2000) provides three reasons used to determine individuals' intentions:

1. Evidential—Engaging in occupation based on an observed piece of evidence (Don is running through the woods because a dog is chasing him).
2. Causal—Engaging in occupation because of cause-and-effect (Barbara is participating in burn care management because she received a burn).
3. Reason-giving—Engaging in occupation based on an application, meaning, or reason (Danielle is volunteering at a children's hospital because she is passionate about working with children).

While Anscombe's evidential and causal explanations for occupational engagement provide a logical rationale as to why someone might engage in an occupation, her third option, reason-giving, focuses on asking a client to *explain* what makes the occupation meaningful. For example, imagine a client, Levi, who has experienced severe physical limitations resulting from a recent stroke. When evaluated by an occupational therapist, Levi indicates that he likes to cook. What is it about cooking that makes this occupation enjoyable to Levi? Is it the mechanics of cooking? Is it the opportunity to feed a family? Is it the ability to socialize with others at a potluck? Looking into the *intentions* of occupational engagement is important because they help occupational therapists identify why occupations are meaningful to clients. Imagine Levi states that cooking is the "dull part" of the activity. If a therapist focuses only on the mechanics of cooking and not on the outcome, there is a good chance Levi will express frustration and opt out of working on this occupation during their treatment session. However, if a therapist helps Levi identify other reasons why cooking is personally motivating, then there is a greater chance of engaging Levi in the therapeutic process. Continuing with this example, let's imagine that the therapist discovers that Levi enjoys making meals for his grandchildren. With this knowledge, a therapist can collaborate with Levi and his extended family to identify options for working toward this goal. Thus, by practicing holistic, client-centered care, the occupational therapist can help Levi increase occupational engagement by identifying the occupations most meaningful to him.

The reasons motivating individuals' engagement in occupations and their intentional actions may not always be observable. Additionally, asking clients to identify their intentions is not always an option due to various types of diagnoses; therefore, it is important for practitioners, researchers, and educators to acknowledge what it is that we still do not know in regard to determining how we can effectively communicate with our clients. Often clients lack self-awareness as to what it is about an occupation that makes it rewarding. Another problem has to do with therapists and clients focusing primarily on declarative knowledge over procedural knowledge. Ryle has written extensively about different types of knowledge, which occupational therapists can apply to their work with clients to achieve better results.

Ryle believed many people confuse "knowing that" and "knowing how" (Ryle, 1949/2009). Ryle defines "knowing that" as the knowledge of a concept, whereas "knowing how" is the ability to perform the activity of the concept (Ryle, 1949/2009). Both types of knowledge are important to learning. A golf player needs to know the rules (knowing that) to play the game. However, a golfer will not excel at the game without repeated practice (knowing how). To apply these two types of knowledge to occupational therapy, let's review a therapy session with Oliver.

Oliver recently underwent an elective posterior hip osteoplasty. As part of the pre-surgical preparatory process, he attended a short class. In the class, he received information about posterior postsurgical hip precautions and watched a video of a person using a reacher, sock aid, and long-handled shoehorn to dress. During his initial evaluation, he correctly stated his posterior hip precautions and explained the process of dressing using adaptive equipment. The occupational therapist believed Oliver had the knowledge to complete lower body dressing on his own, so he asked Oliver to perform the task. Oliver began to use the reacher to remove his socks. He quickly realized that the video made it look a lot easier than it was! As Oliver struggled to slide the prongs of the reacher in place, he bent forward for a better look, temporarily forgetting one of his posterior hip precautions. Although Oliver understood the "rules" of completing lower body dressing (i.e., his posterior hip precautions and use of long-handled adaptive equipment), he had not yet had the opportunity to apply this knowledge to mastering the "knowing how" part of the task. The occupational therapist spent the rest of the session training Oliver to complete the task by going through the process step by step, so that he could master each part of the task. Once Oliver learned how to do it, his performance steadily improved, leading to safe, functional independence in the task.

This scenario with Oliver demonstrates that clients must be given the opportunity to practice new knowledge on a regular basis in order to develop competence and skill. New information, such as hip, cardiac, or sternal precautions, classified by Ryle as "knowing that" must be followed up with multiple training sessions so that "knowing how" can take place. This same idea can also apply to occupational therapy education. All occupational therapy programs provide opportunities for experiential learning so that knowledge learned in a classroom can be applied to lab and fieldwork settings in order to facilitate clinical competence of occupational therapy practitioners.

The philosophical premise behind AP is to further any branch of scientific inquiry by defining problems while looking deeper for answers. A final example of how the philosophical approach of AP has affected our field can be seen in the recent development in occupational therapy education. Specifically, there has been a focus in recent years in occupational therapy curriculum design to define the method used to help students remain centered on learning about the therapeutic use of occupation and other key concepts that make our profession unique from other disciplines in the health care field (Hooper et al., 2015). Hooper et al. (2015) credit Wittgenstein as providing the rationale for clarifying the methods of a professional discipline. Because many outside observers may believe that what occupational therapy practitioners do is simple or even common sense, they may assume that the occupational therapy practice will develop easily or naturally for students. However, occupational therapy educators know that it is important to clearly define methodology in occupational therapy educational programs to critically analyze the success of programs and ensure quality education.

KEY IMPLICATIONS FOR OCCUPATIONAL THERAPY EDUCATION, RESEARCH, AND PRACTICE

The major concepts from both early and contemporary AP provide several avenues for occupational therapy education, research, and practice.

Education

Use of language to improve clarity. Ayer believed that educators should provide checks and balances in learning.

- Use logic models to clarify goals, concepts, and evaluation processes in tracking outcomes.
- Implement checks and balances when teaching formative assessments to meet students' needs using various examples.

Activity-based learning. Ryle believed that "knowing" is more than filling minds with information.

- Improve outcomes by balancing lecture and activity-based learning.

Using models of practice in education. Wittgenstein constructed a model of logic to organize his concept of "language games."

- Integrate models of practice (Person-Environment-Occupation-Performance, Model of Human Occupation, etc.) to guide the curriculum to increase student outcomes.

Research

Evidence-based research. The Vienna Circle used the Principle of Verification to verify concepts.

- Use evidence to ensure that methods are sound and have reliability, validity, and utility.

Teaching evidence-based practice. Anscombe emphasized the provision of evidential reasoning behind intentions.

- Teach students how to find and use evidence to improve outcomes.

Practice

Task analysis. Russell stressed reducing ideas to elemental concepts to seek clarification.

- Help improve client understanding of treatment and learn how to identify deficits.

Interprofessional treatment team. Metaphysical reality stresses the need to collaborate due to departmentalization.

- Help advocate for occupational therapy and increase holistic, client-centered care.

RECOMMENDED READINGS

Anscombe, E. (2000). *Intention* (2nd ed.). Cornell University Press.

Palmer, D. (2016). *Does the center hold?: An introduction to western philosophy* (7th ed.). McGraw Hill.

Schwartz, S. P. (2012). *A brief history of analytic philosophy: From Russell to Rawls.* Wiley.

Searle, J. R. (1999). *Mind, language, and society: Philosophy in the real world.* Basic Books.

REFERENCES

Anscombe, E. (2000). *Intention* (2nd ed.). Cornell University Press. (Original work published 1957)

Anscombe, G. E. M. (1958). Modern moral philosophy. *Philosophy*, *33*(124), 1–19. https://doi.org/10.1017/S0031819100037943

Ayer, A. J. (2002). *Language, truth, and logic* (2nd ed.). Dover.

Hooper, B., Mitcham, M. D., Taff, S. D., Price, P., Krishnagiri, S., & Bilics, A. (2015). Energizing occupation as the center of teaching and learning. *American Journal of Occupational Therapy*, *69*(Suppl. 2), 6912360010p1–6912360010p5. https://doi.org/10.5014/ajot.2015.018242

Johnson, K. R., & Dickie, V. (2019). What is occupation? In B. A. B. Schell & G. Gillen (Eds.), *Willard & Spackman's occupational therapy* (13th ed., pp. 2–10). Wolters Kluwer.

Koetting, J. R., & Malisa, M. (2004). Philosophy, research, and education. In D. Jonassen & M. Driscoll (Eds.), *Handbook of research for educational communications and technology* (2nd ed., pp. 1009–1020). Routledge.

Ozmon, H. A., & Craver, S. M. (2011). *Philosophical foundations of education* (9th ed.). Pearson.

Palmer, D. (2016). *Does the center hold?: An introduction to western philosophy* (7th ed.). McGraw-Hill.

Ryle, G. (2009). *The concept of mind*. Routledge. http://s-f-walker.org.uk/pubsebooks/pdfs/Gilbert_Ryle_The_Concept_of_Mind.pdf (Original work published 1949)

Schwartz, S. P. (2012). *A brief history of analytic philosophy: From Russell to Rawls*. Wiley.

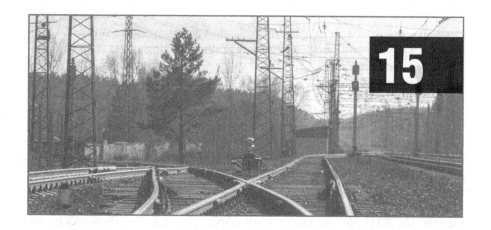

Structuralism
Examining the Interrelationships Around Occupation

Ganesh M. Babulal, PhD, OTD, MSCI, MOT, OTR/L
Jyothi Gupta, PhD, OTR/L, FAOTA

INTRODUCTION

Structuralism asserted that human culture as a phenomenon contains elements or concepts that can be examined and understood as part of a larger system. However, no single element is independent or has intrinsic value; rather, its value is only realized by studying its relationship to other elements and in relation to the larger structure. Structuralism's intellectual itinerary may be compartmentalized into three epochs: a modest beginning in 1900s Europe rooted in semiotics, widespread use and application to the social sciences in the 1950s and 1960s, and laying the foundation for and eventual promulgation of post-structuralism and deconstruction in the 1970s. We limit the focus of this chapter to the first two epochs.

The origin of structuralism is unquestionably tied to the 20th-century Swiss linguist and theorist Ferdinand de Saussure. Although de Saussure himself never published a text about structuralism, notes from students taking his course at the

Taff, S. D. (Ed.). *Philosophy and Occupational Therapy:*
Informing Education, Research, and Practice (pp. 145-153).
© 2021 Taylor & Francis Group.

University of Geneva were compiled and published posthumously in 1916 as *Course in General Linguistics*, thus launching the study of structural linguistics.

MAJOR FACETS OF STRUCTURALISM

De Saussure examined both *langue* and *parole*. *Langue* was the pre-existing under-lying structure of language, while *parole* was the use of language (such as speech). He theorized that language is a social institution constituted of signs, which repre-sent ideas. A *sign* is anything that conveys meaning, and each sign is made up of two parts: a *signifier* (sound-image or word) and the *signified* (a mental concept), which are combined and hence inextricable from each other. De Saussure also proposed two principles: "the arbitrary nature of the sign" and "the linear nature of the signifier" (de Saussure, 2011). He noted that the first principle governs all of linguistics because there is no reason or predetermined rule for why or how a signifier is linked to a sig-nified; hence the arbitrary relationship. For example, the written word and sound for the concept of "daughter" will be pronounced and written differently in two languages (e.g., Dutch, Spanish) but are related to the same signified. Arbitrariness can be present within a single language and across different languages. The second principle regards auditory signifiers (spoken and written words) as being only measurable in time and which cannot be perceived simultaneously. The dimension of time can also change a signifier, either to a different meaning of a sign or to add another layer of meaning. Take, for example, the word "pretty," which has changed connotation from meaning "cunning or crafty" in Old English to "aesthetically pleasing or delicate" in modern use. In other cases, words (loanwords) may be taken from one language and assimilated into another. For example, *pandit* in Hindi is a priest or sagacious scholar, but in the English vernacular, *pundit* (spelled slightly differently) is a critic or learned person. De Saussure contended that language is a system of differences where ideas or signs exist in relation to each other without having positive or negative nature, but one of unprepos-sessing passivity. Most importantly, the ideas and signs cannot exist outside or before the overall structure where "language is form and not a substance" (de Saussure, 2011).

A *sui generis* characteristic of language in structuralism is denoted by how relation-ships are interleaved with essential differences. This is achieved through binary opposi-tions, which argue that a word cannot be understood unless one's observation of it is relative to how it differs from something else or its opposite (e.g., good vs. evil, hot vs. cold). Meaning is not fixed, but exists only relative to the context that creates a system of differences that supports perception and sensation (de Saussure, 2011). As a result, this essential difference subserves consciousness and self-awareness. For example, per-sons understand that they are human through differentiating comparison of other spe-cies or objects, and can further perceive their own identity by comparison again to other humans. More evidence of this system at work is with homophones, which are words that sound the same when spoken (de Saussure, 2011). Take, for example, *cent*, *scent*, and *sent*, which all sound the same when spoken. Yet these signifiers are very dif-ferent when spoken in the context of other signifiers or when they are written out. The overall structure or system of relationships engenders meaning and leads to an infinite permutation as there is no fixed connection between signifier and signified.

APPLICATIONS AND GOALS OF STRUCTURALISM TO CULTURE

The structuralist approach sought to simplify the seemingly irreducible conflux of human innovation and its means originating from the preceding centuries that saw the abolition of slavery, two industrial revolutions, an unprecedented growth in globalization, economic integration, and two world wars (Zinn, 2005). There was an inherent need for an eloquent, underlying theory to explain and connect all of the differences found across the world. The most accessible and unmistakable marker of differences was communication or language, although this demarcation was soon expanded to culture. While the significance of de Saussure's theoretical exposition on semiotics may be challenging to interpret outside of language, its immediate application to other fields was realized in the 1950s and 1960s. Jonathan Culler noted that the application of structuralism to the study of society and culture assumes that society and culture are objects that have meaning (i.e., signs) and that their identity/essence is espoused by a network of relationships (internal and external; Culler, 1975). The means of and production stemming from human innovation have meaning, and those meanings must be rooted in a system of distinction and conventions to make the meaning possible. Among other fields, structuralism lent itself to the fields of sociology and anthropology.

Claude Lévi-Strauss applied de Saussure's theory and posited that culture was a system of symbolic communication where actions are only meaningful in the context of a specific institution, set of conventions, or rules of operation (Lévi-Strauss, 1963). More specifically, Lévi-Strauss suggested that tokens (words, gifts/acts) were exchanged across generations to reproduce and codify the rules of a particular culture. The action of an individual has no particular significance in itself; rather, it belongs to the collective symbolic system to structure specific types of behavior (Lévi-Strauss, 1963). Most notably, meaning is continually reproduced and reified through specific practices or activities, which may include food consumption (preparation/serving), religious practice, rites of passage, games/athletic feats, oral stories, and reading texts. An external observer of one of these practices may be able to provide an objective perspective but cannot grasp the intrinsic meaning. Lévi-Strauss also elaborated that meaning in human thought is fundamentally rooted in binary oppositions (male/female, culture/nature) and their subsequent integration. The underlying structure of social life and engagement is found in the mind. However, it was believed that an uncontaminated form of the human mind could only be found in "primitive" societies, because in more developed societies there are layers of interferences that obscure the central structure.

CORE CONCEPTS

The core belief of structuralism is that all human activities are constructed patterns based on the larger scaffolded institutional systems of language and culture. Structuralism is ahistorical, ignoring context and instead focusing on the fixed patterns and rules underlying the larger system. While application of structuralism is a prominent bedrock of anthropology, it has also been rigorously applied to psychology, literary criticism, and linguistics. Psychoanalysts applied structuralism to understand

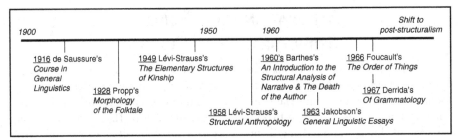

Figure 15-1. Timeline of structuralism by selected published writings.

the unconscious, which was believed to be structured like language, not separate, and as complex as consciousness. In the post-Freudian era, Lacan argued that the unconscious is immersed in signifiers that are connected in a chain to other signifiers, and when traced through psychoanalysis, one can get the fragmented pieces to resurface (Lacan, 2006). In literary criticism and linguistics, Jakobson's analysis and work with persons who had aphasia further defined metaphor and metonymy (Jakobson, 1960). The former means substitution of one sign with another unrelated sign while retaining the same meaning (e.g., angry and red). The latter means using one associated sign with part of another (e.g., crown to represent kingdom). These brief examples demonstrate how the application of sign, signifier, signified, and the role of underlying structures were fundamental in shaping and evolving other fields of study.

Structuralist Thinkers and Their Related Concepts

Similar to other major philosophical schools, structuralism boasted a number of prominent scholars, specifically in its application to other fields, as demonstrated in the prior section and through published works (Figure 15-1). Here we briefly discuss three notable structuralists and concepts associated with their work.

Jacques Lacan used structuralism to revise Freud's tripartite theory of the psyche (id, ego, superego) into the imaginary order, symbolic order, and the real (Lacan, 1978). The *imaginary order* was based on one's visual representation of the world and the origin of seeing differences (including self). The *symbolic order* was using language, specifically words (signifiers) to communicate and understand the world and one's experiences. The *real order* was the unconscious, alinguistic self that encapsulates a sudden reaction that language cannot explain (e.g., flight/fight response or dreams). These concepts were central to delimiting the imperceptible vastness of the unconscious. In literary theory, Roman Jakobson examined the function of language, specifically in verbal communication, and identified six factors: context, addresser, addressee, contact, code, and message (Jakobson, 1960). Briefly, an *addresser* (expressive/emotive) sends a *message* (signifier) to an *addressee* (seeking an effect), which requires a *context* (the signified) that is understandable for the addressee, along with a *code* (shared language) that is shared between both parties across a *contact* (channel/social interaction) among the addresser and the addressee. Jakobson argued that each factor was required in order for successful communication to occur and applied this model to the grammar of poetics (Waugh, 1980). Finally, Roland Barthes critically examined the role of social value systems contributing to myths in general, but applied de Saussure's *sign* to elevate how myths were created. Barthes contended that although myths are signs, there is a deeper level where the sign itself becomes the signifier to which new meaning is added and then becomes the signified (Barthes, 1972). As a result, myths are not arbitrary, but have an underlying reason and represent certain ideologies. Take, for example, the political slogan "Make America Great Again," which was first used in the 1980 presidential campaign and resurfaced in the 2016 U.S. presidential election. The current iteration of this hagiographic image and slogan is presented on a red background, with white text in uppercase font. Barthes noted that all modern myths are created for some reason. This sign was purposefully created as a political slogan to represent one party, summarize its beliefs, and propose an action. At the surface level, the sign implicitly asserts that America has fallen from grace, and for posterity deserves to reclaim what was lost. However, the sign is ahistorical and offers no factual information, no definition of greatness, and no means of how to achieve it other than a vapid suggestion. Further, the definition of *great* in the sign is subjective, leaving it to consumers and viewers to project their own meaning upon it. Nevertheless, the sign was ideologically legitimized by becoming a commodity that was reproduced for profit through mass commercialization of merchandise (shirts, hats, stickers). On this point, Barthes would argue that the sign became a new myth through a second level of signification and could be appropriated for consumer goods as a specific brand. Later on, Barthes also applied structuralism to literature by examining a given work across three levels: functions, actions, and narrative (Barthes & Duisit, 1975). *Functions* are the basic descriptive unit of meaning in writing, which when added together construct an action of a character, which are integrated to become part of the larger narrative. The process of breaking down a work to its lesser constituents affords the reader an opportunity to critically examine the authenticity of a narrative when compared to reality.

IMPACT ON UNDERSTANDING OF OCCUPATION AND OCCUPATIONAL ENGAGEMENT

From a structuralist point of view, humans are self-generating biological systems that self-organize according to uniform principles and processes that create stable structures and behavioral patterns (French, 2011). Human behavior is a biological phenomenon; the nervous system receives sensory input that is analyzed and interpreted, and appropriate behavioral output is generated. As all humans share the same body structure and function, behaviors are also alike. Social interactions are viewed as predictable patterned behavior based on larger scaffolded institutional systems of language and culture (Mayhew, 1980). People engage in certain occupations and perform occupations in a way that is determined by unobservable social structures. An example is gendered occupations across diverse cultures whereby certain "nurturing" occupations are relegated to women; in traditional societies, even today, meal preparation, parenting children, and caring for aging and ailing parents are considered woman's work. Structuralism does not, however, attribute sociological or psychological characteristics to individuals, because the individual is part of a larger system and has no individuality, uniqueness, or agency (Mayhew, 1980). The conflation of roles in the profession's conceptual models and unquestioned tacit acceptance occurs in light of the contested terrain of a gender normative in society.

The identifications of occupation as a pre-existing structure that guides or structures subsequent human behavior (Nelson & Jepson-Thomas, 2003), "specific chunks of activity within the ongoing stream of human behavior which are names in the lexicon of the culture" (Yerxa et al., 1989, p. 5), and "a goal-directed pursuit" (Christiansen et al., 2015, p. 548), align well with structuralism. In contrast, the use of descriptors for occupation such as *unique, meaningful,* and *choice-laden* (Boyt Schell & Gillen, 2019; Hinojosa & Blount, 2009; Hinojosa et al., 2003) is problematic in the structuralist view, as individuals have no agency and meaning is not particular.

The structuralist perspective of society and social phenomena emerges from a system of relationships that determine individual human behavior (Mayhew, 1980). A particular relationship, say a mother, can only be understood in the context of the family structure. Individuality extends as far as pulse rate, height, body weight, metabolic rate, and other physiological factors. Beyond these aspects, the individual's response or behavior is patterned and not unique to the particular individual. Social structures are inherently stratified and distribute power and privilege inequitably. This trickles down to inequitable access and opportunities to resources to engage in a diverse array of enriching occupations (Gupta, 2016). For instance, in the United States, the possibility of achieving the "American Dream" is determined by where one is born and lives; hence the phrase "zip code is destiny." As a result, defining occupation as "a specific individual's personally constructed, non-repeatable experience" (Pierce, 2001, p. 139) is contrary to structuralism. For instance, the concept of bathing or grooming serves the same function for all individuals. Differences in the performance of bathing and grooming are determined by external structures, including sociocultural factors. In other words, there is no unique meaning derived from occupational engagement for a particular individual. Specific meaning, volition, and agency are irrelevant in a structuralist perspective.

Structuralism seeped into occupational therapy in the period spanning 1930–1949 when the profession sought sponsorship from medicine (Reed & Peters, 2006). This entailed adopting a biomedical approach to practice, and subsequently to the mechanistic paradigm prevalent in the 1960s and 1970s (Kielhofner, 2009). Structuralism dominated the practice landscape then and continues to do so today in biomedical settings, especially in organization and language. The structuralist approach is based on the premise that structural dysfunction precedes impaired function. The core constructs of the profession are the rehabilitation of the inner workings of body structures/systems: remediating and restoring the underlying structures restore function, (i.e., improving range of motion, strength, endurance, and motor control results in improved occupational performance). This is not problematic from the stance of scientific structuralism, as body systems and body functions are prerequisites to occupational engagement (Gupta & Taff, 2015). Practice related to physical rehabilitation falls within the purview of structuralism. However, boundaries fall apart philosophically when it comes to espoused views of humans as unique occupational beings who derive particular meaning, identity, and agency through engagement in occupations.

The problem, as noted by Hooper and Wood (2002), is that occupational therapy has adopted a pragmatist view of humans but a structuralist view of knowledge. This contributes to a significant dissonance among the profession's philosophy, theories, and practice. The authenticity of the profession is challenged when practice and espoused values are out of sync (Gupta & Taff, 2015). Although we currently are in the contemporary occupation-based paradigm, structuralist practice is still prevalent in biomedical settings that demand effectiveness, objective evidence, efficiency, uniform protocols, use of modalities, and decontextualized practice.

KEY IMPLICATIONS FOR OCCUPATIONAL THERAPY EDUCATION, RESEARCH, AND PRACTICE

Education

- Structuralism undergirds many foundational disciplines of occupational therapy, particularly the basic sciences. Prerequisites and/or the core curriculum include anatomy, pathophysiology, kinesiology, and neurosciences. This implies that some understanding of the underlying structures, language derivation, and functions of the human body is essential to understanding humans and occupational performance.

- A structuralist approach to education would focus more on teaching the proper order and progressing from simple to complex. Basic science courses are taught prior to introducing conditions, assessment, and interventions. Courses in a curriculum may be sequenced with a developmental approach across the lifespan, in which learning normal development or patterns of movement precedes learning about abnormal development or movements, and simple concepts are introduced as scaffolds for complex conceptual elements.

- Content is presented as deconstructed building blocks. For example, upper extremity movement is taught from anatomy, physiology, and movement-pattern perspectives and then eventually synthesized as a whole for the purpose of clinical reasoning.

Research

- A structuralist approach to inquiry is to represent reality in its true form so that knowledge generated is objective, generalizable, and verifiable by reproducibility.

- Topics of interest are structures and mechanisms, whether the field of study is a specific body system, a whole organism, a population, or a society.

- Knowledge is decontextualized, ahistorical, universally applicable, and timeless.

Practice

- Therapists analyze the demands of an activity or occupation to understand the specific body structures, body functions, performance skills, and performance patterns that are required and to determine the generic demands the activity or occupation makes on the client (American Occupational Therapy Association, 2014).
- Structuralism promotes a developmental and sequential approach—proximal stability (trunk and shoulder) before distal structures (elbow and hand).
- Use of therapeutic modalities such as ultrasound, paraffin bath, transcutaneous electrical nerve stimulation, and iontophoresis creates physiological changes to improve function.

RECOMMENDED READINGS

Culler, J. D. (1975). *Structural poetics: Structuralism, linguistics and the study of literature*. Routledge.

de Saussure, F. (2011). *Course in general linguistics*. Columbia University Press.

Lévi-Strauss, C. (1963). *Structural anthropology* (C. Jacobson & B. G. Schoep, Trans.). Basic Books.

REFERENCES

American Association of Occupational Therapy (AOTA). (2014). Occupational therapy practice framework: Domain and process (3rd ed.). *American Journal of Occupational Therapy, 68*(Suppl. 1), S1–S48. https://doi.org/10.5014/ajot.2014.682006

Barthes, R. (1972). *Mythologies* (A. Lavers, Trans.). Farrar, Straus and Giroux.

Barthes, R., & Duisit, L. (1975). An introduction to the structural analysis of narrative. *New Literary History, 6*(2), 237–272. https://doi.org/10.2307/468419

Boyt Schell, B. A., & Gillen, G. (2019). *Willard and Spackman's occupational therapy* (13th ed.). Lippincott Williams & Wilkins.

Christiansen, C., Baum, M. C., & Bass-Haugen, J. (Eds.). (2005). *Occupational therapy: Performance, participation, and well-being* (4th ed.). SLACK Incorporated.

Culler, J. D. (1975). *Structural poetics: Structuralism, linguistics and the study of literature*. Routledge.

de Saussure, F. (2011). *Course in general linguistics*. New York, NY. Columbia University Press.

French, S. (2011). Shifting to structures in physics and biology: A prophylactic for promiscuous realism. *Studies in History and Philosophy of Biological and Biomedical Sciences, 42*(2), 164–173. https://doi.org/10.1016/j.shpsc.2010.11.023

Gupta, J. (2016). Mapping the evolving ideas of occupational justice: A critical analysis. *OTJR: Occupation, participation and health, 36*(4), 179–194. https://doi.org/10.1177/1539449216672171

Gupta, J., & Taff, S. D. (2015). The illusion of client-centred practice. *Scandinavian Journal of Occupational Therapy, 22*(4), 244–251. https://doi.org/10.3109/11038128.2015.1020866

Hinojosa, J., & Blount, M.-L. (2009). Occupation, purposeful activities, and occupational therapy. In J. Hinojosa & M. L. Blount (Eds.), *The texture of life: Purposeful activities in context of occupation* (3rd ed., pp. 1–19). AOTA Press.

Hinojosa, J., Kramer, P., Royeen, C. B., & Luebben, A. (2003). The core concepts of occupation. In P. Kramer, J. Hinojosa, & C. B. Royeen (Eds.), *Perspectives in human occupation: Participation in life* (pp. 1–17). Lippincott Williams & Wilkins.

Hooper, B., & Wood, W. (2002). Pragmatism and structuralism in occupational therapy: The long conversation. *American Journal of Occupational Therapy, 56*(1), 40–50. https://doi.org/10.5014/ajot.56.1.40

Jakobson, R. (1960). Linguistics and poetics. In T. Sebeok (Ed.), *Style in Language* (pp. 350–377). MIT Press.

Kielhofner, G. (2009). The early development of occupational therapy practice: The pre-paradigm and occupational paradigm period. In G. Kielhofner (Ed.), *Conceptual foundations of occupational therapy practice* (4th ed., pp. 17–30). F. A. Davis.

Lacan, J. (1978). *The four fundamental concepts of psychoanalysis* (A. Sheridan, Trans.). Éditions du Seuil.

Lacan, J. (2006). *Ecrits: The first complete edition in English* (B. Fink, Trans.). W. W. Norton.

Lévi-Strauss, C. (1963). *Structural anthropology* (C. Jacobson & B. G. Schoep, Trans.). Basic Books.

Mayhew, B. H. (1980). Structuralism versus individualism: Part 1, shadowboxing in the dark. *Social Forces, 59*(2), 335–375. https://doi.org/10.1093/sf/59.2.335

Nelson, D., & Jepson-Thomas, J. (2003). Occupational form, occupational performance, and a conceptual framework for therapeutic occupation. In P. Kramer, J. Hinojosa, & C. B. Royeen (Eds.), *Perspectives in human occupation: Participation in life* (pp. 87–155). Lippincott Williams & Wilkins.

Pierce, D. (2001). Untangling occupation and activity. *American Journal of Occupational Therapy, 55*(2), 138–146. https://doi.org/10.5014/ajot.55.2.138

Reed, K. L., & Peters, C. (2006). Occupational therapy: Values and beliefs, part II. The great depression and the war years 1930–1949. *OT Practice* (October), 17–22.

Waugh, L. R. (1980). The poetic function in the theory of Roman Jakobson. *Poetics Today, 2*(1a), 57–82. https://doi.org/10.2307/1772352

Yerxa, E., Clark, F. A., Frank, G., Jackson, J. M., Parham, D., Pierce, D., . . . Zemke, R. (1989). An introduction to occupational science: A foundation for occupational therapy in the 21st century. In J. Johnson & E. Yerxa (Eds.), *Occupational science: The foundation for new models of practice* (pp. 1–17). Haworth Press.

Zinn, H. (2005). *A people's history of the United States: 1492–present.* Harper.

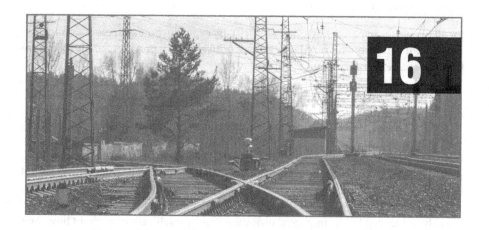

Critical Theory
Resources for Questioning and Transforming Everyday Life

Lisette Farias, PhD, MScOT, Reg. OT
Rebecca M. Aldrich, PhD, OTR/L

INTRODUCTION

Critical theory encompasses a broad group of multifaceted theoretical approaches (e.g., Marxism, work from the Frankfurt school, decolonialism, radical feminism, queer theory) rather than denoting a single overarching theory. These approaches entail reflective and critical assessments of the relationships between social, economic, political, and cultural systems and everyday practices, with a focus on the oppressive consequences of those relationships for certain social groups (Freeman & Vasconcelos, 2010). Critical theory's origins lay within Karl Marx's notions of criticism and social change (Crotty, 2015). Marx argued that social reality was an illusion and that coordinated social structures and practices were intentionally designed to maintain "proper" behavior. Marx's focus on economic hegemony and the struggle of the working class created a legacy for critical theory around monitoring democratic processes and working toward a more just society

Taff, S. D. (Ed.). *Philosophy and Occupational Therapy:*
Informing Education, Research, and Practice (pp. 155-162).
© 2021 Taylor & Francis Group.

for all people (Freeman & Vasconcelos, 2010). By exposing how systems of domination are perpetuated through everyday practices, critical theory provides a basis for liberation and social transformation (Bohman, 2016).

Major Facets of the Philosophy

Critical theory is grounded in the idea that inquiry "must explain what is wrong with current social reality, identify actors to change it, and provide both clear norms for criticism and achievable practical goals for social transformation" (Bohman, 2016, para. 3). Critical theorists see knowledge as partial; value-laden; contextually bound by social, economic, and cultural systems; and created to work for some groups' interests while disadvantaging others (Crotty, 2015). Critical theorists view inquiry as inevitably influenced by the inquirers' own values and are self-reflective about how their knowledge generation practices might maintain or create oppressive structures and power relations. Critical theorists thus focus on how: (1) groups in society (re)produce their own power by disempowering others; (2) society can be improved or altered; and (3) local contexts, knowledge, and interests constrain or support oppressive systems (Cannella & Lincoln, 2009).

General Goals or Intended Outcomes of the Philosophy

Critical theory offers frameworks for examining how the underpinnings of everyday practices (re)produce enduring systems of power and oppression. Consistent with this focus, critical theory aims to expose, illuminate, and/or transform the hidden mechanisms of social inequality (e.g., structures, practices, beliefs, assumptions) by challenging the nature of these mechanisms so as to propel emancipation and social action (Farias & Laliberte Rudman, 2016). Critical theorists are concerned not merely with criticizing the way things are but with identifying how things could and should be different and providing new insights and alternatives to reduce suffering and promote justice (Cannella & Lincoln, 2009). Critical theorists believe new insights can promote social transformation by giving rise to more informed conscious awareness that will lead to action (Farias et al., 2016).

Selected Perspectives, Thinkers, and Key Concepts

The term *critical theory* emerged when German and Western European theorists with a shared interest in Marx's ideas formed the Institute for Social Research, also known as the Frankfurt School, between 1923 and 1933 as an alternative to the traditional or positivist paradigm (Crotty, 2015). The Frankfurt School gave rise to many interpretations and adaptations of Marx's ideas based on social issues that exposed varied dimensions of domination. Prominent first-generation critical theorists included Max Horkheimer, Theodor Adorno, Herbert Marcuse, Walter Benjamin, and Erich Fromm.

Since the 1970s, Jürgen Habermas, Paulo Freire, and other second-generation theorists have developed modern critical theory. Concepts often associated with critical theory include discourse, dialogue, decolonization, emancipation, and conscientization. The rest of this section provides an overview of selected critical theorists and their key ideas rather than a comprehensive exposition of all critical philosophies.

Max Horkheimer directed the Frankfurt School from the early 1930s to the late 1950s. He aimed to show how connecting philosophy with empirical social science could reduce capitalism-related suffering (Berendzen, 2017). Horkheimer set critical theory apart from other philosophies by emphasizing its "historical self-reflexivity and its recognition of the *active* role it plays in reproducing and—potentially—transforming society" (Abromeit, 2018, p. 29). His early work detailed how forms of knowledge, values, and attitudes came to be taken for granted among particular social classes as a result of social, historical, and economic conditions (Abromeit, 2018; Berendzen, 2017). By exposing false assumptions underlying society, Horkheimer believed that critical theorists could identify opportunities for alternative emancipatory forms of social organization (Bohman, 2016).

Herbert Marcuse was one of the most prominent early members of the Frankfurt School. His work framed the gap between ideal conditions for humanity and people's less-than-ideal lived conditions as both a source of alienation and a catalyst for social change. This dialectical characterization of the relationship between ideal and nonideal conditions reflects the ways in which society simultaneously produces dominating and liberatory forces (Bernstein, 2013). In contrast to this two-dimensional way of thinking about domination and liberation as opposite sides of the same coin, one-dimensional thinking does not recognize the simultaneous interplay of these forces and therefore is blind to the contradictions by which society is constituted (Marcuse & Kellner, 1991). For Marcuse, one-dimensional thinking produces administered societies in which domination is internalized, two-dimensional thinking is silenced, and demands for social change are absent.

Jürgen Habermas directed the Frankfurt School from the early 1980s to the early 1990s and is known for his work as a philosopher and public intellectual. He saw public discourse and debate as the highest form of reason and focused on describing how communicative acts manifest the norms that shape everyday life (Henning, 2018). His works were built on "the idea of inclusive critical discussion, free of social and economic pressures, in which interlocutors treat each other as equals in a cooperative attempt to reach an understanding on matters of common concern" (Bohman & Rehg, 2017, p. 2). In general, Habermas helped critical theory move from identifying and eliminating oppressive structures to specifying the conditions of praxis that might realistically foster emancipation given current circumstances (Bohman, 2016).

Paulo Freire was an educationalist who launched literacy programs among peasant people in Brazil in the 1960s. He viewed dialogue as a means to engage with processes that seek to (re)invent knowledge, rather than only as a way to exchange ideas.

> [W]e are communicative beings who communicate to each other as we become more able to transform our reality, we are able to know that we know, which is something more than just knowing . . . Through dialogue, reflecting together on

what we know and don't know, we can then act critically to transform reality. (Shor & Freire, 1987, p. 13)

Freire believed that the marginalization of a certain group in society—what he called a "culture of silence"—is produced by those in power with the aim of oppression and is perpetuated by the absence of reflective participation by those who are disempowered (Freire, 1970). Thus, to break this culture, he argued that people need to be empowered through "conscientization," that is, encouraging individuals to transform their reality through dialogue, reflection, and action.

Boaventura de Sousa Santos is a Professor of Sociology at the University of Coimbra. His work *Epistemologies of the South: Justice Against Epistemicide* (2016) uses the "south" as a metaphor for the suffering, exclusion, and silencing of people and cultures that have been objects of capitalist and colonial violence. According to Santos, colonialism maintains its historical, political, and cultural domination by imposing its ethnocentric knowledge on the world and presenting that version of knowledge as universal. From Santos's perspective, it is urgent to develop new theoretical and political paradigms of social transformation to reinvent emancipation and achieve "cognitive justice." He advocates for different knowledges that have been otherwise made invisible and defined as nonscientific, alternative, or common sense (a process Santos termed "knowledge epistemicide").

Linda Tuhiwai Smith (Ngāti Awa and Ngāti Porou, Māori) is a Professor of Indigenous Education at the University of Waikato and critic of persistent colonialism in academic teaching and research. One of Smith's (2012) most important contributions has been to link the history of European conquest and colonization to the "positional superiority" of scientific knowledge over indigenous knowledge. Smith's works have demonstrated that indigenous epistemologies are no less rigorous than the dominant scientific method and are no less worthy of respect. Her "decolonizing methodologies" demand that research with indigenous peoples and communities should both serve the needs of those communities and be directed by them. Smith argues for legitimizing and respecting other knowledges as parallel ways of knowing to the scientific method.

IMPACT ON UNDERSTANDING OF OCCUPATION AND OCCUPATIONAL ENGAGEMENT

Using critical theory, several authors have highlighted the limits that dominant Eurocentric perspectives impose on our understanding of occupation (Magalhães et al., 2018), such as narrowing the scholarly gaze to center on occupations that make more sense to the Western Anglophone world, framing occupation as solely the product of human action, giving primacy to individuals' abilities to engage in occupations, and neglecting contextual factors that shape occupational experiences (Farias & Laliberte Rudman, 2016). Thus, critical theory has helped reveal what kinds of knowledge about occupation have not been privileged in the existing literature, drawing attention to occupations that have been dismissed or marginalized (e.g., alcoholism, begging, drug abuse, sex work, gang activity) based on Western social expectations and constructs of healthy/unhealthy and proper/improper occupations (Kiepek et al., 2014). This questioning has reinforced the need to explore individual and group engagement in occupation relative to social expectations and contextual influences, focusing on the ways in which cultural, gender-based, generational, socioeconomic, and other factors facilitate or restrict access to occupations; whether engagement in occupations is voluntary or coerced; and who profits from engaging in certain occupations and who is marginalized (Hocking, 2009).

Moving further toward a notion of occupation as situated through and within particular social, political, economic, and other contextual forces (Laliberte Rudman, 2013), critically informed occupational therapists and occupational scientists can consider occupation's relation to social power and the hegemonic or dominant social order. For example, assessing Indigenous parent–infant play using predominant Western standards can increase the likelihood of blaming parents as neglectful, labeling children as "at risk," and perpetuating the dominant social order that has produced systematic social disadvantage through colonialism (Gerlach et al., 2014). Critical theory also encourages scholars and practitioners to take up issues commensurate with critical foci, such as exploring how occupation can perpetuate or transform the hegemonic social order that shapes occupational choices. Galvaan (2015) examined how colonial influences predicted and limited young adolescents' leisure and lifestyle choices, and she used this understanding to create a community-based occupational therapy intervention that targeted the community's internalized oppression. Critically informed scholars and practitioners can explicate not only how occupation is a site where inequality and social difference are constituted (Angell, 2012) but also how occupations have been developed as a means of resistance by minority groups to challenge the majority group's power in society (Pyatak & Muccitelli, 2011; Ramugondo, 2015). By illuminating the multifaceted natures and purposes of occupations such as dressing, playing, creating or listening to music, and watching television, scholars and practitioners can identify points of transformative potential along with the spectra of ways of doing.

Critical theory also raises awareness of the ways in which occupation-centered educational content and processes may perpetuate the dominance of particular views and practices. Educators can adopt a critical stance by ensuring that curricula incorporate global perspectives on occupation (Aldrich, 2015; Dsouza et al., 2017) and provide opportunities for developing critical consciousness and reflexivity (Aldrich & Grajo, 2017; Aldrich & Peters, 2019). Drawing on critical theory, educators can design activities to help students explore the interactions between macro societal structures, local contextual issues, and people's occupational possibilities (Laliberte Rudman, 2010). Overall, drawing upon critical theory can help the profession ensure that its research, education, and practices are open to diverse worldviews, address contested views of occupation, and avoid enacting colonial agendas that perpetuate the dominant social order.

KEY IMPLICATIONS FOR OCCUPATIONAL THERAPY EDUCATION, RESEARCH, AND PRACTICE

Education

- Helps raise awareness of how sociopolitical processes beyond individual control can exclude or prohibit forms of occupational engagement
- Facilitates deeper appreciation for contextualized understandings of occupation
- Supports thinking along a continuum from individual to social/collective levels of action
- Sensitizes learners to the different needs and lived experiences of future clients

Research

- Privileges the need for and inclusion of diverse knowledge-generation methods
- Privileges knowledge co-construction with those affected by oppression
- Focuses research on occupation as a site of survival and resistance against oppression

Practice

- Provides guidance for questioning of assumptions, systems, and structures that shape practice
- Supports the development of a more culturally and socially responsive practice
- Seeks to support people's efforts of resistance and expression of rights
- Disrupts the expert position and traditional practitioner–client power relations

RECOMMENDED READINGS

Best, B., Bonefeld, W., & O'Kane, C. (2018). *The SAGE handbook of Frankfurt School critical theory.* SAGE Publications.

Denzin, N. K., Lincoln, Y. S., & Smith, L. T. (2008). *Handbook of critical and indigenous research methodologies.* SAGE Publications.

Gibson, B. (2016). *Rehabilitation: A post-critical approach.* CRC Press.

REFERENCES

Abromeit, J. (2018). Max Horkheimer and the early model of critical theory. In B. Best, W. Bonefeld, & C. O'Kane (Eds.), *The SAGE handbook of Frankfurt school critical theory* (pp. 19–38). SAGE Publications.

Aldrich, R. M. (2015). Course redesign to promote local and global experiential learning about human occupation: Description and evaluation of a pilot effort. *South African Journal of Occupational Therapy, 45*(1), 56–62. https://doi.org/10.17159/2310-3833/2015/v45n01a10

Aldrich, R. M., & Grajo, L. C. (2017). International educational interactions and students' critical consciousness: A pilot study. *American Journal of Occupational Therapy, 71*(5), 7105230020p1–7105230020p10. https://doi.org/10.5014/ajot.2017.026724

Aldrich, R. M., & Peters, L. (2019). Using occupational justice as a linchpin of educational collaborations. *American Journal of Occupational Therapy, 73*(3), 7303205100p1–7303205100p10. https://doi.org/10.5014/ajot.2019.029744

Angell, A. (2012). Occupation-centered analysis of social difference: Contributions to a socially-responsive occupational science. *Journal of Occupational Science, 21*(2), 104–116. https://doi.org/10.1080/14427591.2012.711230

Berendzen, J. C. (2017). Max Horkheimer. In E. N. Zalta (Ed.), *The Stanford encyclopedia of philosophy* (Fall 2017 ed.). https://plato.stanford.edu/archives/fall2017/entries/horkheimer

Bernstein, R. J. (2013). Marcuse's critical legacy. *Radical Philosophy Review, 16*(1), 59–71. https://doi.org/10.5840/radphilrev20131618

Bohman, J. (2016). Critical theory. In E. N. Zalta (Ed.), *The Stanford encyclopedia of philosophy* (Fall 2016 ed.). https://plato.stanford.edu/archives/fall2016/entries/critical-theory

Bohman, J., & Rehg, W. (2017). Jürgen Habermas. In E. N. Zalta (Ed.), *The Stanford encyclopedia of philosophy* (Fall 2017 ed.). https://plato.stanford.edu/archives/fall2017/entries/habermas

Cannella, G. S., & Lincoln, Y. S. (2009). Deploying qualitative methods for critical social purposes. In N. K. Denzin & M. D. Giardina (Eds.), *Qualitative inquiry and social justice: Toward a politics of hope* (pp. 53–72). Left Coast Press.

Crotty, M. (2015). *The foundations of social research: Meaning and perspective in the research process.* SAGE Publications.

de Sousa Santos, B. (2016). *Epistemologies of the South: Justice against epistemicide.* Routledge.

Dsouza, S. A., Galvaan, R., & Ramugondo, E. L. (2017). *Concepts in occupational therapy: Understanding southern perspectives.* Manipal University Press.

Farias, L., & Laliberte Rudman, D. (2016). A critical interpretive synthesis of the uptake of critical perspectives in occupational science. *Journal of Occupational Science, 23*(1), 33–50. https://doi.org/10.1080/14427591.2014.989893

Farias, L., Laliberte Rudman, D., & Magalhães, L. (2016). Illustrating the importance of critical epistemology to realize the promise of occupational justice. *OTJR: Occupation, Participation and Health, 36*(4), 234–243. https://doi.org/10.1177/1539449216665561

Freeman, M., & Vasconcelos, E. F. S. (Eds.). (2010). Critical social theory: Core tenets, inherent issues. *Critical social theory and evaluation practice: New directions for evaluation, 127*(2010), 7–19 [Special Issue]. https://doi.org/10.1002/ev.335

Freire, P. (1970). *Pedagogy of the oppressed* (M. Bergman Ramos, Trans.). Continuum International Publishing Group.

Galvaan, R. (2015). The contextually situated nature of occupational choice: Marginalized young adolescents' experiences in South Africa. *Journal of Occupational Science, 22*(1), 39–53. https://doi.org/10.1080/14427591.2014.912124

Gerlach, A. J., Browne, A., & Suto, M. (2014). A critical reframing of play in relation to Indigenous children in Canada. *Journal of Occupational Science, 21*(3), 243–258. https://doi.org/10.1080/14427591.2014.908818

Henning, C. (2018). Jürgen Habermas: Against obstacles to public debates. In B. Best, W. Bonefeld, & C. O'Kane (Eds.), *The SAGE handbook of Frankfurt school critical theory* (pp. 402–415). SAGE Publications.

Hocking, C. (2009). The challenge of occupation: Describing the things people do. *Journal of Occupational Science, 16*(3), 140–150. https://doi.org/10.1080/14427591.2009.9686655

Kiepek, N., Phelan, S., & Magalhães, L. (2014). Introducing a critical analysis of the figured world of occupation. *Journal of Occupational Science, 21*(4), 403–417. https://doi.org/10.1080/14427591.2013.816998

Laliberte Rudman, D. (2010). Occupational terminology: Occupational possibilities. *Journal of Occupational Science, 17*(1), 55–59. https://doi.org/10.1080/14427591.2010.9686673

Laliberte Rudman, D. (2013). Enacting the critical potential of occupational science: Problematizing the "individualizing of occupation." *Journal of Occupational Science, 20*(4), 298–313. https://doi.org/10.1080/14427591.2013.803434

Magalhães, L., Farias, L., Rivas-Quarneti, N., Alvarez, L., & Malfitano, A. P. S. (2018). The development of occupational science outside the Anglophone sphere: Enacting global collaboration. *Journal of Occupational Science, 26*(2), 181–192. https://doi.org/10.1080/14427591.2018.1530133

Marcuse, H., & Kellner, D. (1991). *One-dimensional man: Studies in the ideology of advanced industrial society* (2nd ed.). Beacon Press.

Pyatak, E., & Muccitelli, L. (2011). Rap music as resistive occupation: Constructions of Black American identity and culture for performers and their audiences. *Journal of Occupational Science, 18*(1), 48–61. https://doi.org/10.1080/14427591.2011.554154

Ramugondo, E. (2015). Occupational terminology: Occupational consciousness. *Journal of Occupational Science, 22*(4), 488–501. https://doi.org/10.1080/14427591.2015.1042516

Shor, I., & Freire, P. (1987). What is the "dialogical method" of teaching? *Journal of Education, 169*(3), 11–31. https://doi.org/10.1177/002205748716900303

Smith, L. T. (2012). *Decolonizing methodologies: Research and Indigenous peoples* (2nd ed.). Zed Books.

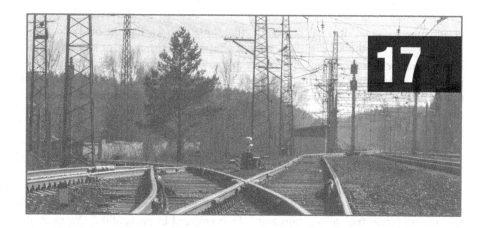

Everyday Hermeneutics

Understanding (the Meaning of) Occupational Engagement

Melissa Park, PhD, MA OT
Aaron Bonsall, PhD, OTR/L
Don Fogelberg, PhD, OTR/L

INTRODUCTION

In this chapter, we draw from three philosophers—Dilthey, Ricoeur, and Gadamer—whose ideas have been used within qualitative health research focused on lived experience or clinical reasoning. All three are known for their contributions to *hermeneutics*, the systematic process of human understanding. We begin with a brief discussion of the critical place that meaning holds in the understanding of occupation. We then introduce key ideas of Wilhelm Dilthey, a 19th-century scholar working at the intersection of philosophy and the emerging discipline of psychology who played a key role in reviving hermeneutics. Finally, we add the perspectives of Paul Ricoeur and Hans-Georg Gadamer, two philosophers who each responded to elements of Dilthey's work. In this chapter, we underscore how hermeneutics underpins key assumptions within occupational therapy as well as

Taff, S. D. (Ed.). *Philosophy and Occupational Therapy:*
Informing Education, Research, and Practice (pp. 163-179).
© 2021 Taylor & Francis Group.

occupational science.[1] It is our contention that those who work in the field of occupational therapy, whether as clinicians, clinical educators, researchers, or students, regularly use a type of "everyday hermeneutics" to reason about what matters to particular persons as they engage in occupation. Thus, in an effort to illuminate this link, we will draw a central concept from each philosopher to explore how everyday hermeneutics plays out or plays into the process of understanding in a particularly illustrative example of a common clinical dilemma.

OCCUPATION AS ENACTED AND EMBODIED MEANING

Our philosophy is deeply tied to our profession's assumptions that occupational engagement is "contributory to the significance and *meaning* of life" (Yerxa, 1967), and that we are "most true to our humanity when engaged in occupation" (Yerxa et al., 1989, p. 7). We are, as Lawlor (2003, p. 432) pointed out, socially occupied beings "*doing something* with *someone* else that *matters,*" whether or not our engagement in occupation is pleasurable (Meyer, 1922; Reilly, 1962) or "frustrating, anxiety provoking or boring" (Yerxa et al., 1989, p. 9). These statements, in turn, underscore how understanding the meaning of engagement in the things that we do is a core concern of both our practice and research in occupational therapy and occupational science. This focus on the quality of engagement in everyday life echoes the work of Dilthey who proposed that *meaning* itself is the unifying force in our experiences: "The connectedness of lived experience in its concrete reality lies in the category of meaning. This is the unity that gathers the sequence of what has been experienced or re-experienced into memory" (1977, pp. 256–257).

What is key is the deep entanglement of meaning with our practical engagements in everyday life and, thus, how the meaning of lived experience is both embodied and enacted. As Dilthey underscores, "meaning does not consist in a unifying point that lies outside lived experience but is contained in these lived experiences and constitutes their connectedness" (Dilthey, 1977, p. 257). The standard definitions of *occupation* that have been developed by occupational therapy's professional and research organizations explicitly incorporate meaning, and thus the term *occupation* is used to denote action of a particular quality. Derived from its Latin root *occupaio,* "to seize or take possession," the term implies action that conveys agency and desire (Yerxa et al., 1989). Rather than something one just happens to stumble into or casually pick up, occupations are actions that carry a sense of purpose and are intimately related to what moves us.

The concept of occupation is invoked as essential both to define therapeutic goals and to select the interventions used to achieve those goals, or to use Gray's (1998) eloquent phrasing, "occupation as ends, occupation as means." If meaning is to be considered a defining characteristic of occupation, then it follows that meaning is central to both the therapeutic efficacy of occupational therapy and in the definition of its desired outcomes. To put it simply, without meaning, we would have neither a therapeutic

---

[1]While we recognize the important distinctions that can be drawn between occupational therapy, a practice carried out primarily within clinical contexts, and occupational science, an academic discipline, in the interests of brevity, we will frequently use the terms interchangeably.

mechanism nor justifiable outcomes. As Reilly (1962) underscored in her Eleanor Clarke Slagle lecture, expertise in "the *meaningful* involvement in problem-solving tasks or creative performances" positioned occupational therapy to be "one of the great ideas of 20th century medicine" (italics added).

Despite the central role that meaning plays in occupation, we often exhort students to *understand* what is meaningful to those with whom we work without teaching the philosophical foundations and systematic rules–based methods for doing so. The types of reasoning (Mattingly, 1991) related to the search for desire (Mattingly, 1998a) and the good (Mattingly, 1998b)—that is, understanding what is most meaningful to particular persons—are implicitly grounded in hermeneutics. Yet such processes are often "underground" (Mattingly, 1998a) and considered illegitimate in clinical contexts (Mattingly & Lawlor, 2001), which paradoxically are the very places where professional graduate students in occupational therapy are expected to learn to understand and interpret what is most meaningful to those with whom they work.

HERMENEUTICS AS A
SYSTEMATIC PROCESS OF UNDERSTANDING

Hermeneutics emerged over time when *philology* (the study of grammar) and *hermeneia* (the art of interpreting) of the Greek poets coalesced into a systematized method to understand theological (and later legal) texts. Dilthey (1996, p. 252) defined hermeneutics as "[t]he theory of the rules of understanding textually fixed objectifications of life." Although traditionally used in the interpretation of written texts, Dilthey applied the logic of hermeneutics to a range of such "objectifications of life," arguing that through "stone and marble, musical notes, gestures, words, and texts, action, economic regulations and constitutions, the same human spirit [as that contained in written texts] addresses us and demands interpretation" (Dilthey, 1996, pp. 236–237). Rather than an end-product of cognitive thought, he considered hermeneutics to be a systematic process "by which we recognize, behind signs given to our senses, that psychic reality of which they are an expression" (p. 319). At the same time, he acknowledged that we cannot stand outside the act of understanding even if the process of understanding "must everywhere have the same characteristics" (Dilthey, 1996, p. 237). This constitutes one of the central dilemmas that hermeneutics as a philosophy raised and has grappled with over time.

Through the process of understanding the meaning of a text or other objectification of life, Dilthey (1996, p. 250) argued that not only is it possible "to understand an author better than he understood himself,"[2] but also that this degree of understanding is the "ultimate goal of the hermeneutic process." How we do that—understand authors better than they might understand themselves (and if it is possible)—may also, ultimately, be central to the study of occupation, which, as Yerxa et al. (1989, p. 10) best encapsulated more than a century later, "requires the study of the person as the author of his or her work, rest, play, leisure, and self-maintenance." Yet, significantly, the formal study of hermeneutics is not routinely included in either our research methods or

---

[2]Dilthey references Schleirmacher for this statement (1996, p. 250).

our professional training. If it is mentioned, it is often defined as an iterative process between text (e.g., transcripts of individual or group interviews), theoretical resources, and/or observations of actions.[3] We rarely clarify what those resources are and/or why they were chosen, define what lived experience actually represents or situate it in any lived contexts, and/or announce our own stance. Yet all of those interpretive moves are central to hermeneutics. Without hermeneutics—a method that focuses on *how* to understand rather than the content of what is understood—we would have neither a systematic method of interpreting lived experience *nor the science upon which the very premise of our profession rests.*

EVERYDAY HERMENEUTICS AND CONTEMPORARY DILEMMAS

Client- or person-centered care is paramount among our professional values. In fact, locating what is meaningful to particular persons in what they do and using those occupations as both ends and means of therapy would ensure that our goals and interventions directly align with what really matters to those with whom we work. Yet, despite our best intentions, professional practice standards and competencies in occupation-based goals and interventions do little to help us understand *how* to understand what is meaningful in what we choose to do, and the ways in which meaning shapes when, where, with whom, and the other nuances of *how* we do what we do. Compared to most medical procedures, occupational therapy requires a greater level of interpersonal engagement to encourage or support engagement in therapeutic activities. Ensuring this double level of engagement (i.e., personal and interpersonal) requires that those activities be meaningful to that particular person—and thus, by our definition of meaningful activities, are occupations. The question then arises: What happens when one's occupation—doing something meaningful—is no longer possible because of an illness or disability?

It is in this gap between a past life and a future one that we often meet the other. We may write about our goals and objectives in terms of function, but to be effective, we must be able to understand what our patients or clients desire. As Cheryl Mattingly's (1998a, p. 107) ethnography clarified, occupational therapists are in search of an object of desire[4] that is—to cite screenwriter guru McKee (1997)—compelling enough to move the patient to action. As Mattingly herself stated, "In my studies of clinical work, I have found that the drive to create a compelling therapeutic plot has less to do with a need to find continuity or coherence than with a need to locate desire." The ability to understand what really matters and its relationship to action and desire through activity and task analysis distinguishes occupational therapy as a professional vocation rather than a technical one. In our attempts to locate desire in our clinical encounters or research projects, the dilemmas we currently face are about the origin of the

---

[3]A rare exception, following Mattingly's work on clinical reasoning, is Alsaker's exemplary use of Ricoeur's hermeneutic process in her analysis of the lived experience of women living with chronic rheumatic conditions.

[4]See, in particular, "The Substance of Story," ch. 7, pp. 135–180.

Table 17-1. Clinical Dilemmas, Concepts in Hermeneutic Philosophy, and Interpretive Strategies		
CLINICAL DILEMMAS	**PHILOSOPHICAL APORIAS**	**KEY CONCEPTS**
How do we understand what really matters to another person (values)?	How do we interpret a text, conversation, experience of another?	*Expressions of Life* (Dilthey)
How do we understand what really matters to our clients when we need to keep our functional objectives in sight?	How do we resolve the tension between explanation and understanding?	*Distanciation* (Ricoeur)
How do we productively use misunderstanding when it emerges?	How can a question of critique in general be accounted for within the framework of a fundamental hermeneutics?	*Prejudice* (Gadamer)

meaning itself, asking us to consider, for example: How do we understand what really matters to another person (values)? How do we understand what persons desire without imposing our own values? How do we understand what really matters to our clients when we need to keep our functional objectives in sight? How do we productively use misunderstanding when it emerges?

Such questions reflect a central challenge to interpretation, one which Dilthey (1996, p. 253) characterized as epistemological:

Each of us is enclosed, as it were, within his own consciousness. This consciousness is individual and imparts its subjectivity to all that we apprehend. . . . The possibility of grasping what is other or alien is one of the most profound epistemological problems. How can an individual bring a sensuously given individual objectification of life to the level of a universally valid objective understanding?

This clash between epistemological stances, or different ways of knowing, has often been described as a conflict between the biomedical model in contrast to the holistic or experiential ways of knowing central to occupational therapy (Hooper, 2006; Kinsella & Whiteford, 2008). Yet the contemporary dilemmas that often emerge in our clinical encounters, research projects, and teaching also reflect *aporias* or the impasses or perplexities first raised by hermeneutic philosophers in their attempt to understand the texts, and then actions, of others—from different historical periods, places, and cultural systems (Table 17-1). This suggests that key concepts—even the most basic—in hermeneutic philosophy could, in turn, illuminate interpretive strategies toward even elementary forms of understanding the other: "One must know what the other is up to" (Dilthey, 1977, p. 125).

In order to show how hermeneutic concepts are used in an often underground and everyday interpretive process, we present data drawn from a participatory research project that explored the challenges and supports to recovery for people living with mental illness. Personal recovery in mental health practice, as put forth by Anthony (1993), is a journey and not a cure (Davidson & Roe, 2007); meaning itself is considered critical in this process (Leamy et al., 2011). The methodology employed in this research project also supported a hermeneutic process, as it mixed narrative-phenomenological (Mattingly, 2010) with dialogical approaches (e.g., Schwartz, 2011), so that our participants as co-researchers brought forward significant or memorable experiences related to providing or receiving care, and then critically reflected upon those moments. The multiple-perspective format of the group brought together—at the same table—four health care providers (occupational therapists, psychiatrist), four people who received mental health services, and two academic researchers with mixed backgrounds in providing and receiving mental health services (Schwartz et al., 2013) and encouraged a hermeneutic process as members grappled with understanding the meaning of recovery as a concept and clinical model.[5]

AN ILLUSTRATIVE CASE

In the following section of a de-identified transcript, Olivia (pseudonym)—a graduate-level occupational therapist—shares "an experience"[6] about a disrupted therapeutic relationship with Chloe, a former client (who was not participating in the research), in the participatory research group, to which Laura, another group member, responds:

Olivia: So my story is about this lady (Chloe) that was referred to me for help with school. She's somebody in one of our clinics and she really wanted to do something in a natural alternative therapy kind of thing. And . . . so when I met with her, she was really, really motivated but uh-, she had-, she was disorganized. Like her thought process, the way she dressed. And I think everybody knew she-, it wasn't a realistic goal for her to go back and do a course where she'd have to work with people and be like a therapist. You know, you need a certain skill . . . and she might have had that but she didn't present it that way. And it was MY job to do whatever tests it would take to kind of increase her self-awareness and make realistic goals with her.

And so I worked with her for a little bit and pushed her to come to group, and she came and she did everything I told her to do . . . OR we collaborated on-, I didn't tell her what to do, I just advised her that she should come. And um, at one point I said, "Well, maybe you should think about volunteering and maybe you should work and maybe THAT'S more realistic for you." Cuz we kept on setting plans and then, aside from coming to the group she couldn't really get herself to go outside in the community. And then at one point she just said, "You know, Olivia, I know that you don't think I can do this, but I'm doing everything you're telling me to do and I really believe that I can do this."

And then I just thought that the obstacle was myself. Maybe, like-, "Am I helping her?" I thought that I was helping her by doing these various exercises to show-, to increase self-awareness, to set realistic goals . . . but I thought,

---

[5]It is notable that this research project preceded new federal policy on recovery in Canada, including a strategic framework (Mental Health Commission of Canada, 2012) and practice guidelines (Chodos et al., 2015).
[6]In narrative-phenomenology, the phrase *an experience* is considered to be a significant experience, one that stands out as an event (Dewey, 1934; Jackson, 2005; Mattingly, 2010).

"Maybe those are just MY values. Maybe she just wants to try it out and . . . who am I to say, 'You can't do it.'" And she actually did enroll in a class and-, it looked like she was able to do it. And . . . my only-, my bigger regret was that had I just let her go and do it and just supported her then-, because our relationship, out interactions stopped after that [. . . .]

Laura: She said what you were thinking. And she figured it out.

Olivia: Yeah. Well she kept saying, "Why do you keep pointing me in the other direction?" And so I said-, and I gave her the evidence that from, you know, what I've seen . . . this, this, this. And then she said-, I guess the moment of-, when I had to think about it was when she said, "I really want to do this!", and then "I thought I was being client-centered. I thought I was being protective of you," and . . . yeah, it was at that moment when she said, "You're not doing what I need you to do."

Stories, as Bruner (1990, 2002) pointed out, are a type of folk psychology, an everyday mode of understanding what someone else is up to, and the "engine" of stories is trouble. For Olivia, her sense-making of Chloe's actions takes on all the characteristics of a story: It is marked by a slippage into present tense, direct citations of what was said during those moments, heightened emotionality, and a troubling experience. She is what Dilthey (1977, p. 133) would characterize hermeneutically as "re-experiencing" the events that led up to a puzzling and even regretful situation in which her relationship with Chloe ends. This re-experiencing or "creation along the line of events" draws us alongside her as she attempts to make sense of what happened that caused this rupture. Thus, it is an ideal exemplar of how such phenomenologically grounded stories afford a particularly potent mode to enter into a particular situation (or text) and follow along with a storyteller's own interpretive process, specifically because we—as the readers—are then also asked to engage in an (everyday) hermeneutic process as we also attempt to make sense of the interactions between Olivia and Chloe, even if our results may differ.

In the following section, we examine Olivia's own reflections in a research setting that cultivated reflection to (1) ground key hermeneutic concepts in actual examples, while (2) making visible how effective interpretive strategies of what really matters affect occupational engagement.

EXPRESSIONS OF LIFE AND PHILOSOPHICAL APORIAS

In an essay entitled "The Understanding of Other Persons and Their Expressions of Life," first published in 1927, Dilthey (1977, p. 123) stated that "understanding opens up a world," and that this world is based upon "both the lived experience and understanding of oneself, and their continuing interaction." His interest in lived experience, however, was less about the individual psychology than how this understanding of lived experience could contribute to what he called "historical knowledge" as the basis of the human sciences:

In this domain [of history,] the given always consists of expressions of life; they occur in the world of the senses, and are the expression of something spiritual

Table 17-2. Expressions of Life as Foci for Understanding		
EXPRESSIONS OF LIFE	CONTEXT	FOCUS OF UNDERSTANDING
Larger structures of thought	Logically perfected	Mere thought-content
Actions	Circumstantially determined	Purpose (rather than communication)
Lived experience	The life context in which a situation is grounded	Motive

and consequently make it possible for us to become acquainted with the latter. I mean here by "expressions of life" not only those expressions which are *intended* to mean or signify something, but also those which, without being intended as the expression of something spiritual, make it understandable to us.

In contrast to the categories used to understand the "natural world," we understand humans through "expressions of life" that emerge from our practical engagements with life itself. Because expressions of life are grounded in our everyday sensory engagement in the world, they give access to those meanings through their very visibility in concepts, actions, and/or lived experience. The excerpt, filled with what we call "experience-near" moments, is an ideal exemplar of practical engagements in which persons re-enter a memory "as if" re-creating or re-experiencing a series of events moving forward in time. This is signaled by slippage into present tense, citing actual phrases that were used, and use of highly metaphoric language to convey the aesthetics or multimodal qualities (or sensory details) of that experience (Mattingly & Lawlor, 2000, 2001; see also Park, 2012).

Dilthey (1977, p. 124) considered three "classes" of life expressions that, much like different types of lenses, foreground different aspects of understanding (Table 17-2). For example, the class of "concepts and value-laden judgments" works well in "logically perfected contexts" or hypothetical situations, and thus lends itself to generalizability. This focus of understanding is readily evident in the backstory when Olivia describes Chloe as "disorganized" in her observations of "thought process, the way she dressed," and thus "not suitable" to be a therapist. As concepts, "disorganization" and "suitability" are also judgments that could pertain to a general type of person (e.g., "patients") that Olivia may have worked with over time. Although highly generalizable, these life expressions lack detail; as Dilthey underscores, "No indication of the peculiarities of life from which it arose is found here."

Olivia's appraisals of the actions, both her own and Chloe's, are equally distant from the particularities needed to deepen understanding. Actions, as a class of life expression, provide more clues to what may be meaningful to a particular person because they are contextually situated. Interpretations of "actions" help us understand motive or purpose, even if it is not explicitly expressed in text or language. The context gives clues to help us understand the person's intentions, to determine what the person may be up to. For example, our interpretation of why someone is cutting wood may be dependent upon whether it is summer or winter, in the city or in the country, even the time of day and/or how the person may be dressed. Olivia, likewise, interprets the degree of commitment that Chloe has to becoming a natural therapist based on her actions. Despite Chloe coming to the occupational therapy group, in other aspects of her life she "kept on setting plans and then . . . she couldn't really get herself to go outside in the community." Thus, Olivia interprets that becoming a natural therapist may not be *that* meaningful to Chloe, as her actions do not seem to indicate that this is a priority or even a possibility. Even in her reflections of her interactions with Chloe, Olivia interprets her own actions (test, increase self-awareness, make realistic goals, collaborate) according to the purpose they serve within the context of her own particular role in the mental health system.

Larger structures of thought—like concepts or values—as well as actions focus understanding on more elemental forms that may lead us to misunderstand the subtleties or complexity of meaning(s). They do not provide Olivia with access to what may really be meaningful to Chloe, leaving Olivia stranded, in a sense, as not being able to anticipate or support what her client really wants to be. Thus, viewing the abstract concepts and interpretation of actions through a clinical or functional lens blurred Olivia's ability to locate what Chloe desires. When Olivia is unable to access or enter more fully into understanding the meaning of being a natural therapist for Chloe, Chloe's engagement in a chosen and hoped-for occupation is compromised. The clinical terms of the mental health context that Olivia uses to interpret Chloe's actions (motivation, disorganization, realistic, self-awareness, evidence) prevent her, as it were, from *experiencing-with* Chloe. Further, Olivia's focus on action *from a functional perspective* within the context of mental health care (lack of skills, not being able to go outside in the community) diminishes the meaning of Chloe's other actions (attendance at occupational therapy group) and leads to Olivia's interpretation that "maybe you [Chloe] should think about volunteering and maybe you should work and maybe THAT'S more realistic for you."

At this point, Olivia enters more fully into the experience-near: She slips into present tense with her "I said," and "she said," and repeatedly anchors their exchange in particular moments in time with her "at one point," "at one point." Then she slips into a reflexive mode as if she is, as Dilthey suggested, re-experiencing rather than merely re-telling events. By focusing on the experience of her actions, she also opens up another level of understanding, which she had not been able to grasp before.

> In introspection that is directed towards our own experiencing, we cannot apprehend the forward movement of the psychic process, for every act of fixation arrests that on which it focuses and gives it a certain duration. But here also the relationship of experiencing, expression, and understanding makes possible a solution. We grasp the expression of an action and we re-experience it. (Dilthey, 1977, p. 251)

Through Olivia's invoking a past experience in the present, she also, in a sense, re-creates the sequence of events in a way that also allows the reader or listener to experience it alongside her. This focus on understanding of lived experience helps her see that those other, more elemental foci might have misled her interpretation of what may have been most meaningful to Chloe: "Maybe those are just MY values." In this sense, Olivia, in her re-creating of the sequence of events from an experience-near perspective, tacking back and forth between what "she said" and what "I said," also (re) experiences her exchanges that lead her to understand how her more "elemental" way of understanding what mattered to Chloe may have "gotten in the way."

Although values are exceedingly useful as an interpretive lens in their relative prox- imity to universal understanding,[7] they are also the most removed from human expe- rience. By focusing on lived experience in its particularities, Olivia also re-creates the past experience as she narrates it; the specific moments or elements of that experience that she includes in her narration, and the specific sequence in which she arranges those moments, enable her to experience the events she is describing anew. Whether it is a resequencing or shift in emphasis on what is recalled, her focus moves from what Chloe was not able to do and opens up another possible interpretation, an alternative vision to the one that she had held at the time: "And she actually did enroll in a class and-, it looked like she was able to do it." In this re-experiencing, understanding is achieved through "interrelatedness and that which is common in them"; "this process presupposes the connection of that which is universally human with individuation" (Dilthey, 1977, p. 231). This could be a rather tricky business as, in essence, we are in- terpreting by projecting our own experiences onto another. Dilthey, however, proposes that the solution lies within our focus on the particularities of individual experiences:

> The material for the solution of this problem comprises all the individual ele- ments which are given, as they are unified inductively. Each is an individual and is so apprehended in the process. It contains a moment which renders possible the apprehension of the individual definiteness of the whole. But the presup- position of the procedure assumes however forms which are developed further and further by immersion into the particular and by comparing these particulars with others. (1977, p. 131)

Generalities prevent Olivia from fully entering into the particularities of Chloe's ex- perience. Although reflexively corrected through her retelling of their interactions, the use of rehabilitation concepts and past clinical experiences led her to prejudge the meaning that Chloe had invested in this goal—however much of a stretch it might have been at a certain point in time—of doing a "natural alternative therapy kind of thing." This misunderstanding results in Olivia feeling a sense of "regret" as she loses the very relationship itself.

This leads us to two additional contemporary conundrums: How do we understand what really matters to our clients when we need to keep our functional objectives in sight? And, further, if we are able to elicit the particularities of experience that can help us more fully understand what really matters to our clients, how do we know that we are not simply projecting our own experiences that may get in the way? We will address these questions in conversation with two articles within our discipline and practice that illustrate the practical relevance of drawing from hermeneutic phi- losophy. Specifically, our reading of Ricoeur's use of *distanciation* and Gadamer's dis- cussion of *prejudice* illustrates how the "systematic process" of hermeneutics also de- veloped across historical time. In other words, Ricoeur and Gadamer explicitly point

---

[7]See, for example, the use of values-based practice as a means to understand experience, which emerged to guide a more "humanistic" approach in the context of evidence-based medicine (Fulford et al., 2011).

out aporias within Dilthey's hermeneutics and then enter into discussion with those impasses. Although not comprehensive of the body of their philosophical oeuvre, the concepts of distanciation and prejudice suggest other avenues for understanding, while the philosophical conversation both mirrors and illustrates how the systematic nature of interpretive processes emerges across time.

THE INFINITE DISTANCE

In one of Yerxa's (2009) articles on occupational science entitled, "The infinite distance between the I and the it," she characterized the challenge of moving back and forth between understanding what really matters *to a subject* (i.e., "I") and a focus on diagnosis, disability, or functional status (e.g., "it"). Although both forms of understanding are necessary and intertwined in our clinical reasoning (e.g., Mattingly, 1991, 1998a; Park, 2008), there is an "infinite distance" between the two. Dilthey graded the interpretation of meaning using classes of life expressions that range from larger structures of thoughts or judgments to lived experience; from more elemental and potentially universal to the most complex and particular. Yerxa's infinite distance refers, however, not to the distance between the universal and the particular, but to the distance between the ways in which we come to understand the world (e.g., "I" and the "it").

Dilthey's (historical) need to establish the legitimacy of a *human* science occurred when a positivist turn toward the natural sciences was viewed as a remedy for the "indulgences" of romanticism. Thus, the infinite difference between the "I" and the "it" represents a precedent that, according to Ricoeur (1981, pp. 9, 111), was characterized by Dilthey as one of mutual exclusion between "the *explanation* of nature and the *understanding* of history," where either you "explain" in the manner of the natural scientist or you "interpret" in the manner of the historian. For Ricoeur, however, Dilthey's distinction between the human and natural sciences—between understanding and explanation—was "disastrous" and the central problem of hermeneutics:

> Explanation has been expelled from the field of human sciences; but the conflict reappears at the very heart of the concept of interpretation between, on the one hand, the intuitive and unverifiable character of the psychologising concept of understanding to which interpretation is subordinated, and on the other hand the demand for objectivity which belongs to the very notion of human science. (1981, p. 1)

The challenge to understanding, Ricoeur (1981, p. 106) suggests, is not objectification, explanation, or even the (infinite) distance between explanation and understanding as ways of knowing. Rather, objectification is essential for understanding to take place; it fulfills this role by creating a necessary distance: "by extricating itself from the immediacy of understanding others," a process that he referred to as *distanciation*. Instead of separating us from understanding, the type of distanciation that comes with explanation is necessary for understanding to take place. For example, Olivia's repetition of the phrase "I thought," three times in quick succession, acts as a distancing mechanism. In this context, the phrase "I thought" creates a sense of separation between the events that she experienced and her understanding of those events. Consider how differently you would interpret the phrases "this assignment is due tomorrow" and "*I thought* this assignment is due tomorrow." The first phrase evokes a sense of certainty; it refers directly to something in the world, whereas the second introduces a differentiation between the world and what the speaker *thinks* about the world. Olivia's repeated invocation of this phrase gives her space to reflect upon herself—not as a subject, but in the third-person perspective. Each repetition of "I thought" creates a space for the reflections that follow to emerge, such as: "*I just thought* that the obstacle was myself," "*I thought* that I was helping her," "*I thought,* 'maybe those are just MY values'."

This distancing, reflective stance from oneself is necessary before one can more fully understand another. Here, Ricoeur directly questions Dilthey's proposal that projecting oneself into the text (i.e., any discourse fixed by thing said, as well as written) is central to the hermeneutic process: "To understand is *not* to project oneself into the text but *to expose oneself* to it; it is to receive an enlarged self from the apprehension of proposed worlds which are the genuine object of interpretation" (Ricoeur, 1981, p. 144 [italics added]). In terms of positionality, Ricoeur turns the process that Dilthey had proposed inside out. Instead of projecting oneself into or behind the text, we expose ourselves by standing in front of the text. Thus, instead of moving forward in the interpretive process, the exposure to text "enlarges" self. Here it is helpful to return to our clinical example to note how Olivia's repetition of thought-thought-thought is quickly followed by a new possibility that had not struck her before: "Maybe those are just MY values." She then, for the first time—in conversation with her "self"—muses about Chloe's own motivations, "Maybe she just wants to try it out and-," to which she then responds, "who am I to say, 'You can't do it.'" In quick succession, Olivia moves from the realization that she may be projecting her own values ("Maybe those are just MY values") to wonder about why Chloe acts as she does. She has, in Ricoeurian terms, placed herself in front of Chloe's story in a way in which she cannot determine what will happen next. It is only by doing this, as Ricoeur (1981, p. 106) suggests, that we can enter into the possibilities afforded by "the world of the work" and, in a sense, make it our own.

> Ultimately, what I appropriate is a proposed world. The latter is not *behind* the text, as a hidden intention would be, but *in front of* it, as that which the work unfolds, discovers, reveals. Henceforth to understand is *to understand oneself in front of the text*. It is not a question of imposing upon the text our finite capacity of understanding, but of exposing ourselves to the text and receiving from it an enlarged self, which would be the proposed existence corresponding in the most suitable way to the world proposed.

By retelling this story of her own encounter with Chloe, Olivia—along with the other seven people in the room, and ultimately everyone reading this chapter—becomes the reader of the text as she retells it. In this sense, she is in front of the text, choosing and telling us the details in present tense, rather than giving us a retrospective view of something the meaning of which has already been determined.

Olivia's interpretive moves are circling around the very thing she is trying to make sense of: that is, her regret that her relationship with Chloe ended. She notes "and . . . my only-, my bigger regret was that had I just let her go and do it and just supported her then-, because our relationship, our interactions stopped after that. . . ." In her unpacking her interpretation of why her relationship with Chloe ended as it did, Olivia understands another potential meaning by opening herself up to the possibilities of Chloe's actions—standing in front of the text—rather than her former reading, which was a form of projecting based on her clinical experience. What is key here is how Olivia then discovers a new interpretive possibility in which she questions her own sense of certainty: "who am I to say, 'You can't do it.'" This is an example of the frequently paradoxical nature of the hermeneutic process summed up so eloquently by Ricoeur's (1981, p. 106) observation that "[a]s a reader, I find myself only by losing myself."

KNOWING FROM WHERE I RESPOND[8]

Dilthey contrasted understanding in the natural sciences, which was guided by categories that had been determined *a priori,* with understanding in the human sciences, which emerges from sensory experiences that coalesce into "expressions of life" that range from larger structures of thought and actions to lived experience itself. Ricoeur, however, suggested that the central impasse or philosophical aporia in hermeneutics could be defined by "*ontological* preoccupations, whereby *understanding* ceases to appear as a simple *mode of knowing* in order to become a *way of being* and a way of relating to beings and being" (1981, pp. 4, 14), crediting Heidegger and Gadamer for leading the turn to "dig beneath the epistemological enterprise." This shift in emphasis from ways of knowing to ways of being underscores the historical nature of knowledge and thus its temporal nature. We come to understand based on our past experiences, and project that forward in anticipation of what will come next: what Mattingly (2010) calls the "anticipatory story." This anticipatory story is a way to discern or prejudge a situation so that one might know how to act next, which requires a reflexive way of being rather than just a way of knowing that verges, in Gadamer's description, on being an ethical stance:

> *The hermeneutical task becomes itself a questioning of things* and is always in part so defined. This places hermeneutical work on a firm basis. A person trying to understand something will not resign himself from the start to relying on his own accidental fore-meanings, ignoring as consistently and stubbornly as possible the actual meaning of the text until the latter becomes so persistently audible that it breaks though what the interpreter imagines it to be. Rather, a person trying to understand a text is prepared for it to tell him something. (1975/2004, p. 271)

Olivia does not shift from a procedural way of knowing ("evidence") into a way of being until Chloe "becomes so persistently audible" in her statements: "Why do you keep pointing me in the other direction?" and "You're not doing what I need you to do."

Gadamer (1975/2004, p. 271) points out the futility of trying to extract oneself from one's own historical circumstance, emphasizing a definition of understanding as "this

---

[8]Please see Zafran's (2019) poetic-political reflections on her own historicity (experiences and fore-meanings) by which she unpacks what cultural humility might look like as an everyday hermeneutic practice in occupational therapy.

kind of sensitivity involves neither 'neutrality' with respect to content nor the extinction of one's self, but the *foregrounding and appropriation of one's own fore-meanings and prejudices*" (italics added). Instead of masking or hiding what we may be thinking based on experience, this way of being asks us "to be aware of one's own bias, so that the text can present itself in all its otherness and thus assert its own truth against one's own fore-meanings" (pp. 271–272).

It is Gadamer who best articulated that the "truth" of any encounter cannot stand outside of "historically effected consciousness" (Gadamer, 1975/2004). Thus, Olivia's judgment of what will happen to Chloe cannot be examined outside Olivia's experiences as a clinician, including its terms and languages, such as "evidence" and "client-centered" and even such concepts as "protective," which stand in for such bioethical values as beneficence:

> I gave her the evidence that from, you know, what I've seen . . . this, this, this. And then she said-, I guess the moment of-, when I had to think about it was when she said, "I really want to do this!", and then "I thought I was being client-centered. I thought I was being protective of you," and . . .

Prior to her self-reflection, however, Olivia's experiences help her understand or prejudge the situation. For Gadamer (1975/2004, p. 272) this is *the* philosophical aporia: "The recognition that all understanding inevitably involves some prejudice gives the hermeneutical problem its real thrust."

Understanding as a recognition that one has misunderstood is what Gadamer calls "an event." Events are experienced as significant experiences or moments that stand out in one's memory, which hold phenomenological importance for interpretation of clinical interaction (see Mattingly, 1998a; Mattingly & Lawlor, 2000) as well as in research methods (e.g., Jackson, 2005; Mattingly, 2010). Olivia marks two "moments" (events). The first occurs when Chloe says, "I really want to do this!" and the second occurs when Chloe says, "You're not doing what I need you to do."

This recognition of misunderstanding is experienced as a moment of disruption and creates a distance between what Olivia thought she knew and what she eventually came to understand. This shift in understanding requires an "openness" that constitutes and is constitutive of what Gadamer describes as insight:

> Insight is more than the knowledge of this or that situation. It always involves an escape from something that had deceived us and held us captive. Thus insight always involves an element of self-knowledge and constitutes a necessary side of what we called experience in the proper sense. (1975/2004, p. 350)

KEY IMPLICATIONS FOR OCCUPATIONAL THERAPY EDUCATION, RESEARCH, AND PRACTICE

- Our understanding of occupational engagement has narrowed as we increasingly focus on functional utility rather than understanding occupations as expressions of embodied and enacted meaning; the contexts in which occupational therapists operate, whether we are delivering clinical services, conducting research, or training occupational therapists, frequently emphasize efficiency and adherence to protocols, concerns that can eclipse the therapeutic instinct to fully understand how meaning operates in the lives of the people we work with.

- Occupational therapists must understand those we work with from two perspectives simultaneously: as recipients of our services (clinical or educational) or research participants, and as autonomous participants with their own lived experience, intentionality, and desires.

- Hermeneutics provides both an in-depth analysis of the phenomenon of understanding and a set of methodologies that can be used to interpret meaning. Focusing on the particularities of lived experience, the actions and the contexts within which those actions occur, and the larger structures of thought expressed can help us to develop more nuanced and complete understanding of those we work with and ourselves. Of these three classes of life expressions (lived experience, actions, and larger structures of thought), lived experience is arguably the most effective avenue for understanding others; unfortunately, it is also the most neglected.

- Creating a "distance" through text (e.g., telling a story, journaling) is a means to open oneself to other possibilities[9] and, thus, interpretations.

- We inevitably bring our previous experiences, including professional training and our own personal and cultural history, to each situation we are attempting to interpret, which increases the likelihood of misunderstandings. Recognizing such misrecognitions when they occur, however, can provide a catalyst for transformation and growth.

RECOMMENDED READINGS

Gadamer, H.-G. (2004). Elements of a theory of hermeneutic experience. In H.-G. Gadamer, *Truth and method* (J. Weinsheimer & D. G. Marshall, Trans., 2nd rev. ed.) (pp. 265–307). Continuum. (Original work published 1975)

Mattingly, C. (1998). *Healing dramas and clinical plots: The narrative structure of experience*. Cambridge University Press.

REFERENCES

Anthony, W. A. (1993). Recovery from mental illness: The guiding vision of the mental health service system in the 1990s. *Psychosocial Rehabilitation Journal, 16*(4), 11–23.

Bruner, J. (1990). *Acts of meaning*. Harvard University Press.

Bruner, J. (2002). *Making stories: Law, literature, life*. Farrar, Straus and Giroux.

Chodos, H., d'Auteuil, S., Martin, N., & Raymond, G. (2015). *Guidelines for recovery-oriented practice: Hope. Dignity. Inclusion.* https://www.mentalhealthcommission.ca/sites/default/files/2016-07/MHCC_Recovery_Guidelines_2016_ENG.PDF

---

[9]For a definitive explanation of how Ricoeur's philosophical work illuminates the narrative practices in occupational therapy, including how the possibilities created through storytelling guide treatment (e.g., see therapeutic employment), please see Mattingly (1998a).

Davidson, L., & Roe, D. (2007). Recovery from versus recovery in serious mental illness: One strategy for lessening confusion plaguing recovery. *Journal of Mental Health, 16*(4), 459–470. https://doi.org/10.1080/09638230701482394

Dewey, J. (1934). Art as experience. In S. D. Ross (Ed.), *Art and its significance: An anthology of aesthetic theory* (3rd ed., pp. 204–220). State University of New York Press.

Dilthey, W. (1977). *Descriptive psychology and historical understanding* (R. M. Zaner & K. L. Heiges, Trans.). Martinus Nijhoff. (Original work published 1927)

Dilthey, W. (1996). The rise of hermeneutics. In R. A. Makkreel & F. Rodi (Eds.), *Hermeneutics and the study of history: Selected works* (Vol. IV, pp. 235–253). Princeton University Press. (Original work published 1900)

Fulford, K. W. M., Caroll, H., & Peile, E. (2011). Values-based practice: Linking science with people. *Journal of Contemporary Psychotherapy, 41*(3), 145–156. https://doi.org/10.1007/s10879-011-9179-z

Gadamer, H.-G. (1975/2004). *Truth and method* (J. Weinsheimer & D. G. Marshall, Trans., 2nd rev. ed.). Continuum.

Gray, J. M. (1998). Putting occupation into practice: Occupation as ends, occupation as means. *American Journal of Occupational Therapy, 52*(5), 354–364.

Hooper, B. (2006). Epistemological transformation in occupational therapy: Educational implications and challenges. *OTJR: Occupation, Participation, and Health, 26*(1), 15–24. https://doi.org/10.1177/153944920602600103

Jackson, M. (2005). *Existential anthropology: Events, exigencies and effects.* Berghahn Books.

Kinsella, E. A., & Whiteford, G. E. (2008). Knowledge generation and utilisation in occupational therapy: Towards epistemic reflexivity. *Australian Occupational Therapy Journal,* 1–10. https://doi.org/10.1111/j.1440-1630.2007.00726.x

Lawlor, M. C. (2003). The significance of being occupied: The social construction of childhood occupations. *American Journal of Occupational Therapy, 57*(4), 424–435. https://doi.org/10.5014/ajot.57.4.424

Leamy, M., Bird, V. J., Le Boutillier, C., Davidson, L., Williams, J., & Slade, M. (2011). Conceptual framework for personal recovery in mental health: Systematic review and narrative synthesis. *British Journal of Psychiatry, 199,* 445–452. https://doi.org/10.1192/bjp.bp.110.083733

Mattingly, C. (1991). What is clinical reasoning? *American Journal of Occupational Therapy, 45*(11), 979–986. https://doi.org/10.5014/ajot.45.11.979

Mattingly, C. (1998a). *Healing dramas and clinical plots: The narrative structure of experience.* Cambridge University.

Mattingly, C. (1998b). In search of the good: Narrative reasoning in clinical practice. *Medical Anthropology Quarterly, 12*(3), 273–297.

Mattingly, C. (2010). *The paradox of hope: Journeys through a clinical borderland.* University of California Press.

Mattingly, C., & Lawlor, M. (2000). Learning from stories: Narrative interviewing in cross-cultural research. *Scandinavian Journal of Occupational Therapy, 7*(1), 4–14. https://doi.org/10.1080/110381200443571

Mattingly, C., & Lawlor, M. (2001). The fragility of healing. *Ethos, 29,* 30–57. https://doi.org/10.1525/eth.2001.29.1.30

McKee, R. (1997). *Story: Style, structure, substance, and the principles of screenwriting.* Harper Collins.

Mental Health Commission of Canada. (2012). *Changing directions, changing lives: The mental health strategy for Canada.* Author.

Meyer, A. (1922). The philosophy of occupational therapy. *Occupational Therapy and Rehabilitation, 1*(1), 1–10.

Park, M. (2008). Making scenes: Imaginative practices for a child with autism in an occupational therapy session. *Medical Anthropology Quarterly, 22*(3), 234–256. https://doi.org/10.1111/j.1548-1387.2008.00024.x

Park, M. (2012). Pleasure, throwing breaches, and embodied metaphors: Tracing transformations-in-participation for a child with autism to a sensory integration-based therapy session. *OTJR: Occupation, Participation and Health, 32*(1 Suppl.), S34–S47. https://doi.org/10.3928/15394492-20110906-05

Reilly, M. (1962). Occupational therapy can be one of the great ideas of 20th century medicine. *American Journal of Occupational Therapy, 16*(1), 1–9.

Ricoeur, P. (1981). *Hermeneutics and the human sciences* (J. B. Thompson, Ed.). Cambridge University Press.

Schwartz, R. (2011). Return to the cave: Exploring barriers to organizational learning in a mental health clinic. *Reflective Practice: International and Multidisciplinary Perspectives, 12*(1), 101–113. https://doi.org/10.1080/14623943.2011.541099

Schwartz, R., Estein, O., Komaroff, J., Lamb, J., Myers, M., Stewart, J., . . . Park, M. (2013). Mental health consumers and providers dialogue in an institutional setting: A participatory approach to promoting recovery-oriented care. *Psychiatric Rehabilitation Journal, 36*(2), 113–115. https://doi.org/10.1037/h0094980

Yerxa, E. J. (1967). 1966 Eleanor Clarke Slagle lecture. Authentic occupational therapy. *American Journal of Occupational Therapy, 21*(1), 1–9.

Yerxa, E. J. (2009). Infinite distance between the *I* and the *It*. *American Journal of Occupational Therapy, 63*, 490–497. https://doi.org/10.5014/ajot.63.4.490

Yerxa, E. J., Clark, F., Frank, G., Jackson, J., Parham, D., Pierce, D., . . . Zemke, R. (1989). An introduction to occupational science, a foundation for occupational therapy in the 21st century. *Occupational Science: The Foundation for New Models of Practice, 6*(4), 1–18. https://doi.org/10.1080/J003v06n04_04.

Zafran, H. (2019). Knowing from where I respond. *Occupational Therapy Now, 21*(4), 18–19.

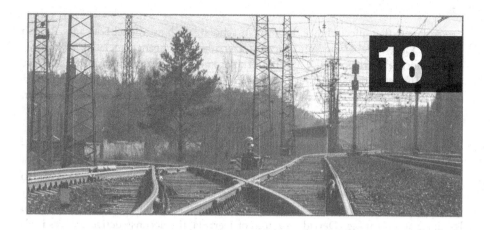

Deconstruction and the Institution of Occupation

Ganesh M. Babulal, PhD, OTD, MSCI, MOT, OTR/L
Anil H. Chandiramani
Steven D. Taff, PhD, OTR/L, FNAP, FAOTA

INTRODUCTION

To define *deconstruction*, one must understand the relationship between its genesis and the historical context that engendered its space. Structuralism dominated French philosophical discussion in the 1950s and 1960s, and deeply permeated the studies of literary theory, linguistics, sociology, psychology, and anthropology, among other fields (Culler, 2008). However, toward the latter end of the 1960s, there was a radical departure from and rejection of structuralism, specifically of its core beliefs. This movement, labeled post-structuralism, critiqued the unidirectional, fixed relationship of the signifier and signified, and a notion of absolute/universal truths (Sarup, 1993). Whereas structuralism views language as shaping world (perception and interaction) and de-emphasizing the subject's autonomy, post-structuralists assert that culture and history ultimately influence how knowledge is produced; they identify the various and intersecting

Taff, S. D. (Ed.). *Philosophy and Occupational Therapy:*
Informing Education, Research, and Practice (pp. 181-188).
© 2021 Taylor & Francis Group.

determinants that affect choice. Prominent scholars such as Michel Foucault, Roland Barthes, Jürgen Habermas, and Jacques Derrida have been associated with post-structuralism (Harrison, 2006). It is important to note that many of these scholars have rejected the label disassociating the movement into pre- and post-epochs. Further, post-structuralism as a movement is not widely recognized in Europe but rather an arbitrary label assigned by American academics (Wood & Bernasconi, 1988).

A key philosopher in this "post-structuralist" movement was Jacques Derrida, whose 1966 lecture at a colloquium at Johns Hopkins, which was intended to clarify and strengthen structuralism, instead expounded on the theoretical limitations of structuralism, including the rigidity of structure and limits of logocentrism or desire to have a center/anchor (Macksey & Donato, 2007). In 1967, Derrida's *Of Grammatology* outlined a method for reading a text and examining the complex relationship between language and meaning (Derrida, 1976). For Derrida, the deconstructive process is always present and occurs during the reading of a text. The progression of deconstruction considers the text as deconstructing itself, rather than the reader or critic doing so—however, as the reader writes, the process of writing (analysis) is also deconstruction (Caputo, 1997a). As a result, there is no single, universal, or correct deconstruction of any text, but rather endless possibilities and interpretations.

DEFINING DECONSTRUCTION AS A NONTRADITIONAL PHILOSOPHY AND ITS MAJOR CONCEPTS

There has been much debate and controversy surrounding the differences between post-structuralism and deconstruction given the proximal emergence of both from the prevailing structuralist milieu. Some theorists lump them together, while others choose to distinguish them based on their foci and connection to structuralism (Honderich, 2005). As a concept, deconstruction is notoriously difficult to define, and many attempts have resulted in diluting the approach from the original texts. Derrida himself took care to delineate deconstruction as not being a method, critique, or analysis in the context of larger philosophy, but the term was contextually chosen in the dominant discourse of structuralism as an "anti-structuralist gesture" (Wood & Bernasconi, 1988). A deconstructive reading interrogates tradition/assumptions and seeks to subvert the text by examining things that contradict the intended meaning and structure (Balkin, 1996).

Deconstruction has commonalities with Heidegger's concept of *Destruktion* (Heidegger, 1962), which was a way of reading or reinterpreting metaphysics in order to reveal the fundamental experiences of the nature of being (Heidegger, 1962). However, *deconstruction* as coined and used by Derrida is an infinite process without a measurable goal that rejects the fixed nature of a text across space and time. In addition to Heidegger, Derrida drew from Nietzsche's and de Saussure's work as motivation but also as context to further develop deconstruction.

To understand major facets of deconstruction, it is important to examine several terminologies that subtend the process. De Saussure contended that language is devoid of substance but has forms that are defined by differences that are external characteristics that compose their internal form and identity (de Saussure, 2011). In semiotics, each element has an identity that is produced by a network of differences that continue to differentiate *ad infinitum*. Binary opposites are a simple example of this form (e.g., light vs. dark, short vs. tall, strong vs. weak, ugly vs. beautiful, life vs. death) and are prominent in discussions of semiotics.

Derrida expanded de Saussure's premise and proposed that a primordial process termed *différance* includes not only language but also ideas/objects (presence) and reality. When meaning or truth is examined, it is not static but differs from itself and is constantly changing or is differed. He argued that *différance* questions time and space. In trying to grasp time, when we think of anything in the present, we cannot grasp it because the present becomes the past and moves away into nothingness (Derrida, 1976). This is the same with the future, because the present comes with future present moments which it is moving toward. Therefore, the differences between these two present(s) become the singular present we perceive. This argument also holds for space, where any object or even thought has an identity by its difference in relation to something else. Related to *différance* is *trace*, or a shadow presence. *Trace* is a shadow surrounding ideas/objects but is not bound by time or space. All ideas and perceptions or objects have the absence of a presence when *différance* operates. This is especially illustrated in the case of binary opposites. The constructs of *différance* and *trace* function simultaneously such that ideas or objects (presence) have no real identities much like signs, just differences. This presence has a trace of other presence(s) joined by a network of relationships that gives the illusion of separation. *Différance* and *trace* suggest that while existence is axiomatic, it is connected through relationships where not a single part is pure or can be identified outside of the others. In effect, the tendency for metaphysics to be concerned with logocentrism via language forces privilege and an arbitrary structure, despite the numerous contradictions that are present in the ambiguity of language.

THE INTENDED OUTCOME OF DECONSTRUCTION

As was previously discussed, Derrida was purposeful in not delimiting the deconstructive process. At its core, this iterative process does not intend to provide answers or ascertain an objective or unifiable truth but rather insists upon examining differences and relationships between presence (ideas/objects; Derrida, 1991). This may seem counter, or even diametrically opposed, to what other philosophies offer. Although deconstruction centered on grammatology and a reading of texts, this process was meant for so much more. Perhaps the most apt quote from Derrida articulating the utility of deconstruction is this:

> The idea behind deconstruction is to deconstruct the workings of strong nation-states with powerful immigration policies, to deconstruct the rhetoric of nationalism, the politics of place, the metaphysics of native land and native tongue . . . The idea is to disarm the bombs . . . of identity that nation-states build to defend themselves against the stranger . . . (Caputo, 1997a, p. 231)

Deconstruction questions the search for identity, the desire to differentiate, and the need to belong to something wholly unique. Whether it is purposeful or subconscious, doing so destabilizes binary relationships and hierarchies of power, but it relegates one to the periphery as undesired and codifies the other as privileged or centered. This is present in modern society across numerous binaries: speech over writing, happiness over sadness, life over death, meaning over meaninglessness, fullness over hunger, or movement/action over inertness/inaction. To deconstruct in the literal sense is to attend to and observe what is included in thinking but also, more importantly, what is excluded (e.g., alterity).

HOW TO DECONSTRUCT?

Derrida considered the Western philosophical tradition (and therefore much of scientific and social thought) problematic due to its unquestioned acceptance of the existence of centers, truth, or ideals (Caputo, 1997b; Derrida, 1976). These fixed concepts contribute to the development of exclusion, ideologies, and oppressive circumstances, and therefore should be questioned and balanced by other perspectives. Deconstruction provides a lens by which to examine assumed truths that facilitate privilege and power differentials in society. The specific elements of deconstruction are: (1) identifying privileged concepts and their marginalized binary opposites; (2) interrogating and destabilizing these binaries; and (3) resituating, or redefining, the concepts in a horizontal and polysemic manner.

At the core of this process, any given concept/text is defined by its reciprocal or binary opposite (e.g., false/true, bad/good, love/hate; Derrida, 1976). Defined largely in contrast with their oppositions, lexical meanings of words and concepts are therefore not fixed. Acknowledging this sets the stage for new interpretations and, consequently, practices. Identifying privilege or hierarchies in any narrative or text essentially involves critical analysis of sources of truth and power contained within terms or concepts. This process requires consideration of the privileging factors for any concept/text and identifying the marginalized, suppressed, or possible reciprocals/binary opposites of the privileged concept (Balkin, 1996).

The second stage of the deconstruction process involves reversing oppressed, marginalized, or alternative concepts, momentarily giving these binary opposites central or preferred status instead of the original privileged terms. This process is intended as a temporary replacement of the privileged concept, which allows the reciprocal concept to gain voice and presence. It is crucial to note that Derrida intended this reversal to be an unmasking that only brings to light the opposite or potential horizons of privileged terms, not a permanent switch in a hierarchy (Derrida, 1976).

Finally, re-situation is a state in which privileged centers and their marginalized binaries interact in a nonhierarchical yet unstable relationship. This instability should not, however, be misconstrued as rationale for complete abandonment of the essence or trace of the original concept. Re-situation places texts or concepts into new contexts where new meanings emerge, which are related to, but different from, previous understandings. Indeed, invention of new terms, concepts, or languages is a fundamentally valid accomplishment in any act of deconstruction.

Impact on Understanding of Occupation and Occupational Engagement

For this exercise, we intend to deconstruct the concept of *occupation*, which is both the lexical center of the profession's name and also the core function of the practice. Occupation has held a privileged status within occupational therapy, but can be subverted to produce a new interpretation that better fulfills the needs of a 21st-century global society. The contemporary concept of occupation originated in the United States Progressive Era of the early 1900s and contains a Western (specifically American) bias that values achievement, efficiency, progress, activity, and independence (McGerr, 2010). The combination of these values alongside an increasing predominance of the medical model has afforded occupation a status that is privileged and seldom questioned. However, the core function of the occupational therapy profession and its assumed benefits are subject to scrutiny when examined in a non-Western or nonmedical model perspective.

We propose that occupational therapy is a sociocultural-medical construct. As a result, we are forced to explore proxies for occupation instead of opposites, which results in modified binaries capable of generating new meanings. The term *occupation* is logically linked to the idea of doing, or being. The term used in English contrasts starkly with the choice made in French and German (*ergo-therapy*), which contains the notion of rehabilitation through activity. There is no term that can be held as a strong binary opposite to *occupation*; however, *activity* or, more specifically, *action* is often used as a proxy. Occupational therapy claims to focus on "beings and doings," but this center of *doing* is hegemonic and is reinforced by how occupational therapy is practiced and reimbursed within the American medical system. This has contributed to limited scholarly examination of the purpose driving the "doing." The opposite of doing is a state of being inert or motionless, a marginalized binary of occupation. Inaction or being sedentary is well-accepted as a negative outcome or consequence because it has direct impact on health, well-being, and perceived quality of life. We assert, however, that this myopic focus on doing/moving/producing can similarly result in compromised health outcomes, increased stress, and decreased quality of life. While productivity and doing are privileged binaries that relate to *occupation*, there are numerous moderating and mediating variables that affect the directional relationship. Though such is implied, "being and doing" does not equate with positive binaries such as happiness, peace, or a healthy life. This fact is evident in annual surveys on quality of life and happiness indices across different nations. The United States consistently ranks in the middle or lower percentiles despite being one of the richest and most productive nations (Helliwell et al., 2019; New Economics Foundation, 2019; *U.S. News & World Report*, 2019). Narrow focus on doing has consequences that are rarely examined, especially when the social fabric of a society is inextricable from work that valorizes productivity. By examining doing as a proxy binary for occupation, deconstruction highlights the trace around doing and inaction and suggests calling attention to being "a-occupation" to fully appreciate the subjective dimension and meaning of *occupation*.

The concept of occupation and positive attributes (being, doing) relationally ascribed by *différance* are partial when asked, "to what end?" Divorced from its roots, the notion of meaning has been firmly fixed as the wellspring that drives "to be" and "to do." This is well established as "occupation" and has become architectonically linked to activities of daily living (ADLs), which, when completed, establish and/or reinforce a sense of meaning. Yet ADLs are determined by experts from biomedical and reimbursement systems (privilege) and assessed through a set of scales that have been standardized. The essential element of creating sets of activities over time that demand engagement and are infused with meaning has been lost in the process. It remains challenging to untangle occupations and activities. Some have suggested that both concepts entail subjectivity in their determination: occupation remains focused on the individual; activities are more culturally defined (Pierce, 2001). One can further argue that occupation is an experience, while activity is an idea; the former remains more sensitive to evolving over time, while the latter is more related to context. Through deconstruction, attempts at differentiation create internal conflict that contradicts, because the identity of these constructs is defined by the absence of others. Although it is clear that the differences between occupation and activity have not been sufficiently addressed in research, understanding the relationship and *trace* between these constructs constitutes a foundational step toward clarifying them in the realm of practice. The deconstruction process suggests redefining these concepts in the absence of privilege and hierarchy, but doing so in an unstable manner to signify the lack of a single truth.

Occupational therapy practice needs to strike a balance between the medical model, which focuses on curing bodily problems, and a sociocultural approach toward addressing individual and collective well-being that it has embraced since its inception. Related concepts such as choice, control, and meaning have not held the center stage for which they were originally intended (Taff et al., 2014). Consequently, the aim of practice remains to restore functional ability as determined by experts working within an inequitable medical insurance system. As a result, occupational therapy has often narrowed its scope to fit medical and scientific paradigms. Recent research in the United States has focused on functional perspectives, albeit with some consideration to quality of life determined according to standardized scales.

In a more wide-ranging view of occupational therapy, we submit that a person's life history, meaning, and engagement are more proximal outcomes that have the potential to redefine the value of occupations. Quantitative, unidimensional outcomes, such as a score on a functioning scale or gaining an extra 10 degrees of range of motion in a joint, radically mute the premise of the profession and potentially propel it toward irrelevance. Instead, the original promise of the profession should be celebrated with fierce attention to persons' lived experiences, subjective meanings they hold to be truths, and new ways of engagement they seek in life.

The importance of such attention is elevated when examined under the macroscope of social forces. Real social forces such as war, racism, discrimination, classism, poverty, abuse, and inadequate access to education, health care, and food are real to a majority of the clients we serve, and the many more not seen by the profession and medicine in general. While these factors may not always be salient, they exist and rest just beneath the surface, affecting daily life and often to the detriment of well-being. Such social forces that innervate reality have been systematically ignored or forgotten, especially in the context of practice in the medical model. Ironically, similar forces engendered the profession a century ago, and as we now face even more complex and dangerous global challenges, it is critical that we remember our history. These same factors also influenced Derrida to critically examine the structure not only of words but also of institutions, objects, and ideas. Our profession can use deconstruction as a powerful tool to literally expose, displace, and redefine these social forces, while continuing to shape the profession's identity for the next century and beyond.

KEY IMPLICATIONS FOR OCCUPATIONAL THERAPY EDUCATION, RESEARCH, AND PRACTICE

Education

- Focus on the dynamic nature of knowledge in curriculum and instructional design.
- Include curricular content that focuses on health care lexicon literacy, where students understand how language (which words are used and how) can affect clinical care, client outcomes, and satisfaction, and the therapist's skill in advocacy.
- Construct learning experiences to intentionally move students toward the stage of contextual knowing, where truths are multiple and individually interpreted.

Research

- In occupational science, continue to expose possible hegemony in the concepts and practices surrounding occupation and occupational engagement.
- Expand use of research designs and methods that highlight subjective aspects of people's everyday experiences.
- Consider underpinning research agendas with a scientific paradigm where multiple realities are accepted as a function of *différance*.

Practice

- Develop and use more ecologically valid clinical assessment tools that focus on client narratives and constructs such as well-being and quality of life.
- Pay more attention to terms and language used in clinical practice and associated professional lexicons such as the *Occupational Therapy Practice Framework* (American Occupational Therapy Association, 2014).
- Provide continuing education for clinicians that hones skills in genuinely client-centered care and being critically reflective practitioners.

RECOMMENDED READINGS

Culler, J. (2008). *On deconstruction: Theory and criticism after structuralism*. Routledge.

Derrida J. (1976). *Of grammatology* (G. C. Spivak, Trans.). Johns Hopkins University Press.

Wood, D., & Bernasconi, R. (1988). *Derrida and différance*. Northwestern University Press.

REFERENCES

American Occupational Therapy Association (AOTA). (2014). Occupational therapy practice framework: Domain and process (3rd ed.). *American Journal of Occupational Therapy, 68*(Suppl. 1), 1–48. https://doi.org/10.5014/ajot.2014.682006

Balkin, J. M. (1996). Deconstruction. In D. M. Patterson (Ed.), *A companion to philosophy of law and legal theory* (pp. 367–374). Blackwell Publishers.

Caputo, J. D. (1997a). *The prayers and tears of Jacques Derrida: Religion without religion.* Indiana University Press.

Caputo, J. D. (1997b). *Deconstruction in a nutshell: A conversation with Jacques Derrida.* Fordham University Press.

Culler, J. (2008). *On deconstruction: Theory and criticism after structuralism.* Routledge.

Derrida, J. (1976). *Of grammatology* (G. C. Spivak, Trans.). Johns Hopkins University Press.

Derrida J. (1991). Letter to a Japanese friend. In P. Kamuf (Ed.), *A Derrida reader* (pp. 270–276). Harvester.

de Saussure, F. (2011). *Course in general linguistics.* Columbia University Press.

Harrison, P. (2006). Post-structuralist theories. In S. Aitken & G. Valentine (Eds.), *Approaches to Human Geography* (pp. 122–135). SAGE Publications.

Heidegger, M. (1962). *Being and time* (J. Macquarrie & E. Robinson, Trans.). Harper.

Helliwell, J., Layard, R., & Sachs, J. (2019). *World happiness report 2019.* Sustainable Development Solutions Network.

Honderich, T. (2005). *The Oxford companion to philosophy.* Oxford University Press.

Macksey, R. A., & Donato, E. (2007). *The structuralist controversy: The languages of criticism and the sciences of man.* Johns Hopkins University Press.

McGerr, M. (2010). *A fierce discontent: The rise and fall of the progressive movement in America.* Free Press.

New Economics Foundation. (2019). *Happy planet index: United States of America.* http://happyplanetindex.org/countries/united-states-of-america

Pierce, D. (2001). Untangling occupation and activity. *American Journal of Occupational Therapy, 55*(2), 138–146. https://doi.org/10.5014/ajot.55.2.138

Sarup, M. (1993). *An introductory guide to post-structuralism and postmodernism.* Pearson Education.

Taff, S. D., Bakhshi, P., & Babulal, G. M. (2014). The accountability–well-being–ethics framework: A new philosophical foundation for occupational therapy. *Canadian Journal of Occupational Therapy, 81*(5), 320–329. https://doi.org/10.1177/0008417414546742

U.S. News & World Report. (2019). *Quality of life ranking.* https://www.usnews.com/news/best-countries/quality-of-life-rankings

Wood, D., & Bernasconi, R. (1988). *Derrida and différance.* Northwestern University Press.

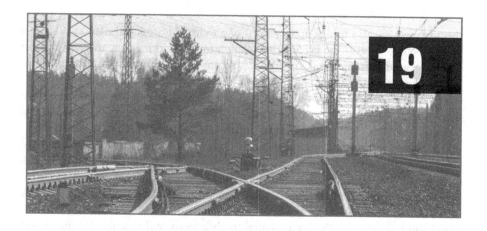

Philosophical Influences on Occupational Therapy in Brazil
A Historical Timeline

Daniel Marinho Cezar da Cruz, PhD, MSc, OT
Daniela da Silva Rodrigues, MSc, OT
Helen Carey, PhD, MSc Adv OT, Dip COT, OTR/L

INTRODUCTION

Creek and Feaver believed that professional philosophy is the system of beliefs and values unique to each profession, which gives its members a sense of identity and exercises control over theory and practice (Creek & Feaver, 1993). Beliefs can determine values, so occupational therapists must first identify unique beliefs regarding the profession of occupational therapy (Mayers, 1990). For Hagedorn (1999), philosophy is a set of beliefs and ideas, the adoption of a particular "world view" accepted by the profession as the basis for academic and professional practice. The principles, values, and practice of the profession must be in accordance with its philosophy. Occupational therapists raise questions and discuss what kind of knowledge occupational therapy uses and uncovers, what science is, and what the limits of each knowledge area are. Hence, they begin an epistemological discussion, which, in questioning the scope, values, and limits of occupational

Taff, S. D. (Ed.). *Philosophy and Occupational Therapy:*
Informing Education, Research, and Practice (pp. 189-199).
© 2021 Taylor & Francis Group.

therapy theories, also brings up questions of a more philosophical nature: What is a human being? What is the profession's relation to the world? What are the values of the profession's existence and knowledge? In "any epistemological discussion rests a philosophical and anthropological decision" (Medeiros, 2003, p. 28).

Historical analysis is important to understand the current state of occupational therapy in a given country. Medeiros (2003) argues that the practice of occupational therapy is "marked by different intervention models and techniques, modified throughout its history as a result of different conceptions of man, health, disease and activity, concomitantly assumed by the sciences that supported it" (Medeiros, 2003, pp. 28–29).

Mayers (1990) summarizes occupational therapy's philosophy as follows: (1) client participation in decision making; (2) the potential to motivate oneself and improve health status; (3) the ability to adapt; (4) look at individual customer needs; (5) meaningful and purposeful activities as central to philosophy and practice; (6) the person is considered as a whole; and (7) recognize the value of roles to the person. More recently, Carey (2017) has categorized contemporary occupational therapy philosophy as comprising: (1) client-centered delivery where the client is the controlling partner, (2) occupational engagement that is fundamental to health and well-being, (3) individualized context, and (4) delivery of therapeutic use of self by the occupational therapist.

The difference between Mayers (1990) and Carey (2017) illuminates how the core philosophy of occupational therapy has remained largely unchanged other than in language and emphasis. Unfortunately, another element that has remained unchanged is the issue of professional identity among occupational therapists internationally (Turner & Knight, 2015). If we have an unchanged belief in our philosophy, then why do we continue to raise and debate identity issues? These issues could be within ourselves as occupational therapists or in how other professions identify us. For many occupational therapists, an occupation-centered paradigm reflects the worldview of the profession, which encompasses philosophy, theories, frameworks, and models for practice (Creek & Feaver, 1993). It could therefore be considered that although we retain the same philosophies, our methods of delivery of those philosophies differ internationally—and perhaps this is not a negative element but rather the ability of our profession to mold to each region's demographic. Kielhofner (2009) suggested three major paradigms in the history of American occupational therapy: the paradigm of occupation (1917–1940s), the mechanistic paradigm (1950s–1970s), and the contemporary paradigm (return to occupation; 1980s–present). However, for this chapter we have chosen to describe select philosophical aspects of Brazilian occupational therapy through some chronological frameworks, rather than classifying them by specific paradigms, because they seem to coexist in Brazil.

HISTORICAL–POLITICAL ROOTS OF OCCUPATION IN BRAZIL AND INITIAL OCCUPATIONAL THERAPY TRAINING

Occupational therapy is a century-old profession in both the United States and the United Kingdom. Its expansion around the world has enabled the production of distinct knowledge and practices influenced by philosophies and the sociohistorical context of each country, as is the case with Brazil. In this country, the profession is commemorating the 50th anniversary of its regulation as a degree in higher education (Oliver et al., 2018). The construction of Brazilian occupational therapy was not based on the sociopolitical contexts of the two great world wars, as occurred in the European and North American countries. In our country, the first indications of occupational therapy began with the treatment of people in psychological distress (i.e., in the field of mental health). With the arrival of the Portuguese royal family to Brazil, the country became a Portuguese colony. As a result, prevailing European ideas of the 19th century regarding psychiatric care profoundly influenced treatment in the country. In 1822, after Brazil's independence, humanitarian approaches gained strength as people with mental illness were liberated from the dungeons and prisons, and hospices and workshops were constructed for distraction and healing (Medeiros, 2003).

At the beginning of the 20th century, the idea of using work to benefit those with mental illness gained strength, and in the 1940s the Occupational Therapy Service of the *Engenho de Dentro* was created. Psychiatrist Nise da Silveira directed the program and taught the first technical courses on occupational therapy beginning in 1948 (Cruz, 2019; Medeiros, 2003; Soares, 1991). She defended the use of activities such as painting and recreation in the psychiatric hospital as a form of expression, and with this practice she showed the improvement of her patients with hands-on experience. As theoretical reference, Nise da Silveira was influenced by the work of Carl Jung (Cruz, 2019; Medeiros, 2003). Polio epidemics and the idea of moral treatment of mental illness are some of the other important milestones in the history of occupational therapy in Latin American countries (Reis & Lopes, 2018). In Brazil, the profession officially emerged in 1956 with the creation of the first training program in Rio de Janeiro, whose characteristics reflected the mechanistic paradigm of rehabilitation. Consequently, the profession began to be practiced in the 1950s, especially within the context of physical rehabilitation, with the aim of restoring the motor and biomechanical functions of individuals with disabilities (Soares, 1991).

From these historical accounts of occupational therapy's origins in Latin America, two major accounts of occupation emerge (Monzeli et al., 2019):

1. As a technology for physical rehabilitation purposes as a response to epidemics in the region
2. As a technical and scientific justification of work that was already taking place in psychiatric hospitals, to give professional form to techniques whose use had already been articulated, to a greater or lesser extent, in the assumptions of moral treatment.

BRAZILIAN OCCUPATIONAL THERAPY DEVELOPMENT AND SOCIAL MOVEMENTS: FROM OCCUPATION TO PRAXIS, HUMAN ACTIVITY, AND CRITICAL OCCUPATIONAL THERAPY

The perspectives, references, models, and approaches used express modes of understanding and action of occupational therapy in line with its time, which may or may not have continuity with the profession's historical course (Galheigo et al., 2018). As discussed earlier in this chapter, across countries we identify the philosophy of the profession in a similar way, but it is recognized that the transfer of theory to practice varies according to political, historical, economic, cultural, and interpretational differences in each country (Carey et al., 2019). The two methods of intervention translated specifically from occupational therapy in Brazil as focused upon mental health are discussed in this section.

The first intervention method, occupational psychotherapy, was founded in the 1970s by Professor Rui Chamone Jorge, in Belo Horizonte—Minas Gerais. This approach, based on the use of expressive activities, sought a new form of care for clients undergoing mental health treatment and prioritized the importance of connection, qualified listening, and humanized care, thereby highlighting occupational therapy's potential as a resource in this process (Mata, 2019). The second intervention method, developed in the early 1980s, is associated with the North American psychodynamic works of Fidlers and Azima, and Canadian theories by Witkower, as well as European psychodynamic works by Legros and Pibarot (French) and Gibertoni and Piergrossi (Anglo-Italian), and enabled discussion on the therapeutic use of activities. Proposed by Maria José Benneton as the theory of associative trails, this approach focused on the relationship between the triad of therapist-patient-activity, and was applied as a procedure of occupational therapy (Benetton, 2006; Nascimento, 1990).

In the 1970s, the field of Brazilian occupational therapy largely departed from Anglo-Saxon works regarding rehabilitation. With this departure, and the impact of both the psychodynamic approach and sociohistorical context, a field of knowledge emerged, adopting the term *activities* and other similar concepts such as action. This changing language further constructed the delivery of occupational therapy (Marcolino et al., 2019). One of the most important historical milestones of this period was the central role that the university began to play in the production of knowledge and practices of occupational therapy in Brazil (Galheigo et al., 2018). At this time, new critical issues confronted the hegemonic biomedical and scientific model, and subsequently the practices of institutions subscribing to these models. Hence, in 1979 the term *occupational therapy* emerged in the social field, proposed by Jussara de Mesquita Pinto, who first applied an intervention to improve the living conditions of young people at the State Foundation for the Welfare of Children (*Fundação Estadual do Bem-Estar do Menor*—FEBEM; Galheigo, 2016).

Later, due to the historical and social insertion of the profession into the health policies of the country, the profession drew influence from a Marxist perspective (Soares, 1991). The epistemological debate regarding Brazilian occupational therapy emerged from the different theories of occupational therapy in Brazil and the conflict generated by the coexistence of different models in professional practice (Medeiros, 2003). As a result, Brazilian occupational therapists set out to think about the profession from the perspectives of philosophy, education, sociology, and anthropology, aiming at the emancipation, participation, and social inclusion of their clients (Cruz, 2018). Still, some historical milestones have provided new interdisciplinary opportunities and practices for Brazilian occupational therapy, such as the creation of the Unified Health System, which is free to the population and based on Marxist theoretical foundations and trends (Gomez et al., 2018). This resulted in Brazilian occupational therapy developing akin to the United Kingdom with its National Health System. The government-funded systems that became accessible to all resulted in the expansion of occupational therapy to address a wide range of occupational barriers, while also managing an increased demand for services. Both Brazil and the United Kingdom have developed priority management systems that serve the government health system as a whole—with safe and effective discharge from inpatient services becoming a priority in order to enable throughput in a highly pressurized service (Wales, 2012).

Other milestones were psychiatric reform and the debate on the deinstitutionalization of Basaglian inspiration (Galheigo et al., 2018), and the appreciation of a profession-specific model of practice: the Gary Kielhofner Model of Human Occupation. Despite the translation of the first four articles of this model in Brazil, it was criticized by occupational therapists, who interpreted some aspects of the model as being closer to a reproduction of reductionism, for example, based on behavioral psychology in general systems theory (Ferrari, 1991; Mângia, 1998; Soares, 1991).

Additional landmarks have also become foundational to the practice of Brazilian occupational therapy. These include sociological, anthropological, and philosophical ideas from author Robert Castel, a French philosopher and sociologist whose relevant works include the exclusion issue and the concept of disaffiliation. His work explored the impact on individuals when social network support is fragile, leading to isolation, economic losses, and deprivation. Other influential ideas came from Adolfo Vázquez, a political philosopher whose works were influenced by Karl Marx. He pointed to the concept of praxis as a political and historical action of transformation and change in society. Other authors, such as Agnes Heller, Paulo Freire, Émile Durkheim, Michel Foucault, Karl Marx, and Franco Basaglia, reflected a movement of resistance among occupational therapists toward a critical occupational therapy foundation that responds to the social demands of its clients, in a movement of transformation for themselves and society (Barros et al., 2007). These milestones were manifested in actions such as the labor insertion of people in psychological distress, community-based rehabilitation, and a social model of occupational therapy that attended to populations previously neglected by the profession, such as street children, people struggling for housing, the LGBTQ population, and socially vulnerable women and children, among others.

Again, some elements of these developments are similar to the development of the social care system in the United Kingdom. Occupational therapists in the United Kingdom have strong intervention delivery services to address occupational barriers directly related to housing, social vulnerability, and inclusion (Wilberforce et al., 2016). Occupational therapy in both Brazil and the United Kingdom has placed, and continues to place, importance on addressing social disadvantage as a major occupational barrier.

Research as a Central Element in the Production of Occupational Therapy Knowledge in Brazil (2000–Present): Human Activity, Occupation, and Social Participation

More than 60 years after the establishment of the first occupational therapy technical course in Brazil, it is still important to explore the paths taken by the profession so as to grasp the structure and development of the field; to decipher connections that the past establishes with the present, in some cases outlining contemporary occupational therapy; and to study the place occupied by the profession in the country (Reis & Lopes, 2018). Despite criticism of the Eurocentric term *occupation* and its associated models in the 1990s, occupational therapy in Brazil has nonetheless incorporated into its practices some Anglo-Saxon perspectives. Examples include the Human Occupation Model instrument: the Occupational Role Identification List (Cordeiro, 2005), the Canadian Occupational Performance Measure from the Canadian Occupational Performance Model (Caldas et al., 2011), the *Occupational Therapy Practice Framework* (American Occupational Therapy Association, 2014), and the Occupational Justice benchmark (Malfitano et al., 2019). All these demonstrate a return to the centrality of "occupation" in research and intervention for Brazilian occupational therapy. In addition, there are currently occupational therapists who base their practice in developmental, neurodevelopmental, and ecological theories and their respective approaches, including sensory integration, normal movement development via the Bobath approach, and others such as the cognitive behavioral, psychoanalytic-dynamic, and socio-interactionist approaches.

This diversity demonstrates both our potency and our fragility. Perspectives and conceptions of subject, society, and worldviews coexist, sometimes with significant substantive, conceptual, and methodological coherence and sometimes with limitations. There is a risk of insufficient discernment of the fundamentals being used, producing a disorderly mixture of concepts, theoretical intake, and production of practices (Galheigo et al., 2018). For example, social inequality is viewed internationally as an occupational barrier. However, the defining construct in the delivery of occupational therapy is to apply such approaches to pure occupational engagement. Where to place the emphasis in the social approach to service delivery remains a controversial debate in Brazilian occupational therapy. This is similar to Europe, where the marked increase in refugee numbers has resulted in significant occupational deprivation and alienation, and thus has been identified as an emergent area of practice through which the profession can make a marked positive change (Trimboli & Halliwell, 2018).

Since about 2000, the universities, largely responsible for the production of knowledge and vocational training, have expanded the discussion of Brazilian occupational therapy, motivated by the creation of public and social policies that allowed for the expansion of occupational therapy professionals into different practice settings. Thus, in 2009 the first graduate program in occupational therapy was created in the country, at the Federal University of São Carlos (UFSCar), with the objective of expanding and developing scientific knowledge in the field. In the following decade, two additional graduate programs in occupational therapy were created: the Master of Occupation Studies at the Federal University of Minas Gerais (Petten et al., 2019), and the Professional Master's of the University of São Paulo (Almeida & Oliver, 2019). Together, these three programs have explored and identified different ways of thinking about knowledge production and the philosophy of occupational therapy, as well as associated questions regarding how the profession serves society.

Brazil, a developing country, still has many socioeconomic inequalities among groups, revealing that health and quality of life are also driven by social determinants of health (economic, social, and political factors), many of which are surprising considering the Brazilian reality. In the most contemporary view of occupational therapy delivery, the focus is on enjoyment in occupational engagement aligned with personalized delivery of intervention (Carey, 2017). The social approach in Brazil considers societal groups in terms of enhancing productive occupational engagement rather than focusing on personalized context. Many occupational therapy clients are deprived of engagement in occupations due to their social condition and because there are only around 17,000 occupational therapists in Brazil, a small number for a country of 200 million people. Perhaps developing more personalized care with fulfilling engagement in productive occupations at its core could be a future paradigm change for Brazil, but a marked growth in the number of occupational therapists would be required to achieve this goal.

Defining the Current Philosophical Context in Brazil

The philosophy of occupational therapy in Brazil seems far removed from the occupation-centered paradigm, although there are some therapists who strive to discuss occupation and use it in their practices and research. Nevertheless, it can be concluded that Brazilian occupational therapy has distinct influences: namely, some characteristics of North American philosophy and, on the other side, a divergent construction of a uniquely Brazilian occupational therapy—a therapy with political and cultural roots focused on citizenship, culture, and education, guided by critically transformative thought for the population that receives its services. There is no consensus among Brazilian occupational therapists, scholars, or practitioners about their philosophical approaches, but we can safely say that the theoretical and philosophical knowledge used to inform their practice is strongly influenced by a political movement of resistance against inequalities and lack of opportunities for participation . . . conditions under which most of the Brazilian population lives.

Today, it can be observed that occupational therapy in Brazil is under the influence of two philosophical approaches. One is based on social changes and occupational justice supported by references to anthropology, sociology, and philosophy. The second is the growing return of occupation-centered practice framed through North American and European theories of occupation. These two philosophical approaches sometimes coexist in research and practice, showing that Brazilian occupational therapists understand occupation as a complex phenomenon that requires holistic and critical thinking to improve their practice according to lived realities.

In particular, the return to the discussion of occupation seems to be related to the need to understand the different meanings of occupation and human activity and to expand this dialogue internationally, for instance, when using concepts such as "meaningful occupation," "occupational justice," or "occupational engagement." Despite the existence of these two philosophical approaches, Brazilian occupational therapists still tend to base their practice on therapeutic techniques rather than embracing occupational therapy models of practice utilized in other countries.

Impact on Understanding of Occupation and Occupational Engagement

The different philosophical approaches adopted by Brazilian occupational therapists and scholars have amplified the scope of the profession in this country. Fields of practice not only include traditional health care delivery but are also expanding to social, educational, and cultural areas. Moreover, critical philosophical theories are guiding perspectives centered on social changes in the contexts where these clients, groups, and populations are living.

None of the thinkers such as Castel, Vázquez, Freire, Heller, Basaglia, and many others were occupational therapists, but they all influenced Brazilian occupational therapists to formulate their practices for deinstitutionalization of their clients, emancipation, inclusion, justice, and social participation. Examples of these approaches are the inclusion of mental health clients in labor activities, community interventions for people with disabilities, occupational therapy intervention with poor adolescents at schools, and work with other populations such as LGBTQ, women who have suffered violence, and people living in the streets.

As a consequence, occupational engagement assumes a key role not only in the performance of basic daily life needs but also the possibility of accessing other meaningful occupations, such as social participation in their communities and a commitment to occupational justice. This is important for the Brazilian people, who have been deprived of many occupations due to social, economic, and political forces and issues.

Key Implications for Occupational Therapy Education, Research, and Practice

Education

- Occupational therapy in Brazil should offer students the possibility to study the similarities and differences in the profession's various philosophies.
- The explicit teaching and connection of theories, models, and practical structures of occupational therapy may contribute to a better understanding of the profession's philosophy.

Research

- Researchers in Brazilian occupational therapy are challenged to study the profession's philosophy, to debate the significance of its beliefs and determine how they contrast with different philosophies in the international context.
- International collaboration in research may be developed by means of research projects that compare philosophies adopted by different countries.

Practice

- The beliefs and values adopted by Brazilian occupational therapists are similar to those adopted in other countries, especially those with nationally funded health care systems, but the practices vary according to local political-cultural differences.
- The social approach is an emerging aspect of popular occupational therapy delivery in Brazil reflecting a wider view of existing occupational barriers.
- Practice communities should discuss the knowledge basis and philosophies of occupational therapy to contribute to the professional identity and for improvement of the services offered by the profession.

RECOMMENDED READINGS

Castel, R. (1988). *The regulation of madness: The origins of incarceration in France.* University of California Press.

Castel, R. (2008). The roads to disaffiliation: Insecure work and vulnerable relationships. *International Journal of Urban and Regional Research, 24*(3), 519–535. https://doi.org/10.1111/1468-2427.00262

Vazquez, A. S. (1977). *The philosophy of praxis* (M. Gonzalez, Trans.; 2nd ed.). Humanistic Press.

REFERENCES

Almeida, M. C., & Oliver, F. C. (2019). Professional master's degree in occupational therapy at the University of São Paulo: Betting on the strength of collective processes. *Brazilian Journal of Occupational Therapy, 27*(2), 233–234. https://doi.org/10.4322/2526-8910.ctoED27022

American Occupational Therapy Association (AOTA). (2014). Occupational therapy practice framework: Domain and process (3rd ed.). *American Journal of Occupational Therapy, 68*(Suppl. 1), 1–48. https://doi.org/10.5014/ajot.2014.682006

Barros, D. D., Lopes, R. E., & Galheigo, S. M. (2007). Terapia ocupacional social [Social occupational therapy]. In M. A. Cavalcanti & C. Galvão (Eds.), *Terapia ocupacional: Fundamentação & prática* [Occupational therapy: foundations and practice] (pp. 348–353). Guanabara Koogan.

Benetton, M. J. (2006). *Trilhas Associativas: Ampliando subsídios metodológicos à clínica da terapia ocupacional* [Associated tracks: Enlarging methodological resources to occupational therapy practice]. Arte Brasil Editora.

Caldas, A. S. C., Facundes, V. L. D., & Silva, H. J. (2011). The use of the Canadian occupational performance measure in Brazilian studies: A systematic review. *Occupational Therapy Journal of the University of São Paulo, 22*(3), 238–244. https://doi.org/10.11606/issn.2238-6149.v22i3p238-244

Carey, H. (2017). *The impact of "doing" for people with motor neurone disease. A case study approach.* University of Wales.

Carey, H., Cruz, D. M. C., & Layne, K. (2019). Proposing possibilities for an international debate in occupational therapy. *Brazilian Journal of Occupational Therapy, 27*(3), 463–466. https://doi.org/10.4322/2526-8910.ctoed2703

Cordeiro, J. R. (2005). *Validade transcultural da lista de papéis ocupacionais para portadores de doença pulmonar obstrutiva crônica [Cross-cultural adaptation of the role checklist for patients with chronic obstructive pulmonary disease].* Dissertação (Mestrado em Ciências Médicas) [master's dissertation in medical sciences]. Universidade Federal de São Paulo.

Creek, J., & Feaver, S. (1993). Models for practice in occupational therapy: Part 1, defining terms. *British Journal of Occupational Therapy, 56*(1), 4–6. https://doi.org/10.1177/030802269305600103

Cruz, D. M. C. (2018). Occupational therapy models and possibilities for practice and research in Brazil: Models of practice in occupational therapy and possibilities for clinical practice and research in Brazil. *Interinstitutional Brazilian Journal of Occupational Therapy, 2*(3), 504–518.

Cruz, D. M. C. (2019). Historical milestones of occupational therapy research in Brazil. *British Journal of Occupational Therapy, 82*(9): 529–531. https://doi.org/10.1177/0308022618820270

Ferrari, M. A. C. (1991). Kielhofner and the model of human occupation. *Occupational Therapy Journal of the University of Sao Paulo, 2*(4), 216–219.

Galheigo, S. M. (2016). Social occupational therapy in Brazil: A historical synthesis of the constitution of a field of knowledge and practice. In R. E. Lopes & A. P. S. Malfitano (Eds.), *Social occupational therapy: Theoretical and practical designs* (pp. 49–68). EdUFSCar.

Galheigo, S. M., Braga, C. P., Arthur, M. A., & Matsuo, C. M. (2018). Knowledge production, perspectives and theoretical-practical references in Brazilian occupational therapy: Milestones and trends in a timeline. *Brazilian Journal of Occupational Therapy, 26*(4), 723–738. https://doi.org/10.4322/2526-8910.ctoAO1773

Gomez, C. M., Vasconcellos, L. C. F., & Machado, J. M. H. (2018). A brief history of worker's health in Brazil's unified health system: Progress and challenges. *Ciência & Saúde Coletiva [Science & Public Health], 23*(6), 1963–1970. https://doi.org/10.1590/1413-81232018236.04922018

Hagedorn, R. (1999). *Foundations for practice in occupational therapy.* Dynamis Editorial.

Kielhofner, G. (2009). *Conceptual foundations of occupational therapy* (4th ed.). F. A. Davis.

Malfitano, A. P. S., de Souza, R. G. da M., Townsend, E. A., & Lopes, R. E. (2019). Do occupational justice concepts inform occupational therapists' practice? A scoping review. *Canadian Journal of Occupational Therapy, 86*(4), 299–312. https://doi.org/10.1177/0008417419833409

Mângia, E. F. (1998). Notes on the field of occupational therapy. *Occupational Therapy Journal of the University of São Paulo, 9*(1), 5–13.

Marcolino, T. Q., Von Poellnitz, J. C., Silva, C. R., Villares, C. C., & Reali, A. M. M. R. (2019). "And a door opens": Reflections on conceptual and professional identity issues in the construction of clinical reasoning in occupational therapy. *Brazilian Notebooks of Occupational Therapy, 27*(2), 403–411. https://doi.org/10.4322/2526-8910.ctoao1740

Mata, C. C. (2019). "Chance para uma Esquizofrênica": Primeiros fundamentos da terapia ocupacional do prof. Rui Chamone Jorge ["Chance for a schizophrenic": First Foundations of Occupational Therapy by Prof. Rui Chamone Jorge]. *Revista Interinstitucional Brasileira de Terapia Ocupacional [Interinstitutional Review of Brazilian Occupational Therapy], 3*(3), 307–315.

Mayers, C. A. (1990). A philosophy unique to occupational therapy. *British Journal of Occupational Therapy, 53*(9): 379–380. https://doi.org/10.1177/030802269005300910

Medeiros, M. H. R. (2003). *Terapia Ocupacional—um Enfoque Epistemológico e Social [Occupational Therapy—An Epistemological and Social Approach].* EdUFSCar.

Monzeli, G. A., Morrison, R., & Lopes, R. E. (2019). Histórias da terapia ocupacional na América Latina: A primeira década de criação dos programas de formação profissional [Histories of occupational therapy in Latin America: The first decade of creation of the education programs]. *Cadernos Brasileiros de Terapia Ocupacional [Notes on Brazilian Occupational Therapy], 27*(2), 235–250. https://doi.org/10.4322/2526-8910.ctoAO1631

Nascimento, B. A. (1990). The myth of therapeutic activity. *Revista de Terapia Ocupacional da Universidade de São Paulo [Occupational Therapy Journal of the University of São Paulo]*, 1(1), 17–21.

Oliver, F. C., Souto, A. C. F., & Nicolau, S. M. (2018). Terapia ocupacional em 2019: 50 anos de regulamentação profissional no Brasil [50th anniversary of occupational therapy regulation in Brazil]. *Revista Interinstitucional Brasileira de Terapia Ocupacional [Brazilian Interinstitutional Journal of Occupational Therapy]*, 2(2), 244–256.

Petten, A. M. V. N. V., Faria-Fortini, I., & Magalhães, L. C. (2019). Um novo mestrado em terapia ocupacional: Perspectivas e desafios [Another masters program in occupational therapy: Perspectives and challenges]. *Cadernos Brasileiros de Terapia Ocupacional [Notes on Brazilian Occupational Therapy]*, 27(2), 231–232.

Reis, S. C. C. A. G., & Lopes, R. E. (2018). O início da trajetória de institucionalização acadêmica da terapia ocupacional no Brasil: O que contam os(as) docentes pioneiros(as) sobre a criação dos primeiros cursos [The beginning of the trajectory of occupational therapy academic institutionalization in Brazil: what professors tell pioneers about the creation of the first courses]. *Cadernos Brasileiros de Terapia Ocupacional [Notes on Brazilian Occupational Therapy]*, 26(2), 255–270.

Soares, L. B. T. (1991). *Terapia ocupacional: Lógica do capital ou trabalho? Retrospectiva histórica da profissão no Estado brasileiro de 1950 a 1980* [Occupational therapy: a capitalistic or work meaning? An historical retrospective of the profession from 1950 to 1980]. Editora Hucitec.

Trimboli, C., & Halliwell, V. (2018). A survey to explore the interventions used by occupational therapists and occupational therapy students with refugees and asylum seekers. *World Federation of Occupational Therapists Bulletin, 74*(2), 106–113. https://doi.org/10.1080/14473828.2018.1535562

Turner, A., & Knight, J. (2015). A debate on the professional identity of occupational therapists. *British Journal of Occupational Therapy, 78*(11), 664–673. https://doi.org/10.1177/0308022615601439

Wales, K. (2012). Occupational therapy discharge planning for older adults: A protocol for a randomized trial and economic evaluation. *British Medical Journal Geriatrics, 12*(34), 1–7. https://doi.org/10.1186/1471-2318-12-34

Wilberforce, M., Hughes, J., Bowns, I., Fillingham, J., Pryce, F., Symonds, E., . . . & Challis, D. (2016). Occupational therapy roles and responsibilities: Evidence from a pilot study of time use in an integrated health and social care trust. *British Journal of Occupational Therapy, 79*(7), 409–416. https://doi.org/10.1177/0308022616630329

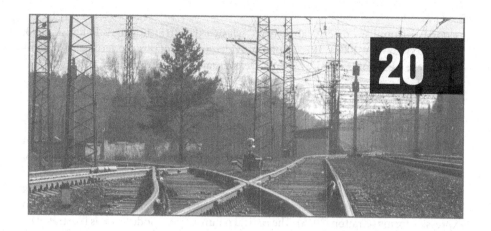

Postmodernism

Foundations for Problematizing and Reimagining Conditions of Possibility

Rebecca M. Aldrich, PhD, OTR/L
Debbie Laliberte Rudman, PhD, OT Reg. (ON)
Aaron Bonsall, PhD, OTR/L

INTRODUCTION

More than a philosophy, postmodernism also encompasses movements in architecture, linguistics, psychology, and visual, literary, and performing arts. Postmodern ideas and practices began to coalesce in the second half of the 20th century to counter and destabilize Western positivist and reductionist approaches. Rejecting the idea that knowledge is absolute, objective, and available through universal truths or unified grand narratives (Aylesworth, 2015; Layder, 2006), postmodern theorists see knowledge as situated and political (Whiteford et al., 2000). Postmodernists are skeptical about how phenomena are represented and link those representations to the exercise of power (Boyne & Rattansi, 1990; Hicks, 2011). Thinkers labeled as postmodernist—such as Jean-François Lyotard, Michel Foucault, Gilles Deleuze, Richard Rorty, Jacques Derrida, and Jean Baudrillard—vary widely and can be linked to other philosophical traditions such

Taff, S. D. (Ed.). *Philosophy and Occupational Therapy:*
Informing Education, Research, and Practice (pp. 201-207).
© 2021 Taylor & Francis Group.

as post-structuralism or critical theory (Aylesworth, 2015; Boyne & Rattansi, 1990; Hicks, 2011; Layder, 2006). This chapter provides a précis of postmodernism as it manifests in the works of Lyotard, Foucault, Deleuze, and Rorty.

MAJOR FACETS OF THE PHILOSOPHY

Postmodernists believe that there is no universally true narrative about the way the world works or how it should be ordered; instead, they argue that different descriptions of "reality" are constructions that reflect particular groups' relative positions of power in society (Aylesworth, 2015; Hicks, 2011). Postmodern philosophers seek to deconstruct dominant representations that foster oppression, with the goal of opening spaces for diverse representations and amplifying previously silenced conceptual and expressive forms (Gratton, 2018). The radical nature of postmodernism is illustrated by its destabilization of a commonly accepted idea: that of the coherent, rational, unified subject or "individual" (Crotty, 2015). In postmodern thinking, the individual—as well as a range of other taken-for-granted ideas—is repositioned as fragmentary, dynamic, situated, constituted within power relations, and the "product of a number of cross-cutting discourses and practices" (Layder, 2006, p. 119).

GENERAL GOALS OR INTENDED OUTCOMES
OF THE PHILOSOPHY

Postmodern thinkers pose "questions about how social relations should be organized and lived, about the social possibilities of our age, and about the social visions it is desirable to underwrite" (Boyne & Rattansi, 1990, pp. 23–24). They support pluralism by aiming to illustrate the relative validity of different principles, perspectives, and values. Postmodernists stress that their ideas are not meant to be taken as fundamental truths, and their reluctance to prescribe detailed ends reflects this emphasis (Aylesworth, 2015). Instead of providing replacements for existing "universal" truths, postmodern philosophers posit strategies for uncovering and deconstructing the metanarratives that shape current conditions. Their larger goal is to inspire collective problematizing that seeks to redistribute power (Aylesworth, 2015; Hicks, 2011).

SELECTED PERSPECTIVES, THINKERS,
AND KEY CONCEPTS

Jean-François Lyotard was a French philosopher and activist who is best known for introducing the term *postmodern* into the philosophical canon in the second half of the 20th century (Gratton, 2018). Lyotard demonstrated a "restless dissatisfaction with established ideas" (Malpas, 2003, p. 6), and his early writings focused on questioning how knowledge is framed, generated, and mobilized through different language "games" (e.g., science, philosophy, economics) that shape societies and experiences (Aylesworth, 2015). Lyotard illuminated the exploitative and colonial uses of metanarratives about reason, and he suggested that justice lay in challenging the hegemony of such narratives (Aylesworth, 2015; Gratton, 2018). Through his celebration of creative and aesthetic forms and the questions they raised about prevailing ways of thinking (Malpas, 2003), Lyotard aimed to disrupt the capitalist commodification of knowledge that (1) narrowed what was "presentable," (2) silenced alternative phrasings, and (3) reduced "the human to modes of efficiency" (Gratton, 2018). Overall, Lyotard advocated for all groups' "rights to employ their own language games (and hence values) to present their points of view" (Malpas, 2003, p. 68).

Michel Foucault was a professor at various French universities from the 1960s through the mid-1980s. His historical explorations were motivated by a concern for marginalized ways of being and doing (Gutting & Oksala, 2019). In constructing histories of the present, Foucault traced backward from present regimes of truth to destabilize taken-for-granted realities and dominant discourses, particularly those related to humans as subjects. He sought to reveal discontinuity in history to demonstrate the precarious, contingent nature of what has come to be viewed as truth and to detail the particular conditions of possibility that sustained the taken-for-granted (Aylesworth, 2015; Chambon, 1999). Foucault also expanded the notion of government beyond the state to encompass diverse social actors whose endeavors aimed to shape the "conduct of conduct" through technologies and practices. He sought to reveal the microdynamics of power involved in the governance of everyday life, attending to the productive ways in which power operates to produce particular "truths" aligned with dominant rationalities. He detailed the discourses, technologies, and practices employed by various types of social agents and institutions, such as health care professionals and educational institutions, to shape how subjects come to understand themselves and how they should act in the world (Chambon, 1999; Layder, 2006). His work aimed to create conditions for transformation by demonstrating that the present is neither natural nor inevitable, thereby opening up spaces for developing alternative ways of being and doing (Chambon, 1999; Laliberte Rudman, 2010).

Gilles Deleuze was a French philosopher and public intellectual who lectured and published from the mid-1950s through the mid-1990s (Smith & Protevi, 2018). He built his philosophy on a conception of difference that critiqued modern representations' assertions of truth-value and unity. Deleuze framed difference as productive or generative (Aylesworth, 2015; Colebrook, 2002), and his work aimed to elucidate how fundamental processes of creation and becoming revealed interconnections, power relations, and possibilities for change (Barlott et al., 2017; Colebrook, 2002). Deleuze opposed the search for essential characteristics, linear thinking, hierarchical ordering systems, and totalizing structures, all of which are common in dominant forms of thought. He instead embraced rhizomatic counterthought, which involves multidirectionality, polymorphous understandings, and attending to the complexities of assemblages. Deleuze emphasized the process of "becoming," which includes adopting rhizomatic thought, as a means to resist and disrupt oppressive ordering systems and create new ways of thinking (Barlott et al., 2017; Holmes & Gastaldo, 2004).

Richard Rorty was an American philosopher whose work spanned from the 1950s through the early 2000s (Ramberg, 2009). Although Rorty's work overlaps with other topics in this book (e.g., pragmatism) and he emphasizes power less than other postmodernists, his critique of the nature of truth most closely aligns with the thinkers featured in this chapter. Rorty (1979) argued that descriptions of the world, and therefore truths about the world, depend on languages: the world on its own, unfettered from descriptions created by humans, cannot be true or false (Rorty, 1989). For Rorty (1979), objectivity should not be conceived of as a representation (or mirror) of external reality but instead as an agreed-upon vocabulary that has been established through past and present argument. Rorty postulated that some vocabularies are better able than others to shape worldviews and determine public understanding in a way that draws societies together through common hopes and comprehensions. He also argued that the revolutionary or abnormal discourse of artists, philosophers, and unfamiliar cultures can enliven societies that have become entrenched in (and hindered by) familiar vocabularies (Rorty, 1979, 1989).

IMPACT ON UNDERSTANDING OF OCCUPATION AND OCCUPATIONAL ENGAGEMENT

Lyotard, Foucault, Deleuze, and Rorty all focused on the ways in which communicative practices reveal, reinforce, and can potentially transform power relations. By showing that language games and vocabularies shape experience and that discourses mobilize power, these postmodern thinkers demonstrated that taking up and mobilizing language in particular ways has consequences. For instance, choosing to take up language that unquestioningly equates science with rationality has the consequence of perpetuating power structures that privilege linear ways of knowing, which are characteristic of—and work for—some cultures but not others. In recognition of these consequences, scholars in occupational therapy have begun to highlight how the language used to name and frame occupations has long been grounded in White, Eurocentric, middle-class ways of knowing that can be limiting for both practitioners and clients (Aldrich et al., 2017; Hammell, 2009). Following these examples, occupational therapy practitioners, educators, and scholars can draw on postmodern resources to excavate their language choices, unearthing how their taken-for-granted communication practices convey particular constructions of experience and occupation that are embedded in social power relations.

Postmodern philosophies can also help create spaces for alternate language practices around occupation. Lyotard's work can be used to foster "attunement to the plurality of opinions" (Gratton, 2018, para. 13), "openness to what is surprising, and attentiveness to the possibilities that [an] event's disruption of established genres might reveal" (Malpas, 2003, p. 106). Kiepek, Beagan, Laliberte Rudman, and Phelan's (2018) questioning of the labeling of occupations as unhealthy, illegal, and deviant exemplifies the plurality, openness, and possibilities that come from attending to language in this way. Foucault's writings can help identify opportunities for questioning the ways of doing and being that come to be expected for particular members of society, such as the notion that aging adults should be productive even in retirement (Laliberte Rudman, 2010). Foucault's work also challenges occupational therapists to be critically reflexive regarding how they are implicated in the circulation of power through their discursive constructions of occupations and the practices that flow from those discursive constructions, in order to guard against unintentionally re-producing occupational inequities (Gerlach et al., 2018). Deleuze's work, both alone and in partnership with Felix Guattari, can help occupational therapists "find the sin-gular conditions under which something new is produced" (Smith & Protevi, 2018, para. 9) and analyze "human occupation acentred from the individual" (Barlott et al., 2017, p. 525). Finally, Rorty (1989) can help occupational therapy practitioners, edu-cators, and scholars understand that people "need to be able to tell themselves a story about how things might get better, and to see no insuperable obstacle to this story's coming true" (p. 86). Rorty's emphasis on vocabularies can be used to understand the process of narrative reasoning through which clients and therapists transform therapy sessions into lived stories that link outcomes to future possibilities (Bonsall, 2012; Mattingly & Fleming, 1994).

Whiteford et al. (2000) suggested that postmodernism "created a social and in-tellectual environment conducive to a renaissance of occupation," (p. 62) given its emphasis on power, situatedness, and diverse ways of knowing. They argued that postmodern perspectives supported "the aims of occupational science to challenge the privileging of one group or perspective over another, and to illuminate the di-verse perspectives, temporality, and situatedness of occupation in its cultural, physi-cal, social, and institutional context" (p. 66). As Carrasco (2018) demonstrated more recently, postmodern ideas are useful for exploring "the role that current knowledge about occupation plays in the specific forms of conduct control of certain individu-als and groups" (p. 516) both within and outside occupational therapy. Postmodern philosophies can thus guide occupational therapists and occupational scientists as they analyze, deconstruct, and reimagine the linguistic and conceptual frameworks that shape their education, research, and practice activities.

KEY IMPLICATIONS FOR OCCUPATIONAL THERAPY EDUCATION, RESEARCH, AND PRACTICE

Education

- Justifies the need to incorporate ongoing critical reflexivity regarding standard/normative occupational therapy knowledge and practices (Hammell, 2009).
- Provides a rationale for incorporating interdisciplinary perspectives on power, such as gender studies, cultural studies, and intersectionality.
- Opens space for dialogue about diverse understandings of occupation (Hocking, 2012).

Research

- Supports thinking about ways researchers "capture, absorb, and appropriate" (Barlott et al., 2017, p. 526) people's occupational experiences, and how such research practices can reinforce or challenge existing power structures.

- Facilitates research that challenges and extends epistemological and methodological boundaries in ways that diversify understandings of occupation (Laliberte Rudman, 2014).
- Enhances attention to historical foundations as a means to reveal tentativeness of taken-for-granted assumptions, particularly when such assumptions result in marginalization (Kantartzis & Molineux, 2012).

Practice

- Highlights the need to attend to how power permeates everyday life, including how people understand themselves and their everyday possibilities for occupation.
- Promotes critical reflexivity about the "truths" that guide occupational therapy practices, and how such truths may unintentionally marginalize alternative ways of doing and being (Carrasco, 2018; Laliberte Rudman, 2010).
- Recognizes a need to understand the various languages and vocabularies that construct ideas of occupations, and the impact of those ideas on the people whom occupational therapists serve (Kiepek et al., 2014; Njelesani et al., 2015).

RECOMMENDED READINGS

Polzer, J., & Power, E. (2016). *Neoliberal governance and health: Duties, risks, and vulnerabilities*. McGill-Queen's University Press.

Sim, S. (2013). *Fifty key postmodern thinkers*. Routledge.

REFERENCES

Aldrich, R. M., Laliberte Rudman, D., & Dickie, V. A. (2017). Resource seeking as occupation: A critical and empirical exploration. *American Journal of Occupational Therapy, 71*(3), 7103260010p1–7103260010p9. https://doi.org/10.5014/ajot.2017.021782

Aylesworth, G. (2015). Postmodernism. In E. N. Zalta (Ed.), *The Stanford encyclopedia of philosophy* (Spring 2015 ed.). https://plato.stanford.edu/archives/spr2015/entries/postmodernism

Barlott, T., Shevellar, L., & Turpin, M. (2017). Becoming minor: Mapping new territories in occupational science. *Journal of Occupational Science, 24*(4), 524–534. https://doi.org/10.1080/14427591.2017.1378121

Bonsall, A. (2012). An examination of the pairing between narrative and occupational science. *Scandinavian Journal of Occupational Therapy, 19*(1), 92–103. https://doi.org/10.3109/11038128.2011.552119

Boyne, R., & Rattansi, A. (1990). The theory and politics of postmodernism: By way of an introduction. In R. Boyne & A. Rattansi (Eds.), *Postmodernism and society* (pp. 1–45). Macmillan Education.

Carrasco, J. (2018). Political dimensions in the actions of health-care practitioners: Reflections for occupational science based on the Chilean psychiatric reform. *Journal of Occupational Science, 25*(4), 509–519. https://doi.org/10.1080/14427591.2018.1519869

Chambon, A. (1999). Foucault's approach: Making the familiar visible. In A. S. Chambon, A. Irving, & L. Epstein (Eds.), *Reading Foucault for social work* (pp. 51–81). Columbia University Press.

Colebrook, C. (2002). *Gilles Deleuze*. Routledge.

Crotty, M. (2015). *The foundations of social research: Meaning and perspective in the research process* (2nd ed.). SAGE Publications.

Gerlach, A. J., Teachman, G., Laliberte Rudman, D., Aldrich, R. M., & Huot, S. (2018). Expanding beyond individualism: Engaging critical perspectives on occupation. *Scandinavian Journal of Occupational Therapy*, 25(1), 35–43. https://doi.org/10.1080/11038128.2017.1327616

Gratton, P. (2018). Jean François Lyotard. In E. N. Zalta (Ed.), *The Stanford encyclopedia of philosophy* (Winter 2018 ed.). https://plato.stanford.edu/archives/win2018/entries/lyotard

Gutting, G., & Oksala, J. (2019). Michel Foucault. In E. N. Zalta (Ed.), *The Stanford encyclopedia of philosophy* (Spring 2019 ed.). https://plato.stanford.edu/archives/spr2019/entries/foucault

Hammell, K. W. (2009). Self-care, productivity, and leisure, or dimensions of occupational experience? Rethinking occupational "categories." *Canadian Journal of Occupational Therapy*, 76(2), 107–114. https://doi.org/10.1177/000841740907600208

Hicks, S. R. C. (2011). *Explaining postmodernism: Skepticisim and socialism from Rousseau to Foucault* (2nd ed.). Ockham's Razor Publishing.

Hocking, C. (2012). Occupations through the looking glass: Reflecting on occupational scientists' ontological assumptions. In G. E. Whiteford & C. Hocking (Eds.), *Occupational science: Society, inclusion, participation* (pp. 54–66). Wiley-Blackwell.

Holmes, D., & Gastaldo, D. (2004). Rhizomatic thought in nursing: An alternative path for the development of the discipline. *Nursing Philosophy*, 5(3), 258–267. https://doi.org/10.1111/j.1466-769X.2004.00184.x

Kantartzis, S., & Molineux, M. (2012). Understanding the discursive development of occupation: Historico-political perspectives. In G. E. Whiteford & C. Hocking (Eds.), *Occupational science: Society, inclusion, participation* (pp. 38–53). Wiley-Blackwell.

Kiepek, N. C., Beagan, B., Laliberte Rudman, D., & Phelan, S. (2018). Silences around occupations framed as unhealthy, illegal, and deviant. *Journal of Occupational Science*, 26(3), 341–353. https://doi.org/10.1080/14427591.2018.1499123

Kiepek, N. C., Phelan, S. P., & Magalhães, L. (2014). Introducing a critical analysis of the figured world of occupation. *Journal of Occupational Science*, 21(4), 403–417. https://doi.org/10.1080/14427591.2013.816998

Laliberte Rudman, D. (2010). Occupational terminology: Occupational possibilities. *Journal of Occupational Science*, 17(1), 55–59. https://doi.org/10.1080/14427591.2010.9686673

Laliberte Rudman, D. (2014). Embracing and enacting an "occupational imagination": Occupational science as transformative. *Journal of Occupational Science*, 21(4), 373–388. https://doi.org/10.1080/14427591.2014.888970

Layder, D. (2006). *Understanding social theory* (2nd ed.). SAGE Publications.

Malpas, S. (2003). *Jean François Lyotard*. Routledge.

Mattingly, C., & Fleming, M. H. (1994). *Clinical reasoning: Forms of inquiry in a therapeutic practice*. F. A. Davis.

Njelesani, J., Teachman, G., Durocher, E., Hamdani, Y., & Phelan, S. K. (2015). Thinking critically about client-centred practice and occupational possibilities across the lifespan. *Scandinavian Journal of Occupational Therapy*, 22(4), 252–259. https://doi.org/10.3109/11038128.2015.1049550

Ramberg, B. (2009). Richard Rorty. In E. N. Zalta (Ed.), *The Stanford encyclopedia of philosophy* (Spring 2009 ed.). https://plato.stanford.edu/archives/spr2009/entries/rorty

Rorty, R. (1979). *Philosophy and the mirror of nature*. Princeton University Press.

Rorty, R. (1989). *Contingency, irony, and solidarity*. Cambridge University Press.

Smith, D., & Protevi, J. (2018). Gilles Deleuze. In E. N. Zalta (Ed.), *The Stanford encyclopedia of philosophy* (Spring 2018 ed.). https://plato.stanford.edu/archives/spr2018/entries/deleuze

Whiteford, G., Townsend, E., & Hocking, C. (2000). Reflections on a renaissance of occupation. *Canadian Journal of Occupational Therapy*, 67(1), 61–69. https://doi.org/10.1177/000841740006700109

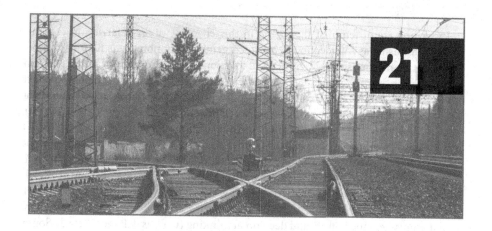

Intersectionality
Feminist Theorizing in the Pursuit of Justice and Equity

Alison Gerlach, PhD, MSc (OT)
Lilian Magalhães, PhD, OT

Introduction

There is no single feminist theory, but all feminist perspectives share a common purpose of political activism toward justice and equity. Historically, in the global North during the 19th and early 20th centuries, dominant feminist thought, often referred to as "first wave feminism," privileged the voices of White, middle-class women who asserted that all women experience oppression. This form of feminist theorizing and political activism, which focused on overcoming sexism and achieving gender equity, failed to recognize the complex realities of women's lives and their experiences of oppression and inequity within diverse historical, geographical, sociocultural, and economic contexts. As Audre Lorde (2007) famously stated: "There is no such thing as a single-issue struggle, because we do not live single-issue lives" (p. 138).

Taff, S. D. (Ed.). *Philosophy and Occupational Therapy: Informing Education, Research, and Practice* (pp. 209-219). © 2021 Taylor & Francis Group.

In writing about feminist theorizing in this chapter, we are referring to contemporary feminisms as intersectional, in which gender as nonbinary is no less or more important than other social identities and locations. Gerlach writes from the position of a European immigrant-settler, cisgender woman in the ongoing colonial context of Canada. As an ally and advocate *with* Indigenous partners on a shared agenda of fostering Indigenous children's health equity (Gerlach, 2018; Gerlach et al., 2018), her work is informed by Black feminist scholarship (Collins, 2009; Collins & Bilge, 2016) and Indigenous feminist perspectives (Anderson, 2016). Magalhães, a Black-descent Brazilian female, writes from a hybrid positionality. The larger part of her academic training and practice as an occupational therapist and professor has been in Brazil. She has also lived and worked for 16 years in Canada, where she received most of her training in qualitative research and critical thought. Her work is mostly influenced by Black feminist, emancipatory, and decolonial thinking (Collins & Bilge, 2016; de Sousa Santos, 2015; Freire, 1985; Zavala, 2013). Her transnational experiences enact a location described by Zavala (2013) as an "outsider within" perspective.

FEMINISMS AS INTERSECTIONAL

In recent decades, North American and Eurocentric feminist scholarship has been critiqued for limiting feminist thinking by reproducing hegemonic generalizations based on the experiences of women who often identify as White, Christian, middle-class, and heterosexual—thus effectively erasing the lived realities and political concerns of women who do not share these social locations and whose experiences of oppression are rooted in a complex nexus of class, race, ethnicity, and sexual identity/expression (hooks, 2000). In response to the challenges experienced by Black women in the United States in "falling through the cracks" of social movements in the 1960s and 1970s that tended to focus on single-issue struggles of race, gender, or class, Black feminist scholars developed the ideas that would come to be conceptualized as *intersectionality* (Collins & Bilge, 2016).

Intersectionality, as developed by Black feminist scholars such as Patricia Hill Collins (2009), bell hooks (2000), and Kimberlé Crenshaw (1989), complicates the analyses of women's lives by embracing a paradigm of race, class, and gender as intersecting systems of oppression that reconceptualize the social relations of domination *and* resistance. *Intersectionality* is defined as:

a way of understanding and analyzing the complexity in the world, in people, and in human experiences. The events and conditions of social and political life and the self can seldom be understood as shaped by one factor. They are generally shaped by many factors in diverse and mutually influencing ways. When it comes to social inequality, people's lives and the organization of power in a given society are better understood as being shaped not by a single axis of social division, be it race or gender or class, but by many axes that work together and influence each other. Intersectionality as an analytical tool gives people better access to the complexity of the world and of themselves. (Collins & Bilge, 2016, p. 2)

Intersectionality therefore challenges the idea that race and gender cannot be treated as mutually exclusive categories of discrimination and analysis (Crenshaw, 1989).

Rather, as an analytical lens, intersectionality seeks to reveal and generate a greater understanding of the complexity of people's lived realities within equally complex societies. This analytical framework emphasizes the *simultaneous* interaction of important social divisions, including race, class, gender, disability, and so forth, with power relations within a society that include racism, class exploitation, sexism, and ableism (Collins & Bilge, 2016). According to Collins and Bilge (2016), intersectionality as an analytical framework brings into focus social inequality, mutually constructed relations of power, the interconnections between social differences, the importance of social context, and the complexity of the world and the solutions needed to address social injustices. This form of critical inquiry is necessarily linked to doing critical social justice work, which we introduce later in this chapter in relation to health inequities and occupational therapy.

THE SITUATED AND CONTEXTUALIZED NATURE OF FEMINIST THEORIZING

Since its inception, intersectionality has continued to evolve through Black activist and feminist, postcolonial, queer, and Indigenous scholarship to contest the assumption that "women" as a fixed category of analysis constitutes a homogenous group (Bunjun, 2010; Collins, 2009; Crenshaw, 1989; van Herk et al., 2011). Ongoing scholarly debates on the issues of the claimed homogeneity of feminist thought and struggle are particularly salient in an era of globalization, growing economic inequality, and single-issue media coverage.

Whether drawing from the experiences of immigrant women living in North America (Huot & Veronis, 2018; Zimmerman, 2015) or unpacking the contradictions of the identity and authenticity of scholarship developed in the South (Connell, 2014), it is evident that a global project of a singular feminism is problematic and ineffective (Pausé et al., 2012). For example, Black-, Arabian-, and Philippine-descent feminists located in the United States have challenged the claims put forward by White feminist scholars, articulating their inconsistencies and rejecting widespread stereotypes about women from peripheral locations (Connell, 2014). Very often these labels are attached to women, despite good intentions, by scholars but also by feminist advocates. For example, from Western values standpoints, Muslim women are portrayed as a homogeneous group, without further elaboration on their diversity around ethnicity, social status, and even religious practices. As such, Muslim women are often perceived as submissive and oppressed while class and cultural contexts, quite essential in these cases, are dismissed (Zimmerman, 2015). Also, as Huff, Laliberte Rudman, Magalhães, and Lawson (2018) highlight, "Africana womanism" challenges Western dualistic conceptualizations of male–female static dichotomies of gender occupations and gender roles. Instead, the authors articulate a situational perspective in which "women can shift in and out of gender depending of context . . . For example, in some East-African tribes, daughters can become an 'honorary son' if the family has no other male-born children, illustrating how female can shift to a traditional male role if needed" (p. 557).

In the context of Latin America, Connell (2014) questions the pervasiveness of Northern colonial thinking, even when revisited by scholars from the South:

> Creative feminist work in the South often involves a critical appropriation of Northern ideas, in combination with ideas that come from radically different experiences. . . . The problem is not that local content is absent from Southern writing, but that local realities are reduced to the status of a "case" framed by metropolitan conceptualizations. (p. 525)

Further, Connell (2014) insists that "feminists researchers in different parts of the world urgently need ways to cross-fertilize, rather than to separate, their work" (p. 522). This also means acknowledging that feminism is not constrained to scholarly work, which presents another opportunity to understand the differences in the praxis of feminist groups across borders. As Paulo Freire suggests, in combination with critical dialogue, people must act together to transform their realities (Freire, 1997).

In the context of settler-colonial nation states, including the United States, Canada, New Zealand, and Australia, colonization had, and continues to have, gendered, classed, and racialized undercurrents (Pausé et al., 2012). Feminist theorizing has tended to obscure Indigenous women's lived experiences of gendered forms of oppression that continue to operate in, and be reproduced through, colonial and patriarchal structures (Arvin et al., 2013). In response, Indigenous women writers, scholars, and activists have advocated for critical feminist theorizing to examine, confront, and transform how Indigenous women's human rights and well-being are constrained by their individual and collective experiences of intersecting forms of oppression, including patriarchy, racism, gender discrimination, and socioeconomic marginalization (Anderson, 2010, 2016; Green, 2017; Huhndorf & Suzack, 2010; Kuokkanen, 2007; LaRocque, 2007, 2009; St. Denis, 2007). Indigenous feminist scholarship has prompted contentious political, cultural, and scholarly debates (Monture-Angus, 1995; Smith, 2009; Suzack et al., 2010). However, a small but growing number of Indigenous feminists, who resist a single or unified definition of Indigenous feminism, are carefully and specifically formulating their own ideologies on a feminist inquiry that foregrounds the commonalities and particularities of Indigenous women's life experiences and circumstances (Huhndorf & Suzack, 2010). Importantly, Indigenous feminism must be shaped and informed by Indigenous women. However, as Huhndorf and Suzack (2010) contend, promoting social change and justice for Indigenous women requires "the engagement, contributions, and support of Indigenous men and non-Indigenous men and women" (p. 4).

Thus, the multiplicity and dynamic interaction of personal, social, and structural factors that shape a person's lived experience—political, religious, age-related, cultural, economic, ethnic, historically and geographically bounded, and linguistic, among others—must be acknowledged as fluid and situational (Huff et al., 2018). From this perspective, the plurality of feminisms foregrounds its potential to generate nuanced understandings and actions toward addressing local and global concerns of social injustice and inequity, grounded in its underpinnings of intersectionality, complexity, and situatedness.

HEALTH, DISABILITY, AND FEMINIST THEORIZING

Feminism is about doing and not only theorizing that is moving toward justice and equity—it is a political movement (Ahmed, 2017). From an intersectionality perspective, injustices such as health and social inequities are never the result of single, discrete factors. "Rather, they are the outcome of intersections of different social locations, power relations and experience" (Hankivsky, 2014, p. 2). Applying intersectionality in health research draws attention to the politics of health and health care, revealing and disrupting the conflation of ahistorical categories of race and ethnicity, the homogenization of distinct populations, and the power structures within society and health care institutions that simultaneously reproduce experiences of privilege and marginalization. Intersectionality is increasingly being taken up by public health stakeholders and health researchers to interrogate and address social injustices, including structural racism and health inequities in diverse global contexts (Bastos et al., 2018; Gkiouleka et al., 2018; Green et al., 2017; Richman & Zucker, 2019; Viruell-Fuentes et al., 2012).

In theorizing about addressing health inequities experienced by Indigenous families and children in the Canadian context, Gerlach draws on the scholarship of Cree Métis scholar Anderson (2016) to elucidate how relational early childhood practices with Indigenous families can provide a critical counternarrative to "a negative Native female identity" (p. 92) reproduced by historical and contemporary colonial policies and discourses (Gerlach, Browne, et al., 2017, 2018). In this context, Anderson's (2016) theorizing provides an analytical framing of and language for how early childhood programs can support Indigenous women in resisting "negative definitions of being" and "reclaiming" their agency as Indigenous women and mothers.

Employing feminist theorizing in disability-focused services, including occupational therapy, requires attending to the many facets of the social identities and experiences of marginalization and oppression of people with disabilities. The prevalence and experience of diverse disabilities are shaped by multiple factors, including an individual's gender, education, class, and age, as the individual interacts with power relations and systems within society. For example, youth with disabilities who identify as lesbian, gay, bisexual, or transgender frequently experience prejudice and discrimination in mainstream institutions and the broader society as a result of their sexual gender identity/expression (Bucik et al., 2017; Duke, 2011). As noted by Mann and Patterson (2016), integrating ability/disability as a category of analysis into feminist theorizing "does not obscure our critical focus on the registers of race, sexuality, ethnicity, or gender, nor is it additive. Rather, considering disability shifts the conceptual framework to strengthen our understanding of how these multiple systems intertwine, redefine, and mutually constitute one another" (p. 295).

As an analytical lens, intersectionality generates a nuanced and deeper understanding of the complex and mutually compounding effects of multiple identities and processes of marginalization and exclusion experienced by people with disabilities. From this perspective, and consistent with critical disability scholarship, the construct of "dis/ability" (similar to other social identities) is viewed as a continuum, rather than a binary, and as fluid and highly contextual (Ben-Moshe & Magaña, 2014). For example, using this lens to interpret national survey data in South Africa in order to better understand the relationship between disability and poverty elucidates how disability—as it intersects with gender, age, and race—results in negative outcomes in education, employment, and income for all people with disabilities. However, these effects are compounded for women and particularly for Black women with disabilities, who experience "a triple burden" (Moodley & Graham, 2015). These results also highlight the ongoing impact of racism on educational and employment opportunities in post-apartheid South Africa, with Black men *without* disabilities faring worse than White women *with* disabilities, thereby challenging common assumptions about the relationship between disability and poverty (Moodley & Graham, 2015).

Thus, feminist theorizing can produce complex, nuanced, and inclusive understandings of the differences and connections of the multiple social positionings and lived realities of people with disabilities (Hirschmann, 2013). This analytical foundation has the potential to inform the design and delivery of health care that is inclusive and socially responsive, and explicitly addresses discrimination in all its intersecting forms, including homophobia, heterosexism, patriarchy, ableism, and racialization.

THINKING, BEING, AND DOING OCCUPATIONAL THERAPY IN A FEMINIST WAY

Not dissimilar to the roots of feminism, occupational therapy is rooted in and dominated by knowledges and theories that privilege individualistic, Euro-Western, White, English-speaking, Christian, and female values, with assumptions and preferences related to human occupation and the professionalization of occupational therapy (Frank, 1992; Guajardo et al., 2015; Hammell, 2009; Hocking, 2012). In response to concerns about the theoretical imperialism inherent in occupational therapy (Hammell, 2011), critically oriented occupation-focused discourses increasingly emphasize the need to expand occupational therapy theorizing beyond its epistemological roots to become inclusive of and responsive to the realities and complexities of social and occupational injustices and health inequities in diverse global contexts (Farias et al., 2016; Gerlach, 2015; Olivares-Aising, 2018). This scholarship echoes earlier calls for occupational therapy to acknowledge feminism as an "important force for change" (Black et al., 1992; Frank, 1992). However, despite being a female-dominated profession with strong social justice roots and aspirations of occupational justice, feminist occupational theorizing has yet to be fully utilized (Gerlach, 2015; Pollard & Walsh, 2000).

Practicing and researching at the interface of occupation and oppression requires attending to issues such as power, subjectivity, trust, and motives. Critical reflexivity is a guiding principle of occupational therapy with clients who experience structural forms of oppression and marginalization (Gerlach, 2015) and of feminist research methodologies (Leavy & Harris, 2019). Moreover, employing feminist intersectionality in occupational therapy expands research, education, and practice beyond individualistic perspectives and works toward aspirations of social transformation, occupational justice, and health equity (Angell, 2012; Gerlach, Teachman, et al., 2017; Sakellariou &

Pollard, 2017). This theoretical orientation reveals how everyday occupations can (re) produce social relations of power and represent sites of occupational agency or oppression. As noted by Angell (2012):

> Difference is not only produced in occupation, it is also used to reify the categories it creates, "proving" the inferiority of certain groups for participation in certain activities. These processes occur daily and simultaneously through occupation. Occupation, then, can be a structural means through which gender, race, or class are regulated. (p. 7)

From this perspective, participation in specific occupations is shaped by a complex confluence of individual and broader social factors, the latter of which are often beyond an individual's immediate environment or control (Galvaan, 2015; Gerlach, Teachman, et al., 2017; Laliberte Rudman, 2013). For example, feminist theorizing of play in the context of Indigenous children in Canada highlights how dominant and taken-for-granted constructions of this childhood occupation in occupational therapy erase the multifaceted impacts of colonization on children's occupational opportunities and inadvertently reproduce colonial stereotypes of "poor mothering" or "at-risk" children (Gerlach et al., 2014). Employing a feminist analysis of Latin American migrant female workers in Spain reveals how their class, gender, and ethnicity shape how they experience and negotiate their way through occupational opportunities on a daily basis and highlight how occupational injustices are produced and perpetuated (Rivas-Quarneti et al., 2018). Thus, "knowing and doing" occupational therapy that aspires to be socially transformative requires "attuning our eyes to the interlocking nature of oppression and its often invisible influence on occupational opportunities" (Angell, 2012, p. 10).

KEY IMPLICATIONS FOR OCCUPATIONAL THERAPY EDUCATION, RESEARCH, AND PRACTICE

Education

- For educational curricula to include topics on the global underpinnings of gender inequities in order to generate nuanced understandings of human occupations and experiences of disability beyond the global North.
- For educational programs to provide opportunities for students to critically consider the complex context in which individual and collective occupations and experiences of agency and disability are shaped by, and can be oppressed through, the complex intersection of diverse social identities and broader structural factors.

Research

- For researchers to be self-reflexive and understand the complexities of social categories and intersecting forms of oppression and discrimination.

- For researchers to engage with policy makers early on and throughout the research process in order for findings to be successfully utilized and translated into practical benefits.
- For researchers to use mixed-methods in order to capture the context and complexity of research participants' lived realities.

Practice

- For occupational therapists/scientists to critically reflect on their social location within broader relations of power within their society and how these locations influence their being, knowing, and doing.
- For occupational therapists/scientists to reflect on ways to question and disrupt the gendered and subjective nature of taken-for-granted occupations.
- For occupational therapists/scientists to enact social conversations to give visibility to how relations of power shape occupational opportunities.

RECOMMENDED READINGS

Angell, A. M. (2012). Occupation-centered analysis of social difference: Contributions to a socially responsive occupational science. *Journal of Occupational Science, 21*(2), 104–116. https://doi.org/10.1080/14427591.2012.711230

Collins, P. H., & Bilge, S. (2016). *Intersectionality*. Polity Press.

Gerlach, A. J. (2015). Sharpening our critical edge: Occupational therapy in the context of "marginalized populations." *Canadian Journal of Occupational Therapy, 82*(4), 245–253. https://doi.org/10.1177/0008417415571730

Huff, S., Laliberte Rudman, D., Magalhães, L., & Lawson, E. (2018). "Africana womanism": Implications for transformative scholarship in occupational science. *Journal of Occupational Science, 25*(4), 554–565. https://doi.org/10.1080/14427591.2018.1493614

Leavy, P., & Harris, A. (2019). *Contemporary feminist research from theory to practice*. The Guildford Press.

TED TALKS

Adichie, C. (2009, July). *The danger of a single story* [Video]. TED Conferences. https://www.ted.com/talks/chimamanda_adichie_the_danger_of_a_single_story

Crenshaw, K. W. (2016, October). *The urgency of intersectionality* [Video]. TED Conferences. https://www.ted.com/talks/kimberle_crenshaw_the_urgency_of_intersectionality

REFERENCES

Ahmed, S. (2017). *Living a feminist life*. Duke University Press.

Anderson, K. (2010). Affirmations of an Indigenous feminist. In C. Suzack, S. M. Huhndorf, J. Perreault, & J. Barman (Eds.), *Indigenous women and feminism: Politics, activism, culture* (pp. 82–91). UBC Press.

Anderson, K. (2016). *A recognition of being: Reconstructing Native womanhood* (2nd ed.). Sumach Press.

Angell, A. M. (2012). Occupation-centered analysis of social difference: Contributions to a socially responsive occupational science. *Journal of Occupational Science, 21*(2), 104–116. https://doi.org/10.1080/14427591.2012.711230

Arvin, M., Tuck, E., & Morrill, A. (2013). Decolonizing feminism: Challenging connections between settler colonialism and heteropatriarchy. *Feminist Formations, 25*(1), 8–34. https://doi.org/10.1353/ff.2013.0006

Bastos, J. L., Harnois, C. E., & Paradies, Y. C. (2018). Health care barriers, racism, and intersectionality in Australia. *Social Science and Medicine, 199*, 209–281. https://doi.org/10.1016/j.socscimed.2017.05.010

Ben-Moshe, L., & Magaña, S. (2014). An introduction to race, gender, and disability: Intersectionality, disabilities studies, and families of color. *Women, Gender, and Families of Color, 2*(2), 105–114. https://doi.org/10.5406/womgenfamcol.2.2.0105

Black, R. H., Loukas, K. M., Froehlich, J., & MacRae, N. (1992). Feminism: An inclusive perspective. *American Journal of Occupational Therapy, 46*, 967–970. https://doi.org/10.5014/ajot.46.11.967

Bucik, A., Ptolemy, A., & Simpson, A. (2017). *Canada: Discrimination and violence against LGBQTI2S persons with disabilities.* https://tbinternet.ohchr.org/Treaties/CEDAW/Shared%20Documents/CAN/INT_CEDAW_NGO_CAN_25380_E.pdf

Bunjun, B. (2010). Feminist organizations and intersectionality: Contesting hegemonic feminism. *Atlantis: A Women's Studies Journal, 34*(2), 115–126.

Collins, P. H. (2009). *Black feminist thought: Knowledge, consciousness, and the politics of empowerment* (2nd ed.). Routledge.

Collins, P. H., & Bilge, S. (2016). *Intersectionality.* Polity Press.

Connell, R. (2014). Rethinking gender from the South. *Feminist Studies, 40*(3), 518–539. https://www.jstor.org/stable/10.15767/feministstudies.40.3.518?seq=1

Crenshaw, K. W. (1989). Demarginalizing the intersection of race and sex: A Black feminist critique of antidiscrimination doctrine, feminist theory and antiracist politics. *University of Chicago Legal Forum, 1989*(8), 138–167.

de Sousa Santos, B. (2015). *Epistemologies of the South: Justice against epistemicide.* Routledge.

Duke, T. (2011). Lesbian, gay, bisexual, and transgender youth with disabilities: A meta-synthesis. *Journal of LGBT Youth, 8*(1), 1–52. https://doi.org/10.1080/19361653.2011.519181

Farias, L., Laliberte Rudman, D., & Magalhães, L. (2016). Illustrating the importance of critical epistemology to realize the promise of occupational justice. *OTJR: Occupation, Participation and Health, 36*(4), 234–243. https://doi.org/10.1177/1539449216665561

Frank, G. (1992). Opening feminist histories of occupational therapy. *American Journal of Occupational Therapy, 46*, 989–999. https://doi.org/10.5014/ajot.46.11.989

Freire, P. (1985). *The politics of education: Culture, power, and liberation.* Greenwood Publishing Group.

Freire, P. (1997). Cultural action and conscientization. *Harvard Educational Review, 68*(3), 499–521. https://doi.org/10.17763/haer.40.3.h76250x720j43175

Galvaan, R. (2015). The contextually situated nature of occupational choice: Marginalized young adolescents' experiences in South Africa. *Journal of Occupational Science, 22*(1), 39–53. https://doi.org/10.1080/14427591.2014.912124

Gerlach, A. J. (2015). Sharpening our critical edge: Occupational therapy in the context of "marginalized populations." *Canadian Journal of Occupational Therapy, 82*(4), 245–253. https://doi.org/10.1177/0008417415571730

Gerlach, A. J. (2018). Thinking and researching relationally: Enacting decolonizing methodologies with an Indigenous early childhood program in Canada. *International Journal of Qualitative Methods, 17*(1), 1–8. https://doi.org/10.1177/1609406918776075

Gerlach, A. J., Browne, A. J., Sinha, V., & Elliot, D. E. (2017). Navigating structural violence with Indigenous families: The contested terrain of early childhood intervention and the child welfare system in Canada. *International Indigenous Policy Journal, 8*(3), 1–23. https://doi.org/10.18584/iipj.2017.8.3.6

Gerlach, A. J., Browne, A. J., & Suto, M. J. (2014). A critical reframing of play in relation to Indigenous children in Canada. *Journal of Occupational Science, 21*(3), 243–258. https://doi.org/10.1080/14427 591.2014.908818

Gerlach, A. J., Browne, A. J., & Suto, M. J. (2018). Relational approaches to fostering health equity for Indigenous children through early childhood intervention. *Health Sociology Review, 27*(1), 104–119. https://doi.org/10.1080/14461242.2016.1231582

Gerlach, A. J., Teachman, G., Laliberte Rudman, D., Huot, S., & Aldrich, R. (2017). Expanding beyond individualism: Engaging critical perspectives on occupation. *Scandinavian Journal of Occupational Therapy, 25*(1), 35–43. https://doi.org/10.1080/11038128.2017.1327616

Gkiouleka, A., Huijts, T., Beckfield, J., & Bambra, C. (2018). Understanding the micro and macro politics of health: Inequalities, intersectionality & institutions: A research agenda. *Social Science & Medicine, 200,* 92–98. https://doi.org/10.1016/j.socscimed.2018.01.025

Green, J. (2017). *Making space for Indigenous feminism.* Fernwood.

Green, M. A., Evans, C. R., & Subramanian, S. V. (2017). Can intersectionality theory enrich population health research? *Social Science & Medicine: Medical Anthropology, 178,* 214–216. https://doi.org/10.1016/j.socscimed.2017.02.029

Guajardo, A., Kronenberg, F., & Ramugondo, E. L. (2015). Southern occupational therapies: Emerging identities, epistemologies and practices. *South African Journal of Occupational Therapy, 45*(1), 3–10. https://doi.org/10.17159/2310-3833/2015/v45n01a2

Hammell, K. W. (2009). Sacred texts: A sceptical exploration of the assumptions underpinning theories of occupation. *Canadian Journal of Occupational Therapy, 76,* 6–13. https://doi.org/10.1177/000841740907600105

Hammell, K. W. (2011). Resisting theoretical imperialism in the disciplines of occupational science and occupational therapy. *British Journal of Occupational Therapy, 74,* 27–33. https://doi.org/10.4276/03 0802211X12947686093602

Hankivsky, O. (2014). *Intersectionality 101.* San Francisco University.

Hirschmann, N. J. (2013). Disability, feminism, and intersectionality: A critical approach. *Radical Philosophy Review, 16*(2), 649–662. https://doi.org/10.5840/radphilrev201316247

Hocking, C. (2012). Occupations through the looking glass: Reflecting on occupational scientists' ontological assumptions. In G. Whiteford & C. Hocking (Eds.), *Occupational science: Society, inclusion, participation* (pp. 54–66). Wiley-Blackwell.

hooks, b. (2000). *Feminist theory: From margin to center* (2nd ed.). South End Press Classics.

Huff, S., Laliberte Rudman, D., Magalhães, L., & Lawson, E. (2018). "Africana womanism": Implications for transformative scholarship in occupational science. *Journal of Occupational Science, 25*(4), 554–565. https://doi.org/10.1080/14427591.2018.1493614

Huhndorf, S. M., & Suzack, C. (2010). Indigenous feminism: Theorizing the issues. In C. Suzack, S. M. Huhndorf, J. Perreault, & J. Barman (Eds.), *Indigenous women and feminism: Politics, activism, culture* (pp. 1–17). UBC Press.

Huot, S., & Veronis, L. (2018). Examining the role of minority community spaces for enabling migrants' performance of intersectional identities through occupation. *Journal of Occupational Science, 25*(1), 37–50. https://doi.org/10.1080/14427591.2017.1379427

Kuokkanen, R. (2007). Myths and realities of Sami women: A post-colonial feminist analysis for the decolonization and transformation of Sami society. In J. Green (Ed.), *Making space for Indigenous feminism* (pp. 72–92). Fernwood.

Laliberte Rudman, D. (2013). Enacting the critical potential of occupational science: Problematizing the "individualizing of occupation." *Journal of Occupational Science, 20,* 298–313. https://doi.org/10.108 0/14427591.2013.803434

LaRocque, E. (2007). Métis and feminist: Ethical reflections on feminism, human rights and decolonization. In J. Green (Ed.), *Making space for Indigenous feminism* (pp. 53–71). Fernwood.

LaRocque, E. (2009). Reflections on cultural continuity: Contuinuity through Aboriginal women's writings. In G. G. Valaskakis, E. Guimond, & M. D. Stout (Eds.), *Restoring the balance: First Nations women, community, and culture* (pp. 149–174). University of Manitoba Press.

Leavy, P., & Harris, A. (2019). *Contemporary feminist research from theory to practice.* The Guildford Press.

Lorde, A. (2007). Learning from the 60s. In A. Lorde (Ed.), *Sister outsider: Essays & speeches by Audre Lorde* (p. 138). Crossing Press.

Mann, S. A., & Patterson, A. S. (2016). *Reading feminist theory: From modernity to postmodernity.* Oxford University Press.

Monture-Angus, P. (1995). *Thunder in my soul: A Mohawk woman speaks.* Fernwood.

Moodley, J., & Graham, L. (2015). The importance of intersectionality in disability and gender studies. *Agenda, 29*(2), 24–33. https://doi.org/10.1080/10130950.2015.1041802

Olivares-Aising, D. (2018). Occupational justice and human scale development: A theoretical integration approach. *Journal of Occupational Science, 25*(4), 474–485. https://doi.org/10.1080/14427591.2018.1513780

Pausé, C. J., Powell, K., Waitere, H., Wright, J., & Gilling, M. (2012). We say what we are and we do what we say: Feminisms in educational practice in Aotearoa New Zealand. *Feminist Review, 102*(1), 79–96. https://doi.org/10.1057/fr.2011.50

Pollard, N., & Walsh, S. (2000). Occupational therapy, gender and mental health: An inclusive perspective? *British Journal of Occupational Therapy, 63*(9), 425–431. https://doi.org/10.1177/030802260006300904

Richman, L. S., & Zucker, A. N. (2019). Quantifying intersectionality: An important advancement for health inequality research. *Social Science, 226,* 246–248. https://doi.org/10.1016/j.socscimed.2019.01.036

Rivas-Quarneti, N., Movilla-Fernández, M. J., & Magalhães, L. (2018). Immigrant women's occupational struggles during the socioeconomic crisis in Spain: Broadening occupational justice conceptualization. *Journal of Occupational Science, 25*(1), 6–18. https://doi.org/10.1080/14427591.2017.1366355

Sakellariou, D., & Pollard, N. (2017). *Occupational therapies without borders: Integrating justice with practice* (2nd ed.). Elsevier.

Smith, A. (2009). Indigenous feminism without apology. In U. Minnesota (Ed.), *Reflections and resources for deconstructing colonial mentality: A sourcebook compiled by the Unsettling Minnesota collective* (pp. 159–161). September.

St. Denis, V. (2007). Feminism is for everybody: Aboriginal women, feminism and diversity. In J. Green (Ed.), *Making space for indigenous feminism* (pp. 33–52). Fernwood.

Suzack, C., Huhndorf, S. M., Perreault, J., & Barman, J. (Eds.). (2010). *Indigenous women and feminism: Politics, activism, culture.* UBC Press.

van Herk, K. A., Smith, D., & Andrew, C. (2011). Examining our privileges and oppressions: Incorporating an intersectionality paradigm into nursing. *Nursing Inquiry, 18,* 29–39. https://doi.org/10.1111/j.1440-1800.2011.00539.x

Viruell-Fuentes, E. A., Miranda, P. Y., & Abdulrahim, S. (2012). More than culture: Structural racism, intersectionality theory, and immigrant health. *Social Science & Medicine: Medical Anthropology, 75,* 2099–2106. https://doi.org/10.1016/j.socscimed.2011.12.037

Zavala, M. (2013). What do we mean by decolonizing research strategies? Lessons from decolonizing, Indigenous research projects in New Zealand and Latin America. *Decolonization: Indigeneity, Education & Society, 2*(1), 55–71.

Zimmerman, D. D. (2015). Young Arab Muslim women's agency challenging Western feminism. *Affilia, 30*(2), 145–157. https://doi.org/10.1177/0886109914546126

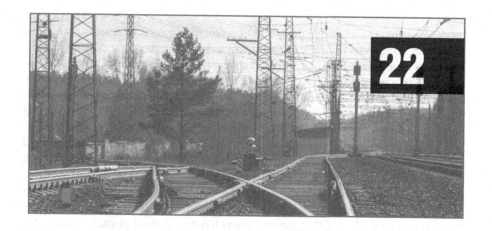

Capable *and* Occupied

How the Capabilities Approach Can Enrich the "Occupation" Discourse

Ganesh M. Babulal, PhD, OTD, MSCI, MOT, OTR/L
Parul Bakhshi, PhD, DEA (MPhil)
Jean-Francois Trani, PhD, MSc, MPhil

INTRODUCTION

The Capabilities Approach (CA) is positioned broadly in the traditional schools of thought of social justice as well as human rights. However, it also firmly states that it is an "approach": a framework that aims to provide a space and a lexicon that encourages policy discussions and dilemmas linked to the operationalization of values of equality and equity. In the 1979 Tanner Lectures, Amartya Sen, the originator of the approach, asked the fundamental question, "Equality of what?" (Sen, 1979), as an invitation to consider values and entitlements with a specific focus on questions of social justice. In the 1990s, Sen, alongside another economist, Mahbub ul Haq, proposed the Human Development Report (HDR) to be published each year to gauge the progress that has been made in development. The aim was to contest neoliberal utilitarian views that posit economic growth as the goal or end of development, with human progress being a means to achieve

Taff, S. D. (Ed.). *Philosophy and Occupational Therapy:
Informing Education, Research, and Practice* (pp. 221-231).
© 2021 Taylor & Francis Group.

monetary gains. The utilitarian perspective presented economic indicators, such as the gross domestic product (GDP), as the main yardstick to establish a ranking of individuals or nations. The HDR contended that people should be at the center of development and that questions of equality should be assessed in considerations of progress. Recognizing that to counter the GDP there is a need for a quantifiable and qualifiable measure, the HDR presented the Human Development Index, which is composed of both a measure of economic growth and also a measure of health and education to take into account issues of equality. However, Sen also strongly advocated for the need to engage in complex discussions around human flourishing and well-being through critical dialogue and debate. As a result, the literature around the CA, its relevance, and its operationalization have been ongoing in bodies such as the Human Development and Capabilities Association, as well as in international policies and programs. In the past 5 years, the OXFAM (2019) annual report has documented in stark numbers the yawning chasm between the increasingly deprived majority and the minuscule group controlling global economic wealth. The relevance of the CA is indisputable in addressing basic inequities (in health and education) as well as the new challenges that must be addressed, such as climate chaos.

CAPABILITIES APPROACH IN OCCUPATIONAL THERAPY

Occupational therapy celebrated its centennial anniversary in 2017, and with more than a century's growth, occupational therapy practice is now challenged to meet the novel and complex demands of a more integrated and global community of patients, clients, and stakeholders. The field is tasked with balancing questions of individualistic vs. collectivistic well-being and how to navigate a paradigm shift in reframing itself from a largely medical model identity and foci toward more socially and context-sensitive practices within communities. The field recognizes the challenge of moving beyond curing physical problems through traditional rehabilitation to address more distal and universal constructs such as well-being, equity, and multidimensional meaning. Occupational therapy's locus is occupation, where activities "occupy" time and structure the foundation of daily routine. Occupation as a seminal construct is arcuate and has lexically been referred to as a noun, verb, adjective, and adverb, and used interchangeably to describe participation, activities, and engagement. The amorphous nature of occupation has led to a lack of a clear definition, misunderstanding, and misappropriation, in particular around philosophical considerations and practical use. As a result, the application of occupation in dynamic cultural, social, religious, and political environs remains limited. Some recent philosophical discourses outside of the United States have begun examining the application of the CA to help occupational therapy transcend its internal limitation to reach broader communities by incorporating and applying core concepts of the CA (Hammell, 2015; Taff et al., 2014).

MAIN CONCEPTS OF THE CAPABILITIES APPROACH

The Fundamentals: Capabilities and Functionings

At the very core of the CA is the value placed on human well-being, which is viewed as "freedoms" that constitute the end purpose of development and progress rather than a mere means for reaping economic benefits. In the 1990s, as international institutions moved toward viewing progress solely in terms of neoliberal capitalism, the need to put human beings at the center of discourses became not just an academic impetus but a social justice necessity (Sen, 2000a). As a consequence, the CA provided a valuable space within which to defend the rights of vulnerable people and groups in order to construct the scaffolding for holding governments and other institutions accountable for principles of equity and social justice. However, there has been much debate about the scope of these concepts.

It is often stated that capabilities are "beings and doings that people have reason to value" (Sen, 1999). This definition is stated in a number of papers as the essence of the CA. However, the distinction between capabilities and functionings, which is at the very core of the approach, presents many nuances and raises essential questions of validity and relevance in various contexts. The first distinction that must be noted is that a "functioning" is fundamentally different from a "commodity" as viewed in traditional welfare economics, because a functioning represents a choice, or "freedom," in the capabilities lexicon (Robeyns, 2005). The choice is made through the process of reasoning and placing value on choices. The "capability" represents the various choices that are plausible for an individual at a given time.

Beyond the theoretical rhetoric, this distinction is paramount to considerations of operationalization for policy and assessment. It is argued that social policies should remain focused on expanding choices or capabilities and not on selected functionings that are predefined. In terms of assessment, the debates around application of the CA in measurement have been ongoing. Amartya Sen has refused to predefine any set of capabilities that could be viewed as universal and constitutive of a good human life. Pushing back, Martha Nussbaum has proposed a list of central capabilities that can be used as a yardstick for evaluation in most contexts. The literature around "well-being," "satisfaction," and "happiness" has proliferated through the construction of various scales and measures. However, it is not always possible to define the extent to which these perspectives have influenced effective policy.

Finally, the concept of "basic capabilities" has been specified as "the freedom to do some basic things that are necessary for survival and to avoid or escape poverty" (Sen, as cited in Robeyns, 2005, p. 93). The basic capabilities are also instrumental in achieving other, more complex capabilities that may be valued. For example, health and adequate nutrition are foundational in achieving social affiliation. However, in terms of assessment, tools and methods often remain focused on achieved functioning, especially in situations of extreme deprivation, without attempting to gauge the wider capabilities.

Agency and Adaptive Preferences: Challenges for Assessment and Accountability

If the individual is central to the development process, then the yardstick for assessment must reflect human flourishing in terms of choice or freedoms. The latter requires agency, which ensures that people "are engaged in actions that are congruent with their values" (Alkire, 2008, p. 31) and are seen as the main decision-makers in their own lives. Agency is thus the reflection of not just the chosen functioning, but also the freedom to make that choice within a larger capability set. Agency allows individuals to pursue goals that they have reason to value; it also constitutes an assessment nightmare, as it cannot simply be observed. As a consequence, well-being and satisfaction are often considered to be proxies for agency, even though the essence of the concept is often lost in assessment efforts.

For comprehensive consideration of the challenges of operationalizing the CA for assessment and accountability, it is important to include and understand the concept of adaptive preferences (APs), which can help somewhat to nuance the discussions and move them out of purely theoretical realms. APs are constrained choices that are made in restricted contexts that undermine freedoms. There is a real danger in confusing the two concepts—APs and choice based on agency—within the assessment space: most assessment endeavors fail to make the distinction and compound the two.

Especially in disability discourses, the clarification of terms requires special attention. "Unfavourable social and economic circumstances as well as lifelong habituation to adverse environment might induce people to accept current negative situations" (Teschl & Comim, 2005, p. 230). Sen claims that adaptation is closely linked to questions of identity and associated social arrangements. One example of this is the traditional roles that women and men are assigned and how these shape the perception of well-being in many societies. Distinguishing APs from choices based on agency requires a profound understanding of cultural norms and social practices, as well as awareness that valued achieved functionings can often be compounded with collective expectations. For example, assessments of self-esteem as inherent to individual well-being are based on a belief that self-esteem is valued as an individual trait. However, in reality, self-esteem may not be a highly valued trait in societies where the collective supersedes the individual.

Collective Capabilities and Social Exclusion: A Need to Expand Concepts

Although Sen recognized that many capabilities are socially based, he stopped short of defining collective capabilities (CCs). However, some authors have stated that there is inherent utility in defining CCs that are valued not by individuals but by groups that share social identities and goals. The argument put forth is that these CCs are not merely an aggregation of individual capabilities but instead constitute freedoms that are different in nature (e.g., the constitution of women's self-help groups enables them to advocate for rights; Evans, 2002; Ibrahim, 2006). CCs are especially relevant to groups that have faced deprivation and exclusion, as they are essential for building collective agency and empowerment.

Social exclusion provides a collective lens through which to examine collective processes that lead to poverty and deprivation. Sen also puts forth the argument that social exclusion is a dimension of capability deprivation and constitutes a denial of basic human rights (Sen, 2000b). By situating social exclusion not as a question inherent to welfare theories but as a factor within capabilities, space is made for an essential framing of challenges: the onus to "include" vulnerable people and groups is placed on social structures and not on individuals (Klasen, 1999, p. 2). The argument for the value of diversity thus also becomes central to the ability to make use of opportunities provided within a context. Within the field of disability, these discussions become of utmost importance, especially when considering persons with severe and/or mental forms of disability (Dubois & Trani, 2009; Terzi, 2005). In terms of operationalizing the CA for people whose capabilities have been systematically denied, it is essential to consider CCs as a means for creating a space where the most vulnerable can gain a voice.

Changing the Discourse of "Productivity" and "Outcomes" to "Well-Being" and "Meaning"

A central aim of occupational therapy practice remains to restore functional ability, as determined by therapists who have received specialized training and work within an inequitable medical insurance system. The occupational therapy profession largely functions like many other medical professions, rendering treatment services and receiving compensation: a *sine qua non* for the intersection of capitalism and medicine. As a result, occupational therapy has inadvertently narrowed its reach to fit medical and scientific paradigms, and recent research in the United States has focused on functional perspectives with limited consideration of quality of life as determined through standardized scales. Moreover, the illusory concept of participation, as redefined within the medical model, has also been stripped of its philosophical origins of empowerment and challenge to existing power dynamics to be used as a limited outcome through predefined measures that determine achievement (Taff et al., 2014). This progression is an expected development, given the overarching system and reimbursement model, but it becomes untenable when the same occupational therapy practice is applied in contexts that differ from the usual. As discussed earlier, the key barrier occupational therapy needs to surmount is moving beyond merely quantifiable outcomes and increasing demands to demonstrate higher productivity, and instead realigning or recalibrating its focus onto well-being and meaning. The field must evolve and adopt concepts from the CA that synergistically align with its core principles and redefine "occupation" for the new context.

Human Rights and Dignity as the Goal

The CA closely mirrors human rights concerns: both focus closely on questions of dignity. Maintenance of human dignity requires a will to engage with the complexity of human lives, diversity, and inclusion and oppose the prevalence of simplistic utilitarian analyses. The CA is concerned with "capabilities as a space where inequalities should be evaluated" (Fukuda-Parr, 2011, p. 76). Moreover, "the combination of human rights and capabilities could build a pragmatic framework for international accountability for ending poverty" (Vizard, 2007, p. 248). Authors argue here that instead of using a language of outcomes, it is essential to sharpen the focus on entitlements and obligations that value human dignity. Although the capabilities literature does not always clearly define or delineate the concept of "dignity," Nussbaum uses it as the foundation for proposing a list of central basic capabilities that determine a good human life (Nussbaum, 2000). She also posits that dignity should not be just an elusive ideal but a complex attribute of human existence that encompasses questions of respect, agency, and equality (Claassen, 2014). Discourses pertaining to human dignity are essential for the most vulnerable and disempowered and do require more consideration by policy makers and implementers. Without in-depth argumentation, any action will have the potential to be paternalistic, charity-based, and reflective of a handout where dignity is assumed to ensue with a minimal provision of basic needs at best and as a proxy for crossing monetary thresholds at worst. Meeting the goal of preserving and strengthening human dignity calls for respect for agency and commitment to entitlements provided by social groups and collective engagement. A very plausible answer to Sen's question "equality of what?" could be "human dignity."

Dangers of Instrumentalization of a Philosophy

In a number of contexts of practice, such as occupational therapy in the United States, philosophy is often used as a proxy for superficial ethical questions, which themselves are often prompted by considerations that are mostly linked to legal questions with minimal discussion of ethics. The spaces for influence, and the discussions of the fundamental underlying values, are being curbed even within influential spheres of academia. The formats (for funding of research) and the need to be "efficient" in academic discussion and teaching (1-hour formats) have contributed to the weakening and contraction of spaces for argumentation. Complex concepts (such as well-being and empowerment) are thus boxed into five-point, Likert-type scales, and human dignity is at best implied. This reduction of complex philosophical dilemmas leads to a plethora of buzzwords that maintain the illusion that values are mainstreamed when, in reality, they have been stripped of their inherent meanings and are being utilized to serve a predefined agenda (Cornwall, 2007). The concept of "participation" as that word is used in medical assessment is one example of this (Babulal et al., 2015). The danger of this phenomenon, aside from a lack of humility, lies in its failure to ensure that the most deprived populations do not just receive services but are empowered to be agents of change in their own lives.

OPPORTUNITIES FOR OPERATIONALIZING OCCUPATIONAL THERAPY THROUGH A CAPABILITIES LENS

Natural Synergies Between Occupational Therapy and the Capabilities Approach

There has been extensive research and academic discussion pertaining to how the CA can serve as a grid for gauging occupational injustice, deprivation, and even apartheid (Hammell & Beagan, 2017; Pollard et al., 2005). First, let us acknowledge the broader commitment of occupational therapy to concerns of social justice and equity, even though the discipline does not use the Human Rights lexicon (especially in the United States), although the synergies are evident: "occupational rights [are] rights of an individual to experience meaning and enrichment in one's occupations: to participate in a range of occupations for health and social inclusion; to make choices and share decision-making power in daily life; and to receive equal privileges for diverse participation in occupations" (Townsend & Wilcock, 2004, p. 80). Most of the discussions have, however, remained in the domain of morality and values (Hocking, 2017). In terms of operationalization, Nussbaum's list of central capabilities has been viewed as foundational in the occupational justice discourse and with most disempowered groups (Mousavi et al., 2015). At its origins, occupational therapy focused on "doings" and "beings" (capabilities) as well as "becoming" (agency; Wilcock, 1999). However, we argue that the CA has not been analyzed with regard to its aim to influence policy, nor in rethinking assessment beyond predefined outcomes. There is an opportunity to design assessment in the light of a person's agency, as well as awareness of constrained choices or APs, which would more obviously embrace the goals of human dignity and equity. Finally, the CA will be crucial in addressing the new challenges that human societies face: mental illness, growing inequality, and changing human behaviors concerning the urgent dangers of climate change. The CA can also enable discussions around preventive and collective occupations rather than following intervention mentalities (i.e., disaster management).

Capabilities Approach and the Sustainable Development Goals: Where Does Occupational Therapy Fit in?

The transition from the Millennium Development Goals (MDG 2000–2015) to the Sustainable Development Goals (SDG 2015–2030) constituted a profound paradigm shift from the simplistic to the complex, from the individual to the collective, and from siloed views toward comprehensive multidimensional perspectives of life that include not just human lives but also extend to other forms of life. This shift was not merely an ideological one but was also ushered in by a failure to address equality. The example of SDG 4 reflects the evidence-based process behind moving from an overt focus on simplistic outcomes (MDG looked only at access to schools) toward engaging in questions of quality and inclusion. SDG 4 also decisively moves the goalposts from the instrumental value of education as a capability toward an intrinsic recognition of its inherent value in human flourishing. However, the connection between occupational therapy and SDGs has been minimal and should be explored further in order for occupational therapy to remain relevant and connected in an increasingly globalized world.

IMPACT ON UNDERSTANDING OF OCCUPATION AND OCCUPATIONAL ENGAGEMENT

Both the CA and occupational therapy have been accused of using confusing jargon. One of the reasons for the confusion lies in the fact that both have borrowed terms used in lay language and assigned specific functional meanings to them: namely, *capabilities* and *occupations*. The former is closely related to freedom of choices, whereas the latter aims to broaden the understanding of everyday activities by including the meanings that these activities hold for individuals. The capabilities lexicon has been in the past and continues to be debated not just by economists and social policy experts but also by philosophers and grass-roots organizations. However, the term *occupation* has not been sufficiently scrutinized. Few papers discuss definitions, but the majority of definitions use the term itself to explain its meaning; discussions about the underlying philosophical concepts that influence occupational therapy are, for the most part, ignored by practitioners and to some extent by educators. As a consequence, the occupational therapy dialogue occurs for the most part in an academic echo chamber and outside of the specialist views, in lay language, where assumptions are allowed to remain and proliferate.

It is also essential to state that occupational engagement has to be defined not just within a space of individual choices but also with regard to ethical responsibility and accountability. Most often, in terms of practice specifically, though occupational therapists promote advocacy and self-advocacy, the onus for the latter is left to individual choice. However, in high-income countries outside the United States, occupational therapy is shaped within universal health care systems and, as a consequence, can engage more visibly with questions of inequality and discrimination at a collective level.

The new challenges posed by a rapidly changing world will demand more in-depth discussion about values and principles and compel us to focus more closely on ethics and accountability. Climate catastrophe will force debates around collective occupations, moving away from individualistic client-centered perspectives. The proliferation of nationalist governments headed by demagogues across the globe is threatening democratic principles that were thought to be the law of the land. Occupational therapy will need to return to some of the original discussions that gave it its strength, most notably community-based understanding of collective action. "Engagement" will have to move toward empowerment and real participation. For this to occur in the profession, occupational therapists who recognize that part of their job is to fight inequality and injustice will need to leave their comfort zones and delve into politics and policy.

KEY IMPLICATIONS FOR OCCUPATIONAL THERAPY EDUCATION, RESEARCH, AND PRACTICE

Education

- Recognize the nonsustainability and irrelevance of teaching occupational therapy as a "technique" without using a social justice lens to focus on equity, especially in the United States.

- Carve out space within overtechnical curriculums for critical discourses on social injustice, so that the next generation can challenge practices and devise new pathways to address these crucial challenges.

Research

- Reduce the hypocrisy of evidence-based practice and policy. The research gold standard, which considers randomized controlled trials and meta-analyses to be the most useful for producing information that can be relevant for action, is a fallacy and a false promise, as well as a complete negation of human rights and a failure to address inequalities and inequities. This main challenge in research is not limited to occupational therapy but applies as well to other medical and social service professions. Qualitative narratives, mixed-methods, and systems thinking must be promoted as crucial means toward ensuring that research is not viewed as just an academic exercise but as a way to find relevant solutions to messy social problems.

- Revise the funding system for U.S.-based occupational therapy, which currently largely excludes research of qualitative community-based perspectives. It is time to look outside to see what can we learn from lower- and middle-income countries where resources (financial and human) are scarce and where community-based initiatives have been in place for some time. Research funding is required for this. However, there is also an opportunity for humility through promoting dialogues with countries that have contextually defined occupational therapy.

Practice

- Overcome the resistance to examining collective capabilities and collective occupations, and to imagining that sometimes individual well-being cannot be the center of attention. Climate-change chaos will force occupational therapy to adapt or become obsolete.

- Incorporate social justice and human rights and work in collaboration with other professions. There can be no sustainable occupational therapy without this. The refugee crisis, for instance, calls for a multidimensional approach that includes medical experts, legal experts, and persons from relevant social services. The roles each of these can play will transcend the boundaries of their profession, and allow them to devise innovative ways to fight human rights violations.

- Put the question of the identity of occupational therapists to the test in coming decades. A willingness to engage in larger social debates and assume definite positions will be demanded; the excuse of being "client-centered" will just not be acceptable anymore.

RECOMMENDED READINGS

Hammell, K. W. (2015). Quality of life, participation and occupational rights: A capabilities perspective. *Australian Occupational Therapy Journal, 62*(2), 78–85. https://doi.org/10.1111/1440-1630.12183

Mousavi, T., Forwell, S., Dharamsi, S., & Dean, E. (2015). The historical shift towards human rights in occupational therapy with special reference to the capabilities approach and its implications. *World Federation of Occupational Therapists Bulletin, 71*(2), 81–87. https://doi.org/10.1179/2056607715Y.0000000005

Sen, A. (1999). *Development as freedom.* Oxford University Press.

Taff, S. D., Bakhshi, P., & Babulal, G. M. (2014). The accountability–well-being–ethics framework: A new philosophical foundation for occupational therapy. *Canadian Journal of Occupational Therapy, 81*(5), 320–329. https://doi.org/10.1177/0008417414546742

REFERENCES

Alkire, S. (2008). Using the capability approach: Prospective and evaluative analyses. In F. Comim, M. Qizilbash, & S. Alkire (Eds.), *The capability approach: Concepts, measures and applications* (pp. 26–50). Cambridge University Press.

Babulal, G. M., Bakhshi, P., Kopriva, S., Ali, S. A., Goette, S. A., & Trani, J.-F. (2015). Measuring participation for persons with mental illness: A systematic review assessing relevance of existing scales for low and middle income countries. *BMC Psychology, 3*(1), 36. https://doi.org/10.1186/s40359-015-0093-0

Claassen, R. (2014). Human dignity in the capability approach. In M. Düwell, J. Braarvig, R. Brownsword, & D. Mieth (Eds.), *The Cambridge handbook of human dignity: Interdisciplinary perspectives* (pp. 240–249). Cambridge University Press.

Cornwall, A. (2007). Buzzwords and fuzzwords: Deconstructing development discourse. *Development in Practice, 17*(4–5), 471–484. https://doi.org/10.1080/09614520701469302

Dubois, J. L., & Trani, J. F. (2009). Extending the capability paradigm to address the complexity of disability. *ALTER European Journal of Disability Research, 3*(3), 192–218. https://doi.org/10.1016/j.alter.2009.04.003

Evans, P. (2002). Collective capabilities, culture, and Amartya Sen's development as freedom. *Studies in Comparative International Development, 37*(2), 54–60. https://doi.org/10.1007/BF02686261

Fukuda-Parr, S. (2011). The metrics of human rights: Complementarities of the human development and capabilities approach. *Journal of Human Development and Capabilities, 12*(1), 73–89. https://doi.org/10.1080/19452829.2011.541750

Hammell, K. W. (2015). Quality of life, participation and occupational rights: A capabilities perspective. *Australian Occupational Therapy Journal, 62*(2), 78–85. https://doi.org/10.1111/1440-1630.12183

Hammell, K. W., & Beagan, B. (2017). Occupational injustice: A critique/L'injustice occupationnelle: une critique. *Canadian Journal of Occupational Therapy, 84*(1), 58–68. https://doi.org/10.1177/0008417416638858

Hocking, C. (2017). Occupational justice as social justice: The moral claim for inclusion. *Journal of Occupational Science, 24*(1), 29–42. https://doi.org/10.1080/14427591.2017.1294016

Ibrahim, S. S. (2006). From individual to collective capabilities: The capability approach as a conceptual framework for self-help. *Journal of Human Development, 7*(3), 397–416. https://doi.org/10.1080/14649880600815982

Klasen, S. (1999). Social exclusion, children and education: Conceptual and measurement issues. *European Studies, 3*(4), 1–24. https://doi.org/10.1080/14616690120112208

Mousavi, T., Forwell, S., Dharamsi, S., & Dean, E. (2015). Occupational therapists' views of Nussbaum's practical reason and affiliation capabilities. *Occupational Therapy in Mental Health, 31*(1), 1–18. https://doi.org/10.1080/0164212X.2014.1003265

Nussbaum, M. (2000). *Women and human development: The capabilities approach.* Cambridge University Press.

OXFAM International. (2019). *5 shocking facts about extreme global inequality and how to even it up.* https://www.oxfam.org/en/5-shocking-facts-about-extreme-global-inequality-and-how-even-it

Pollard, N., Alsop, A., & Kronenberg, F. (2005). Reconceptualising occupational therapy. *British Journal of Occupational Therapy, 68*(11), 524–526. https://doi.org/10.1177/030802260506801107

Robeyns, I. (2005). The capability approach: A theoretical survey. *Journal of Human Development, 6*(1), 93–114. https://doi.org/10.1080/146498805200034266

Sen, A. (1979). Equality of what? The Tanner lecture on human values. https://tannerlectures.utah.edu/_documents/a-to-z/s/sen80.pdf

Sen, A. (1999). *Development as freedom.* Oxford University Press.

Sen, A. (2000a). A decade of human development. *Journal of Human Development, 1*(1), 17–23. https://doi.org/10.1080/14649880050008746

Sen, A. (2000b). *Social exclusion: Concept, application, and scrutiny.* https://www.adb.org/sites/default/files/publication/29778/social-exclusion.pdf

Taff, S. D., Bakhshi, P., & Babulal, G. M. (2014). The accountability–well-being–ethics framework: A new philosophical foundation for occupational therapy. *Canadian Journal of Occupational Therapy, 81*(5), 320–329. https://doi.org/10.1177/0008417414546742

Terzi, L. (2005). A capability perspective on impairment, disability and special needs. *Theory and Research in Education, 3*(2), 197–223. https://doi.org/10.1177/1477878505053301

Teschl, M., & Comim, F. (2005). Adaptive preferences and capabilities: Some preliminary conceptual explorations. *Review of Social Economy, 63*(2), 229–247. https://doi.org/10.1080/00346760500130374

Townsend, E., & Wilcock, A. (2004). Occupational justice and client-centred practice: A dialogue in progress. *Canadian Journal of Occupational Therapy, 71*(2), 75–87. https://doi.org/10.1177/000841740407100203

Vizard, P. (2007). Specifying and justifying a basic capability set: Should the international human rights framework be given a more direct role? *Oxford Development Studies, 35*(3), 225–250. https://doi.org/10.1080/13600810701514787

Wilcock, A. A. (1999). Reflections on doing, being and becoming. *Australian Occupational Therapy Journal, 46*(1), 1–11. https://doi.org/10.1046/j.1440-1630.1999.00174.x

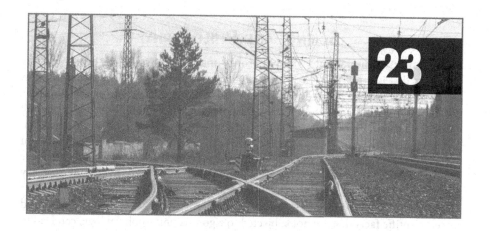

How Philosophy Can Support Occupational Therapy's Relevance in the 21st Century

Steven D. Taff, PhD, OTR/L, FNAP, FAOTA
Moses N. Ikiugu, PhD, OTR/L, FAOTA
Jyothi Gupta, PhD, OTR/L, FAOTA

INTRODUCTION

Occupational therapy is a practice discipline. As such, occupational therapy practitioners value "doing" as their primary *modus operandi*, particularly given that their principal focus is the enhancement of occupational participation. For some time now, coupled with this value of doing has been the profession's push for evidence-based practice, as occupational therapy practitioners strive for acceptance among other highly skilled health care professions (American Occupational Therapy, 2019). Given this focus of the profession on establishing itself as a science-informed profession by emphasizing practice that is supported by research evidence, why should philosophy matter? After all, in the day-to-day work of therapists, philosophy will not inform a practitioner on how to perform specific intervention procedures, nor whether those procedures are effective in producing desired results.

Taff, S. D. (Ed.). *Philosophy and Occupational Therapy:*
Informing Education, Research, and Practice (pp. 233-243).
© 2021 Taylor & Francis Group.

SCIENCE AND PHILOSOPHY

To answer the important "why philosophy matters" question, we begin with the argument that it is not possible to have a science that is not informed by philosophy. In the first place, it is philosophy that enables us to raise questions about possibilities of a future reality, which then, at the right time, can be tested through scientific experimentation (Payne, 2015). For example, questions raised by Darwin and even earlier by Aristotle and others about the genesis of organisms, which were in the realm of metaphysics, were not answerable until many years later when the genetic structure was discovered (Pray, 2008). Therefore, a profession that is limited to scientific inquiry is very much stifled and not in a position to explore "possibilities which enlarge our thoughts and free them from the tyranny of custom" (Payne, 2015, p. 8). In the second place, scientific facts that are not subjected to rigorous philosophical logic can lead to wrong conclusions. Philosophical logic demands that sound conclusions about reality be based on true premises. Scientific inquiry provides those premises. However, those premises must be plausible in order to lead to valid conclusions. For example, if we examine the proposition that participation in human occupation leads to good health and well-being, the logical argument could be presented as follows:

a. People who participate in salutogenic occupations are healthy and feel good

b. Javier participates in salutogenic occupations

c. Therefore, Javier is healthy and feels good

Scientifically, we can test this proposition by having Javier participate in an occupation and then measuring Javier's health and well-being. If Javier is healthy and experiences (or reports a feeling of) well-being after participating in that occupation, scientifically we can make a case that our proposition about the connection of meaningful occupations to well-being is supported. However, this conclusion would be predicated on the assumption that we determine and measure "salutogenic occupations," "health," and "well-being" correctly (so that the premise is true). Only then can our conclusions have validity. Such analysis, including how we arrive at what is "meaningful," is in fact based on philosophical inquiry. That is why for many years, philosophy and science were indistinguishable, and in fact, science was referred to as "natural philosophy" (Massimi, 2009). This was the case until after Immanuel Kant's philosophical epoch, when science and philosophy split, with each becoming a specialized area of inquiry. Therefore, even a practice discipline such as occupational therapy cannot dispense with philosophy. If we situate inquiry without a foundational philosophy, we run the risk of using science to answer the wrong questions, thus producing evidence that does not support the validity of the profession.

This argument leads to the conclusion that there are many ways in which the various branches of philosophy can help occupational therapy raise fundamental questions that are critical to the identity of the profession. Ontologically, philosophical inquiry can help us define ourselves clearly as a profession by answering questions such as: What is our essence as a profession? Why do we exist? Why/How are we different from any other profession? Epistemologically, we can explore questions such as: What is the nature of knowledge in our professional perspective? How are we to acquire relevant professional knowledge? Ethical questions with which we struggle and, therefore, can be informed by philosophy could be: What value do we add to human existence? What ought we to do as professionals? What ought we not to do as professionals?

AN ONTOLOGICAL PERSPECTIVE OF OCCUPATIONAL THERAPY

Who are we as a profession? Many scholars have struggled to answer this question over the years of our existence as a profession. Hooper and Wood (2002) trace the alternating priorities the profession has placed on structuralist and pragmatist philosophical approaches to guide research and practice since its inception in 1917. Within this context, occupational therapy continues to be influenced in many ways by the medical model, and thus has taken to science as the defining foundation of the profession. Science, as rooted in a realist and objectivist paradigm, is—and should remain—a foundational aspect of occupational therapy. In other words, we see ourselves primarily as a science-based profession. However, science alone is not sufficient to improve the human condition or to differentiate us from other professional disciplines such as physical therapy or social work. Science is precise, rigorous, and yields impressive results. Nevertheless, as Ortega y Gasset (1960) observes, "science wins these admirable qualities at the cost of maintaining itself on a plane of secondary problems . . . science is only a meager portion of the mind and the organism" (p. 65). Something more than the purely empirical truth of science is needed: an element which illuminates the subjectively human aspects of everyday life. Again, Ortega y Gasset (1960) is instructive in arguing that what we need is a "complete perspective, with foreground and background, not a partial landscape, not a horizon from which the lure of the great distances has been cut away. Lacking a set of cardinal points, our footsteps would lack direction" (p. 66). Here we suggest that philosophy provides those cardinal points which offer guidance to approaching life on a daily basis, to improving the human condition through embracing and using science and philosophy together to provide a more complete and true understanding of the reality of humans as occupational beings.

Put simply, as argued earlier in this chapter, science *needs* philosophy. Science advances through revolutions, or paradigm shifts, that fundamentally alter its nature and priorities (Kuhn, 1962/1996). Paradigms are essentially ways of understanding the world and are inherently philosophical in nature (Artigas, 2001), exploring possibilities that may not have been tested through scientific inquiry. Therefore, it is clear that philosophy is an equally valuable form of inquiry to inform scientific insights and is key to the development of the science of occupational therapy itself. However, what is the value of philosophy to the profession in more practical terms as situated-in-the-world? We suggest that philosophy can serve as a driving force supporting the *relevance* of occupational therapy, particularly as we move forward in an era defined by rapid change and uncertain future, shifting perspectives of knowledge, and focus on the distinct value of competing professions.

Dunning (1973) suggested that the "argument for excellence" (p. 18) in occupational therapy consists of the delivery of high-quality services, continuous improvement in practice and theory, and reconciliation between theories. Philosophy, Dunning contends, contributes to both professional excellence and perhaps its very survival. In the modern landscape of health care, professions must also demonstrate their distinct value to the people and populations they serve. A key contributor to sustaining a profession is society's perception of *relevance*. Coville (2014) defines relevance as a combination of thinking (functionality), sensory appeal (optics and feel), community (social perception), and values. Relevance is no longer a matter of merely being practical or useful; one must make an experiential and emotional connection. Styrlund and Hayes (2014) offer an alternative composition of relevance comprised of authenticity, mastery, empathy, and action. These four elements constitute our further discussion of relevance and how each of these individually is enhanced through the use of philosophy.

Authenticity is the foundation of relevance, in the sense of "being true to self and real to others" (Styrlund & Hayes, 2014, p. 64). Connected closely to philosophical questions of ontology, developing authenticity requires that we build our self-awareness of who we are and what we value. This self-awareness helps us understand our capabilities and guides our ethics and actions. Being authentic requires self-critique and demands accountability to self and others. The philosophical school of existentialism has much to say about what it means to live an authentic life (Babulal et al., 2018), or ontologically, to live one's essence. In this regard, our philosophical position is that the choices we make in everyday life construct the people we become, as Sartre (1947/2007) would argue. In addition, these seemingly personal choices affect everyone in the world. Occupational therapy can enhance its authenticity by consistently engaging in self-critique and building systems to hold itself accountable to practitioners, clients, and its espoused values and philosophy. Authenticity would, therefore, address the ontological question of who we are as a profession and our distinct identity when compared with other professions. Such clarity of self-definition can only come from exhaustive philosophical, not scientific, inquiry (Ikiugu & Schultz, 2006).

THE EPISTEMOLOGY OF OCCUPATIONAL THERAPY

Habermas (1971) offers a tripartite view of knowledge, which includes three categories: technical, practical, and emancipatory. Technical knowledge (similar to Ryle's *knowing that*) is analytical and empirical, providing information and explanation. Practical knowledge—*knowing how*—relies on the social sciences as a foundation and focuses on the application in the solution of everyday occupational issues. Emancipatory knowledge is "informed by a social justice schema which values awareness, critique of the status quo and transformational action or change" (Taff & Babulal, 2016, p. 20). Habermas's inclusion of an emancipatory form of knowledge is critical for achieving mastery; being excellent at what one does in the service of others is the pinnacle of relevance because it is the ultimate expression of a meaningful life (Frankl, 2000; Ikiugu & Pollard, 2015). Each role in occupational therapy can be enhanced through mastery in one or all of these knowledge domains. In all aspects of the profession, there exist opportunities to build knowledge and skills; the key consideration is to what end that knowledge and skills are developed. Framing all of our professional "becoming" within a mindset of service to clients and society establishes the ultimate "why" of our professional development. However, service to clients also requires that we foster mastery in collaborating with them, which means we have to be their teachers, partners, and guides, imparting to and exploring with them knowledge about living life to the fullest. Such knowledge can only be gained experientially, as Dewey (1981) stated, through doing. This epistemological perspective can be viewed as the basis of occupational therapy practitioners' endeavor to provide opportunities for occupational participation rather than relying on talking or language alone.

ETHICS OF OCCUPATIONAL THERAPY

Axiology is the branch of philosophy that informs occupational therapy's principles, values, and ethics. Immanuel Levinas's (1998) ethics of "the other" is closely connected to empathy, which refers to the stance of taking another person's perspective, which is itself an ethical act. For Levinas, if an action has no basis in the good it provides for others, then it should not occur. Thus, ethics is a "first philosophy," both as a means and as an end, which can serve as a professional compass as we evolve in a rapidly changing global environment. Building solidarity and expanding the goals and methods of occupational therapy to include multiple cultural perspectives are examples of approaches whose central elements are closely aligned with empathy (Taff et al. 2014). Expanding even further, empathy denotes an interest in justice or, more specifically, according to the occupational therapy lexicon, occupational justice. That means that if we accept the premise that participation in meaningful occupations is necessary for health and well-being, occupational therapy practitioners should advocate for the ability of every citizen of the world to participate in personally meaningful and required occupations. In other words, we need to do everything that we can as a profession to eliminate barriers to participation that may result in any of the many forms of occupational injustice, such as occupational deprivation, alienation, deprivation, apartheid, marginalization, and imbalance (Kronenberg & Pollard, 2005; Townsend & Polatajko, 2013).

Philosophical Constructs That Enhance the Relevance of Occupational Therapy

One of the qualities that occupational therapy practitioners try to develop in clients is mastery. By *mastery* is meant not just competence in specific skills such as how to maintain balance during ambulation, or how to don a shirt, but more holistically in the task of adaptation in general, which makes it possible to live life fully, doing things that one wants or needs to do every day. Thus, mastery refers to harnessing and developing existing talents to become truly excellent in what we are committed to doing (Styrlund & Hayes, 2014). Mastery requires us to abandon imitating others and to focus on our discrete array of strengths, knowledge, and skills. Styrlund and Hayes (2014) suggest five habits of mastery, which we must develop: discipline, proactivity, focus, ordered priorities, and courageous clarity. Mastery is intimately linked to the idea of distinct value and important in every role, not only in our clients' lives but also in the profession. The question of mastery ushers in the notion of intersection between ontology and epistemology of occupational therapy.

Empathy is another construct that can be understood as defining the essence of occupational therapy. In order to assist clients in living meaningful and fulfilling lives through participation in desired occupations, occupational therapy practitioners attempt to enter their clients' life-worlds so that they can understand how the clients experience the world. This ability to see the world through another person's eyes is the definition of empathy (Brown et al., 2010; Ikiugu, 2007). In essence, empathy allows us to view the world from another person's perspective. Developing empathy is "rooted in our belief that we are here on this planet to serve others and have a positive impact on them" (Styrlund & Hayes, 2014, p. 107). Understanding others' needs and resulting behaviors allows us to connect what we do to those we serve. Empathy facilitates building relationships and establishing ethical norms, which are crucial for the practice of occupational therapy.

Finally, occupational therapy is defined by the idea of **doing**. Doing denotes action, which leads to actualization of our being and becoming (Wilcock, 2006). Action is the catalyst of relevance and "carries us from potential to significance in the world" (Styrlund & Hayes, 2014, p. 150). Inert knowledge is minimally useful; however, using knowledge in the service of others or for the collective good is a hallmark of relevance. Framed in philosophical terms, action as praxis echoes Freire (1970/2018) insofar as the action transforms the world for the better in some way. Hannah Arendt (1958/1998) goes even further, suggesting that engaging in everyday praxis is the defining feature of humanity. *Doing*, or *praxis*, is fundamental to occupational therapy's identity and process but can be overlooked outside of the therapeutic encounter. Therefore, occupational therapy should consider planning its professional agenda and structure in an occupation-centered manner.

EMBRACING PHILOSOPHICAL INQUIRY IN PROFESSIONAL DISCOURSE AND ACTION

What, then, must the profession do to support its ontological, epistemological, and axiological substance—in other words, its philosophical integrity? The science of occupational therapy needs to mature and incorporate an increasing proportion of qualitative methods accepted as equally valid evidence. Our practice needs to be truly client-centered (Gupta & Taff, 2015; Hammell, 2013), focusing on prevention and promoting everyday wellness defined as so much more than the absence of disease. Occupational therapy education must provide active, engaged, and transformative learning experiences that prepare future practitioners to be agents of change in the "wicked" (Hanstedt, 2018) contexts of modern health care. Top-down action (legislation, policy change, reimbursement reform) is certainly necessary. However, we believe that the key to shifting the professional paradigm lies within a lower-case philosophical mindset as described in Chapter 1. The concept of *philosophizing* represents a distinctly lower-case approach, one that establishes a culture and occupational habit of philosophizing in all three major areas of occupational therapy.

Philosophizing can be thought of broadly as "the art of rational conjecture" (Russell, 1955/2014, p. 1). This art requires developing specific skills, including the ability to think about humanity in its entirety instead of just oneself and associated social networks. Additional skills necessary for philosophizing include formulating and asking questions (Russell, 1959/1989), a consistent habit of critiquing the status quo, and "negative training," the ability to consider the opposite of one's beliefs and defend those perspectives (Russell, 1955/2014). Perhaps counterintuitively, philosophizing is further developed through leaving the "cult of efficiency" behind and taking the time to think, to bask in leisurely wonder for its own sake (Russell, 1935/1996). This sort of perceived idleness is not typically valued in contemporary societies. However, Russell (1935/1996) advocates that "[p]erhaps the most important advantage of 'useless' knowledge is that it promotes a contemplative habit of mind. There is in the world too much readiness, not only for action without adequate previous reflection but also for some action on occasions on which wisdom would counsel inaction" (p. 24). The component skills and cognitive habits required of philosophizing, while present in all of us, may not be developed fully to offer the most significant impact. They must be explicitly identified, taught, and practiced.

It is important here to make a distinction between *teaching philosophy* and *teaching to philosophize* (Pihlgren, 2008). Nelson (1965) refers to this as "the art not of teaching about philosophers but of making philosophers of the students" (p. 1). To be clear, teaching about philosophy and philosophers is valuable and has benefits to the profession, particularly in terms of research (Hooper et al., 2018). What we suggest here, however, is that occupational therapy should make philosophers out of its educators, clinicians, scientists, policymakers, and leaders. Integrating this concept into entry-level curricula and continuing education opportunities is a start, but philosophizing is a habit that requires consistent use in everyday life. Philosophizing is an occupation that develops us as lower-case philosophers, and, as Adler (1990) notes, is available for us all as indicated in the following statement:

> Whether we know it or not, we are all philosophers. We all think—well or sloppy, enthusiastically or inattentively. The slightest sense perception—a falling leaf, a twinkling star, a smiling child—awakens our minds as well as arouses our feelings and forces us to ask: Why? What? Whence? Whither? (Adler, 1990, p. 230)

SHIFTING PARADIGMS, ENHANCING RELEVANCE

Where is occupational therapy in terms of philosophical influences as we enter the third decade of the 21st century? Within the global professional community, the influences become much more local, strongly affected by culture, traditions, and alternate explanatory models of health and well-being. To be sure, the current philosophies informing occupational therapy internationally are not clear-cut and include a wide variety such as pragmatism, humanism, and existentialism (Ikiugu & Schultz, 2006; Schwartzberg, 2002). Despite these numerous coexisting philosophies, we suggest that a combination of post-analytic realism with hints of neopragmatism remains prominent (particularly in the United States) and guides thoughts about health, reimbursement structures, and the latitude to provide genuinely client-centered care (Gupta & Taff, 2015). To better meet the needs of global populations, we suggest that occupational therapy must shift the core of its philosophical underpinnings to a position where narrative subjectivities and critical social awareness balance the historical emphasis on

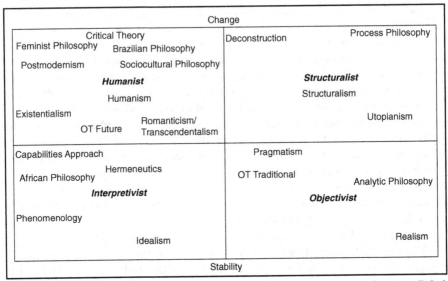

Figure 23-1. Landscape of philosophical thought in occupational therapy. (Adapted from Burrell, G., & Morgan, G. [1979]. *Sociological paradigms and organisational analysis.* Heinemann Educational Books.)

biomedical reductionism and efficiency (Figure 23-1). The question which then logically follows is: "How can this be accomplished?" To this end, we suggest the following strategies as a start:

- Create a globally inclusive charter clearly stating the philosophical (ontological, epistemological, and axiological) foundations and associated professional values as a guiding document to which local organizations should develop accountability mechanisms
- Expand and/or reframe the roles occupational therapists play in promoting prevention, health, and well-being rather than a response to episodic disease management
- Emphasize qualitative, participatory, and community-based research designs to balance the reductionist focus in occupational therapy science
- Ensure that clinical outcomes include patient report and client perceptions of value
- Have professional organizations develop explicit infrastructure, processes, and policies to regularly critique reimbursement mechanisms, practice trends, and educational accreditation and examination standards to ensure inclusivity, equity, and occupational justice

- Continue to explore and redefine the concepts of occupation and participation to include focus on individual capabilities merged with collective needs.
- Work to unify occupational therapy and occupational science and to utilize philosophy as an organizing framework to guide education, research, and practice
- Explicitly add philosophical modes of thinking, or philosophizing, to all occupational therapy educational, research, and clinical processes: What epistemological assumptions are at play? What core values must be evoked? How can actions be guided by the belief in the nature of humans as ever-changing in dynamic environments?
- Include applied philosophy in occupational therapy curricula as a core content area that is integrated with science and evidence-informed practice
- Include evidence of philosophical thinking, preferably as integrated into clinical situations, in certification examinations and educational accreditation standards
- Train students to be "philosopher-clinicians" and continue to support this approach through career-spanning education and opportunities to philosophize

This philosophical shift can result in sustained relevance and expansion of the profession while—most importantly—guiding authentic services that enhance the health, well-being, and quality of life of people and populations worldwide. As the profession moves through its second century, we should all strive to live and work as philosophers in our unique ways. To ignore this opportunity is to the profession's detriment and a disservice to the people and populations with which we partner. Our hope is that this professional paradigm shift will support philosophy as part and parcel of the culture of occupational therapy and consideration in everything we do as educators, scientists, clinicians, policy makers, and leaders. Philosophizing prompts the realization that occupational therapy is so much more than the techniques we use for assessment and intervention. Consistent philosophizing in our professional roles can also transform the very essence of those roles so that they are increasingly influential in shaping a more just and equitable world.

Philosophy and Occupational Therapy: Informing Education, Research, and Practice was imagined to serve two purposes: to introduce readers to a wide variety of philosophical perspectives that can inform the profession, and to spark a professional culture of philosophizing that translates upper-case philosophical ideas into occupationally informed relevance that both sustains the profession and serves the world's occupational needs. Dunning (1973) reminds us how philosophy impacts the very core of our profession:

> Is it not the purpose of occupational therapy to help the client gain a sense of identity and wholeness as he strives not only against physical and emotional disability but also against dehumanizing forces? If occupational therapy is more than a medical technology, then it has to function as a spokesman for the individual and as an agent of societal change. (p. 21)

Dunning's call-to-action is needed now more than ever and is a message echoed throughout this book. Philosophy matters!

REFERENCES

Adler, M. J. (1990). *Reforming education: The opening of the American mind*. Collier Books.

American Occupational Therapy Association (AOTA). (2019). *Evidence-based practice & research*. https://www.aota.org/Practice/Researchers.aspx

Arendt, H. (1998). *The human condition*. University of Chicago Press. (Original work published 1958)

Artigas, M. (2001). *The mind of the universe*. Templeton Foundation Press.

Babulal, G. M., Selvaratnam, A., & Taff, S. D. (2018). Existentialism in occupational therapy: Implications for practice, research, and education. *Occupational Therapy in Health Care, 32*(4), 393–411. https://doi.org/10.1080/07380577.2018.1523592

Brown, T., Williams, B., Boyle, M., Molloy, A., McKenna, L., Molloy, L., & Lewis, B. (2010). Levels of empathy in undergraduate occupational therapy students. *Occupational Therapy International, 17*, 135–141. https://doi.org/10.1002/oti.297

Burrell, G., & Morgan, G. (1979). *Sociological paradigms and organisational analysis*. Heinemann Educational Books.

Coville, A. (2014). *Relevance: The power to change minds and behavior and stay ahead of the competition*. Bibliomotion.

Dewey, J. (1981). My pedagogical creed. In J. J. McDermott (Ed.), *The philosophy of John Dewey* (pp. 442–454). Chicago University Press.

Dunning, R. E. (1973). Philosophy and occupational therapy. *American Journal of Occupational Therapy, 27*(1), 18–23.

Frankl, V. E. (2000). *Man's search for ultimate meaning*. Beacon Press.

Freire, P. (2018). *Pedagogy of the oppressed* (4th ed.) (M. Bergman Ramos, Trans.). Continuum. (Original work published 1970)

Gupta, J., & Taff, S. D. (2015). The illusion of client-centred practice. *Scandinavian Journal of Occupational Therapy, 22*(4), 244–251. https://doi.org/10.3109/11038128.2015.1020866

Habermas, J. (1971). *Knowledge and human interests*. Beacon Press.

Hammell, K. W. (2013). Client-centred practice in occupational therapy: Critical reflections. *Scandinavian Journal of Occupational Therapy, 20*(3), 174–181. https://doi.org/10.3109/11038128.2012.752032

Hanstedt, P. (2018). *Creating wicked students: Designing courses for a complex world*. Stylus.

Hooper, B., Gupta, J., Bilics, A., & Taff, S. D. (2018). Balancing efficacy and effectiveness with philosophy, history, and theory-building in occupational therapy education research. *The Open Journal of Occupational Therapy, 6*(1), 1–9. https://doi.org/10.15453/2168-6408.1347

Hooper, B., & Wood, W. (2002). Pragmatism and structuralism in occupational therapy: The long conversation. *American Journal of Occupational Therapy, 56*, 40–50. https://doi.org/10.5014/ajot.56.1.40

Ikiugu, M. N. (2007). *Psychosocial conceptual practice models in occupational therapy: Building adaptive capability*. Elsevier/Mosby.

Ikiugu, M. N., & Pollard, N. (2015). *Meaningful living across the lifespan: Occupation-based intervention strategies for occupational therapists and scientists*. Whiting & Birch.

Ikiugu, M. N., & Schultz, S. (2006). An argument for pragmatism as a foundational philosophy of occupational therapy. *Canadian Journal of Occupational Therapy, 73*(2), 86–97. https://doi.org/10.2182/cjot.05.0009

Kronenberg, F., & Pollard, N. (2005). Overcoming occupational apartheid: A preliminary exploration of the political nature of occupational therapy. In F. Kronenberg, S. Algado, & N. Pollard (Eds.), *Occupational therapy without borders: Learning from the spirit of survivors* (pp. 59–86). Elsevier-Churchill Livingstone.

Kuhn, T. (1996). *The structure of scientific revolutions* (3rd ed.). University of Chicago Press. (Original work published 1962)

Levinas, I. (1998). *Entre nous: On thinking-of-the-other* (M. B. Smith & B. Harshav, Trans.). Columbia University Press.

Massimi, M. (2009). Philosophy and the sciences after Kant. *Royal Institute of Philosophy Supplement*, 65, 275–311. https://doi.org/10.1017/S1358246109990142

Nelson, L. (1965). *Socratic method and critical philosophy: Selected essays*. Dover.

Ortega y Gasset, J. (1960). *What is philosophy?* (M. Adams, Trans.). W. W. Norton.

Payne, W. R. (2015). *An introduction to philosophy*. https://commons.bellevuecollege.edu/wrussellpayne/an-introduction-to-philosophy

Pihlgren, A. S. (2008). *Socrates in the classroom: Rationales and effects of philosophizing with children*. Elanders Sverige.

Pray, L. (2008). Discovery of DNA structure and function: Watson and Crick. *Nature Education*, 1(1), 100.

Russell, B. (1989). *Wisdom of the west*. Crescent Books. (Original work published 1959)

Russell, B. (1996). *In praise of idleness and other essays*. Routledge. (Original work published 1935)

Russell, B. (2014). *The art of philosophizing and other essays*. Rowman & Littlefield. (Original work published 1955)

Sartre, J. P. (2007). *Existentialism is a humanism* (C. Macomber, Trans.). Yale University Press. (Original work published 1947)

Schwartzberg, S. L. (2002). *Interactive reasoning in the practice of occupational therapy*. Prentice Hall.

Styrlund, P., & Hayes, T. (2014). *Relevance: Matter more*. Mary Mae & Sons.

Taff, S. D., Bakhshi, P., & Babulal, G. M. (2014). The accountability–well-being–ethics framework: A new philosophical foundation for occupational therapy. *Canadian Journal of Occupational Therapy*, 81, 320–329. https://doi.org/10.1177/0008417414546742

Taff, S. D., & Babulal, G. M. (2016). Constructing personal philosophies of practice using Habermasian knowledge domains. *Irish Journal of Occupational Therapy*, 44(2), 19–22.

Townsend, E., & Polatajko, H. (2013). *Enabling occupation II: Advancing an occupational therapy vision for health, well-being, & justice through occupations* (2nd ed.). CAOT.

Wilcock, A. (2006). *An occupational perspective of health* (2nd ed.). SLACK Incorporated.

FINANCIAL DISCLOSURES

Dr. Rebecca M. Aldrich has no financial or proprietary interest in the materials presented herein.

Dr. Ganesh M. Babulal has no financial or proprietary interest in the materials presented herein.

Dr. Parul Bakhshi has no financial or proprietary interest in the materials presented herein.

Dr. Aaron Bonsall has no financial or proprietary interest in the materials presented herein.

Dr. Helen Carey has no financial or proprietary interest in the materials presented herein.

Anil H. Chandiramani has no financial or proprietary interest in the materials presented herein.

Dr. Charles H. Christiansen has no financial or proprietary interest in the materials presented herein.

Dr. Daniel Marinho Cezar da Cruz has no financial or proprietary interest in the materials presented herein.

Ronald R. Drummond has no financial or proprietary interest in the materials presented herein.

Dr. Madeleine Duncan has no financial or proprietary interest in the materials presented herein.

Dr. Aaron M. Eakman has no financial or proprietary interest in the materials presented herein.

Dr. Brad E. Egan has no financial or proprietary interest in the materials presented herein.

Dr. Lisette Farias has no financial or proprietary interest in the materials presented herein.

Dr. Don Fogelberg has no financial or proprietary interest in the materials presented herein.

Dr. Alison Gerlach has no financial or proprietary interest in the materials presented herein.

Dr. Marna Ghiglieri has no financial or proprietary interest in the materials presented herein.

Dr. Jyothi Gupta has no financial or proprietary interest in the materials presented herein.

Dr. Barb Hooper has no financial or proprietary interest in the materials presented herein.

Dr. Moses N. Ikiugu has no financial or proprietary interest in the materials presented herein.

Dr. Elizabeth Anne Kinsella has no financial or proprietary interest in the materials presented herein.

Dr. Lilian Magalhães has no financial or proprietary interest in the materials presented herein.

Dr. Wanda J. Mahoney has no financial or proprietary interest in the materials presented herein.

Dr. Rose McAndrew has no financial or proprietary interest in the materials presented herein.

Dr. Thuli Mthembu has no financial or proprietary interest in the materials presented herein.

Dr. Whitney Lucas-Molitor has no financial or proprietary interest in the materials presented herein.

Dr. Bernard A. K. Muriithi has no financial or proprietary interest in the materials presented herein.

Dr. Anna J. Neff has no financial or proprietary interest in the materials presented herein.

Dr. Ranelle M. Nissen has no financial or proprietary interest in the materials presented herein.

Dr. Melissa Park has no financial or proprietary interest in the materials presented herein.

Lauren Putnam has no financial or proprietary interest in the materials presented herein.

Daniela da Silva Rodrigues has no financial or proprietary interest in the materials presented herein.

Dr. Debbie Laliberte Rudman has no financial or proprietary interest in the materials presented herein.

Arun Selvaratnam has no financial or proprietary interest in the materials presented herein.

Dr. Steven D. Taff has no financial or proprietary interest in the materials presented herein.

Dr. Jean-Francois Trani has no financial or proprietary interest in the materials presented herein.

Dr. Richard L. Whalley has no financial or proprietary interest in the materials presented herein.

Dr. Valerie A. Wright-St Clair has no financial or proprietary interest in the materials presented herein.

INDEX

Abbot, Francis Ellingwood, 14, 18
activity theory, 103–104
Addams, Jane, 9, 17–18, 20, 70, 86
Adorno, Theodor, 156
African philosophy, 111–125
  African ethno-philosophy, 118–121
    impact, 121
  communitarianism, 115
  concepts, 115–117
  divination, 114
  facets, 113–115
  "humanness," 115
  implications, 121–122
    education, 121–122
    practice, 122
    research, 122
  person, 116–117
  personhood, 117
  shamans, 113
  sorcery, 114
  Tutu, Desmond, Archbishop, 115
  Ubuntu, 115
  "whole-ness of be-ing," 115
  witchcraft, 114
Africana womanism, 211
Age of Reason, 9
alcoholism, critical theory, 158–159
American intellectual tradition, 9–11
  Age of Reason, 9
  Bhagavad Gita, 9
  Byron, Lord, 9
  Emerson, Ralph Waldo, 10
  Enlightenment, 9
  Fuller, Margaret, 10
  Goethe, Johann Wolfgang von, 9
  Hinduism, 9
  Native American tribe displacement, 10
  Romanticism, 10
  sacred texts, 9
  Schelling, Friedrich, 9
  Schiller, Friedrich, 9
  Thoreau, Henry David, 10
  Transcendental Club, 10
  Unitarianism, 9
  Upanishads, 9
  Wordsworth, William, 9
analytic philosophy, 135–143
  Anscombe, Elizabeth, 139
  Ayer, A. J., 138
  Carnap, Rudolph, 138
  consequentialism, 139
  definition, 135–136
  early phase, 136–137
  Einstein, Albert, 138
  facets, 136

Feigl, Herbert, 138
Frege, Gottlob, 138
goals, 137
Hume, David, 137
impact, 139–141
implications, 141–142
  education, 141–142
  practice, 142
  research, 142
Kaufmann, Felix, 138
Locke, John, 137
Popper, Karl, 138
recent developments, 137
Russell, Bertrand, 138
Ryle, Gilbert, 138–139
Schlick, Moritz, 138
thinkers, 138–139
Vienna Circle, 138
Wittgenstein, Ludwig, 138
Anscombe, Elizabeth, 137, 139, 142
aporias expressions, hermeneutics, 169–173
Arendt, Hannah, 238
Aristotelian thought, 24
Aristotle, 11, 34, 234
Arnold, Matthew, 67
Arts and Crafts Movement, 8, 71, 86
Ayer, A. J., 138, 141

Bacon, Francis, 47, 63, 76, 85
Bacon, Roger, 63
Bakhtin, M. M., 102, 104–105
Barthes, Roland, 148, 149, 182
Basaglia, Franco, 193, 196
Baudrillard, Jean, 201
"being-in-the-world," 54, 57
Bellamy, Edward, 16
Benjamin, Walter, 156
Bergson, Henri, 46, 130
Berkeley, George, 24–26, 137
Bhagavad Gita, 9
Bhaskar, Roy, 34, 38
Bliss, W. D. P., 9, 17–18
Bradley, Francis Herbert, 25–26
Brazil, philosophical influences, 189–199
  Basaglia, Franco, 193
  Castel, Robert, 193
  context, 195–196
  da Silveira, Nise, 191
  de Mesquita Pinto, Jussara, 192
  Durkheim, Émile, 193
  Foucault, Michel, 193
  Freire, Paulo, 193
  Heller, Agnes, 193
  historical roots, 191
  impact, 196

implications, 196
    education, 196–197
    practice, 197
    research, 197
Jorge, Rui Chamone, 192
Jung, Carl, 191
Marx, Karl, 193
political roots, 191
social movements, 191–193
social participation, 194–195
training, 190–191
Vázquez, Adolfo, 193
Brentano, Franz, 53
Bruno, Giordano, 35
Buddhism, 130
Byron, Lord, 9

Camus, Albert, 54
capabilities approach, 221–231
    adaptive preferences, 224
    capabilities, 223
    collective capabilities, 224–225
    concepts, 223–226
    dignity, 225–226
    discourse, 225
    human rights, 225–226
    impact, 228
    implications, 229–230
        education, 229
        practice, 229–230
        research, 229
    instrumentalization, dangers of, 226
    Millennium Development Goals, 227
    operationalizing, 227–228
        sustainable development goals,
            227–228
        synergies, 227–228
    Sen, Amartya, 221–225
    social exclusion, 224–225
Carnap, Rudolph, 138
Carus, Paul, 15
Castel, Robert, 193
Cavell, Stanley, 2
Chicago School of Civics and Philanthropy,
    86
Christian Humanism, 47
Christian Labor Union, 17
Christian socialism, 16–19
    Abbot, Francis Ellingwood, 18
    Addams, Jane, 17–18
    Bellamy, Edward, 16
    Bliss, W. D. P., 17–18
    Christian Labor Union, 17
    Christian socialism, 17–19
    de Saint-Simon, Henri, 16
    Engels, Friedrich, 16
    Fiske, John, 18–19
    Fourier, Charles, 16
    Gladden, Washington, 18
    Marx, Karl, 16

Metaphysical Club, 18
Owen, Robert, 16
Peabody, Francis, 18
Progressive Era, 19
Rauschenbusch, Walter, 18
Riis, Jacob, 17
Social Gospel Movement, 17–19
Society of Christian Socialists, 17
Spencer, Herbert, 18
Strong, Josiah, 18
Taylor, Graham, 17
"utopian socialism," 16
Collins, Patricia Hill, 210, 211
communitarianism, 115
communities of individuals, 28
Comte, Auguste, 9, 13–16, 18
consequentialism, 139
constructive realism, 37
contextualized nature, 211–212
Copernicus, 35
creative works, 65–69
critical realism, 38
critical theory, 155–162
    Adorno, Theodor, 156
    alcoholism, 158–159
    Benjamin, Walter, 156
    drug abuse, 158–159
    facets, 156
    Freire, Paulo, 157–158
    Fromm, Erich, 156
    gang activity, 158–159
    goals, 156
    Habermas, Jürgen, 157
    Horkheimer, Max, 156–157
    impact, 158–159
    implications, 160
        education, 160
        practice, 160
        research, 160
    Institute for Social Research, 156
    Marcuse, Herbert, 156–157
    Marx, Karl, 155–156
    perspectives, 156–158
    Santos, Boaventura de Sousa, 158
    Smith, Linda Tuhiwai, 158
    understanding, 158–159

da Silveira, Nise, 191
Darwin's theory of evolution, 35
de Beauvoir, Simone, 54
de Mesquita Pinto, Jussara, 192
de Saint-Simon, Henri, 13, 16, 77–78
de Saussure, Ferdinand, 145–149, 182–183
deconstruction, 181–188
    Barthes, Roland, 182
    Derrida, Jacques, 182–183
    ergo-therapy, 185
    Foucault, Michel, 182
    impact, 185–187
    implications, 187

education, 187
  practice, 187
  research, 187
intended outcome, 183–184
methodology of, 184
as nontraditional philosophy, 182–183
origins of, 181–182
post-structuralism, 181–182
structuralism, 181–182
understanding, 185–187
defining philosophy, 1–6
  Cavell, Stanley, 2
  derivation of term, 1
  Durant, Will, 3
  Greek philosophers, 1
  James, William, 2
  Kant, Immanuel, 3
  lovers of wisdom, 1
  "lower-case" philosophy, 5
  ontology, 3
  question, answering, 2–5
  Rorty, Richard, 4–5
  Russell, Bertrand, 2
  "upper-case" philosophy, 4–5
  West, Cornel, 2
  Wiredu, Kwasi, 2
Deleuze, Gilles, 1, 3 201–205
Derrida, Jacques, 148, 182–184, 187, 201
Descartes, René, 24, 26, 28, 54, 63, 116
developmental influences, 7–22
  Addams, Jane, 9
  American intellectual tradition, 9–11
  Arts and Crafts Movement, 8
  Bliss, W. D. P., 9
  Christian socialism, 16–19
    Abbot, Francis Ellingwood, 18
    Addams, Jane, 17–18
    Bellamy, Edward, 16
    Bliss, W. D. P., 17–18
    Christian Labor Union, 17
    Christian socialism, 17–19
    de Saint-Simon, Henri, 16
    Engels, Friedrich, 16
    Fiske, John, 18–19
    Fourier, Charles, 16
    Gladden, Washington, 18
    Marx, Karl, 16
    Metaphysical Club, 18
    Owen, Robert, 16
    Peabody, Francis, 18
    Progressive Era, 19
    Rauschenbusch, Walter, 18
    Social Gospel Movement, 17–19
    Society of Christian Socialists, 17
    Spencer, Herbert, 18
    Strong, Josiah, 18
    "utopian socialism," 16
  Comte, Auguste, 9
  Emerson, Ralph Waldo, 9
  Fuller, Margaret, 9

Harris, William Torrey, 8
James, William, 9
Mach, Ernst, 9
Mathews, Shailer, 9
Mill, John Stuart, 7, 9
Peirce, Charles Sanders, 9
positivism, 13–16
  Abbot, Francis Ellingwood, 14
  Carus, Paul, 15
  Comte, Auguste, 13
  Eliot, C. W., 14
  Fiske, John, 14
  Industrial Age, 16
  James, William, 14–15
  Machine Age, 15
  Mead, George Herbert, 14
  Metaphysical Club, 14
  Mill, John Stuart, 14
  Peirce, Charles Sanders, 14
  pragmatism, similarities, 14–15
  Progressive Era, 14, 16
  Vienna Circle, 15
  Wright, Chauncey, 14
pragmatism, 11–13
  Aristotle, 11
  Dewey, John, 11, 13
  firstness, phenomenological
    category, 11
  James, William, 11–13
  Mead, George Herbert, 11
  Metaphysical Club, 11
  Peirce, Charles Sanders, 11–13
  secondness, phenomenological
    category, 11
  Socrates, 11
  thirdness, phenomenological
    category, 11
  Wright, Chauncey, 11
Progressive Era, 7
Settlement House Movement, 8
Thoreau, Henry David, 9
transcendentalism, 9–11
  Age of Reason, 9
  Bhagavad Gita, 9
  Byron, Lord, 9
  Emerson, Ralph Waldo, 10
  Enlightenment, 9
  Fuller, Margaret, 10
  Goethe, Johann Wolfgang von, 9
  Hinduism, 9
  Native American tribe
    displacement, 10
  Romanticism, 10
  sacred texts, 9
  Schelling, Friedrich, 9
  Schiller, Friedrich, 9
  Thoreau, Henry David, 10
  Transcendental Club, 10
  Unitarianism, 9
  Upanishads, 9

Wordsworth, William, 9
Wright, Chauncey, 9
Dewey, John, 8, 11, 13, 19, 40, 85–88, 120, 130, 237
dialogism, 104–105
dignity, 225–226
Dilthey, Willhelm, 163–165, 167, 169–175
divination, 114
Douglass, Frederick, 69–70
drug abuse, critical theory, 158–159
Durant, Will, 3
Durkheim, Émile, 193
dystopia, 75

Einstein, Albert, 138
Eliot, C. W., 14
embodied meaning, occupation as, 164–165
Emerson, Ralph Waldo, 9–10, 67–68, 70
empathy, 238
engaging with world, 57–58
Engels, Friedrich, 16, 77
Enlightenment, 9
epistemological realism, 36
epistemology, 26, 236–237
Erasmus, 47, 48
ergo-therapy, 185
ethics, 237–238
ethno-philosophy, African, 118–121
    impact, 121
evolution, Darwin's theory of, 35
existentialism, 53–60
    "being-in-the-world," 54, 57
    Brentano, Franz, 53
    Camus, Albert, 54
    de Beauvoir, Simone, 54
    engaging with world, 57–58
    epistemologically, 54
    ethically, 54–55
    Heidegger, Martin, 55–58
    Husserl, Edmund, 53, 56
    implications, 58–59
        education, 58
        practice, 59
        research, 58–59
    Marcel, Gabriel, 54
    ontologically, 54
    ontology, 56–57
    Sartre, Jean-Paul, 54–58
    Solomon, Robert, 58
    structures of temporality, 57
    Stumpf, Carl, 53

Feigl, Herbert, 138
feminist theory, 209–219
    "Africana womanism," 211
    Collins, Patricia Hill, 210
    contextualized nature, 211–212
    disability, 213–214
    first wave feminism, 209
    health, 213–214

hooks, bell, 210
    implications, 215–216
        education, 215
        practice, 216
        research, 215–216
    intersectional feminisms, 210–211
        Collins, Patricia Hill, 210
        intersectionality, defined, 210
    intersectionality, defined, 210
    Lorde, Audre, 209
    methodology, 214–215
    situated nature, 211–212
Fichte, Johann Gottlieb, 63–64
first wave feminism, 209
firstness, phenomenological category, 11
Fiske, John, 14, 18–19
Foucault, Michel, 148, 182, 193, 201–202, 203, 204
Fourier, Charles, 16, 77–78
Frankfurt School. *See* Institute for Social Research
Frege, Gottlob, 138
Freire, Paulo, 157–158, 193, 212, 238
Fromm, Erich, 156
Fuller, Margaret, 9, 10, 70

Gadamer, Hans-Georg, 163, 172–173, 175–176
Galileo, 35
gang activity, critical theory, 158–159
Gladden, Washington, 17–18
Goethe, Johann Wolfgang von, 9, 65–66
Greek philosophers, 1

Habermas, Jürgen, 157, 182, 236
Harris, William Torrey, 8
Hartshorne, Charles, 130
Hegel, Georg Wilhelm Friedrich, 7–8, 11, 24–27, 63–64, 85, 102
Heidegger, Martin, 54–58, 92–95, 97, 175, 182,
Heller, Agnes, 193, 196
Heraclitus, 37, 130
hermeneutics, 163–179
    aporias expressions, 169–173
    Dilthey, Willhelm, 163–165, 167, 169–170, 173–175
    embodied meaning, occupation as, 164–165
    everyday hermeneutics, 166–168
    Gadamer, Hans-Georg, 163, 172–173, 175–176
    implications, 176–177
    infinite distance, 173–175
    life expressions, classes of, 170
    Mattingly, Cheryl, 166
    Ricoeur, Paul, 163, 173
    task of, 175–177
    understanding, 165–166
Hinduism, 9

Hirsch, Emil G., 86
hooks, bell, 210
Horkheimer, Max, 156–157
Hull House, 86
humanism, 45–52
    Bacon, Francis, 47
    Bergson, Henri, 46
    Christian Humanism, 47
    education, 50
    Erasmus, 47
    impact, 49
    implications, 50–51
    Maslow, Abraham, 47–49
    Mill, John Stuart, 46
    Petrarch, Francesco, 47
    practice, 51
    research, 50–51
    Rogers, Carl, 47–49
    Russell, Bertrand, 47
    Third Force Psychology, 47
"humanness," 115
Hume, David, 137
Husserl, Edmund, 53–54, 56, 93, 94, 95

idealism, 23–31
    Aristotelian thought, 24
    Berkeley, George, 24–26
    Bradley, Francis Herbert, 25–26
    epistemology, 26
    ethics, 26
    Hegel, Georg Wilhelm Friedrich, 25
    implications, 30
        education, 30
        practice, 30
        research, 30
    Kant, Immanuel, 2, 25
    occupation, 26–27
        communities of individuals, 28
        dualism, mental/physical, 28
        experience, 29
        meaning, 27
        person, holistic view, 28
        subjective perspective, 29
    philosophical, 23–30
    Plato, 24
imaginary order, 148
Industrial Age, 16
infinite distance, hermeneutics, 173–175
Institute for Social Research, 156
instrumentalism, 83–90
    Addams, Jane, 86
    Arts and Crafts Movement, 86
    Bacon, Francis, 85
    Chicago School of Civics and
        Philanthropy, 86
    Dewey, John, 85
    Hegel, Georg Wilhelm Friedrich, 85
    Hirsch, Emil G., 86
    Hull House, 86
    implications, 88–89

        education, 88
        practice, 88–89
        research, 88
    James, William, 84
    Lathrop, Julia, 86
    Meyer, Adolf, 85–86
    Moral Treatment Movement, 86
    Peirce, Charles Sanders, 83–84
    Slagle, Eleanor Clark, 86
instrumentalization, dangers of, 226
intellectual tradition, 9–11
    Age of Reason, 9
    Bhagavad Gita, 9
    Byron, Lord, 9
    Emerson, Ralph Waldo, 10
    Enlightenment, 9
    Fuller, Margaret, 10
    Goethe, Johann Wolfgang von, 9
    Hinduism, 9
    Native American tribe displacement, 10
    Romanticism, 10
    sacred texts, 9
    Schelling, Friedrich, 9
    Schiller, Friedrich, 9
    Thoreau, Henry David, 10
    Transcendental Club, 10
    Unitarianism, 9
    Upanishads, 9
    Wordsworth, William, 9
intended outcome, deconstruction, 183–184
intentional community, 78
intersectional feminisms, 209–219.
    See also feminist theory
    Collins, Patricia Hill, 210
    hooks, bell, 210
    intersectionality, defined, 210
intersectionality, defined, 210

Jakobson, Roman, 148–149
James, William, 2, 8–9, 11–15, 40, 84–85, 87,
    88, 130
Jorge, Rui Chamone, 192
Jung, Carl, 191

Kant, Immanuel, 3, 11, 24, 25, 26, 34, 63, 64,
    116, 234
Kaufmann, Felix, 138

Lacan, Jacques, 148
language, structure of, 145–146
Lathrop, Julia, 86
Leontiev, Aleksei, 102–107
Lévi-Strauss, Claude, 147–148
Levinas, Immanuel, 237
LGBTQ community, 196
life expressions, classes, 170
literary utopia, 76–77
Locke, John, 137
Lorde, Audre, 209
lovers of wisdom, 1

"lower-case" philosophy, 5
Lyotard, Jean-François, 201–204

Mach, Ernst, 9, 15
Machine Age, 15
Marcel, Gabriel, 54
Marcuse, Herbert, 156–157
Marx, Karl, 16, 77, 155–156, 193
Maslow, Abraham, 47–49
mastery, 237–238
Mathews, Shailer, 9, 17
Mattingly, Cheryl, 92, 166, 175,
MDG. *See* Millennium Development
    Goals
Mead, George Herbert, 11, 14
Merleau-Ponty, Maurice, 54, 94, 95
Metaphysical Club, 11, 14, 18
methodology, 214–215
Meyer, Adolf, 85–86
Mill, John Stuart, 7, 9, 14, 15, 46
Millennium Development Goals, 227
mind-independence, 34
Moral Treatment Movement, 86
More, Thomas, 76
music, romanticism in, 69

Native American tribe displacement, 10
Newton, Isaac, 63

ontological perspective, 235–236
ontology, 3, 56–57
order
    imaginary, structuralism, 148
    real, structuralism, 148
    symbolic, structuralism, 148
Ortega y Gasset, Jose, 235
Owen, Robert, 16, 78

painting, romanticism in, 69
Peabody
    Elizabeth Palmer, 70
    Francis, 18
Peirce, Charles Sanders, 8–9, 11–15, 40,
    83–85
personhood, African philosophy, 111–125
    African ethno-philosophy, 118–121
        impact, 121
    communitarianism, 115
    concepts, 115–117
    divination, 114
    facets, 113–115
    "humanness," 115
    implications, 121–122
        education, 121–122
        practice, 122
        research, 122
    person, 116–117
    personhood, 117
    shamans, 113
    sorcery, 114

Tutu, Desmond, Archbishop, 115
Ubuntu, 115
"whole-ness of be-ing," 115
witchcraft, 114
Petrarch, Francesco, 47
phenomenology, 91–100
    concepts, 94–95
    defining, 92–93
    for educators, 95–96
    facets, 93
    foundations, 92–95
    Heidegger, Martin, 94–95
    Husserl, Edmund, 94
    impact, 95–98
    implications, 98
        education, 98
        practice, 98
        research, 98
    Merleau-Ponty, Maurice, 95
    philosophical concepts, 93–94
    for practitioners, 97–98
    for researchers, 96–97
    thinkers, 94–95
Plato, 24, 26, 33–34, 40–42
Popper, Karl, 138
positivism, 13–16
    Abbot, Francis Ellingwood, 14
    Carus, Paul, 15
    Comte, Auguste, 13
    Eliot, C. W., 14
    Fiske, John, 14
    Industrial Age, 16
    James, William, 14–15
    Machine Age, 15
    Mead, George Herbert, 14
    Metaphysical Club, 14
    Mill, John Stuart, 14
    Peirce, Charles Sanders, 14
    pragmatism, similarities, 14–15
    Progressive Era, 14, 16
    Vienna Circle, 15
    Wright, Chauncey, 14
possibility, reimagining, 201–207.
    See also postmodernism
post-structuralism, 181–182
postmodernism, 201–207
    Baudrillard, Jean, 201
    Deleuze, Gilles, 201, 203–204
    Derrida, Jacques, 201
    facets, 202
    Foucault, Michel, 201, 203–204
    goals, 202
    impact, 204–205
    implications, 205–206
        education, 205
        practice, 206
        research, 205–206
    Lyotard, Jean-François, 201–204
    perspectives, 202–204
    Rorty, Richard, 201–205

understanding, 204–205
pragmatism, 11–13, 83–90
  Addams, Jane, 86
  Aristotle, 11
  Arts and Crafts Movement, 86
  Bacon, Francis, 85
  Chicago School of Civics and
    Philanthropy, 86
  Dewey, John, 11, 13, 85
  firstness, phenomenological category, 11
  Hegel, Georg Wilhelm Friedrich, 85
  Hirsch, Emil G., 86
  Hull House, 86
  impact, 86–87
  implications, 88–89
    education, 88
    practice, 88–89
    research, 88
  James, William, 11–13, 84
  Lathrop, Julia, 86
  Mead, George Herbert, 11
  Metaphysical Club, 11
  Meyer, Adolf, 85–86
  Moral Treatment Movement, 86
  Peirce, Charles Sanders, 11–13, 83–84
  secondness, phenomenological category,
    11
  Slagle, Eleanor Clark, 86
  Socrates, 11
  thirdness, phenomenological category, 11
  Wright, Chauncey, 11
prehension, 130
process philosophy, 127–133
  Bergson, Henri, 130
  Buddhism, 130
  concepts, 129–130
  education, 132
  facets, 128
  Hartshorne, Charles, 130
  Heraclitus, 130
  impact, 131–132
  implications, 132
  practice, 132
  prehension, 130
  research, 132
  thinkers, 130
  understanding, 131–132
  Whitehead, Alfred North, 130
Progressive Era, 7, 14, 16, 19

Rauschenbusch, Walter, 18
real order, 148
realism, 33–44
  Bhaskar, Roy, 38
  Bruno, Giordano, 35
  Copernicus, 35
  critical realism, 38
  Darwin's theory of evolution, 35
  Dewey, John, 40
  Galileo, 35

Heraclitus, 37
  implications, 40–42
    education, 40–41
    practice, 42
    research, 41
  James, William, 40
  mind-independence, 34
  objective, 38–39
  occupation, 39–40
  Peirce, Charles Sanders, 40
  Plato, 40–42
  varieties of, 35–38
    constructive realism, 37
    epistemological realism, 36
    scientific realism, 35
    semantic realism, 36
    situational realism, 37–38
    structural realism, 36
relevance, 233–243
  Arendt, Hannah, 238
  empathy, 238
  epistemology, 236–237
  ethics, 237–238
  Levinas, Immanuel, 237
  mastery, 237–238
  ontological perspective, 235–236
  Ortega y Gasset, Jose, 235
  paradigm shift, 239–241
  professional discourse, 238–239
  relevance, 237–238
  science, 234–235
Ricoeur, Paul, 163, 172–175
Riis, Jacob, 17
Rogers, Carl, 47–49
romanticism, 10, 61–74
  Arnold, Matthew, 67
  Arts and Crafts Movement, 71
  Bacon, Francis, 63
  Bacon, Roger, 63
  creative works, 65–69
  Descartes, René, 63
  Douglass, Frederick, 69–70
  Emerson, Ralph Waldo, 67
  Fichte, Johann Gottlieb, 63–64
  Fuller, Margaret, 70
  Goethe, Johann Wolfgang von, 65–66
  impact, 71–72
  implications, 72–73
    education, 72
    practice, 73
    research, 72
  music, romanticism in, 69
  Newton, Isaac, 63
  painting, romanticism in, 69
  Peabody, Elizabeth Palmer, 70
  Rousseau, Jean-Jacques, 63
  Schiller, Friedrich, 66–67
  Schlegel, Friedrich, 66
  Settlement House Movement, 71
  social movements, momentum of,

64–65
Thoreau, Henry David, 68
transcendental social reforms,
    69–70
Whitman, Walt, 68–69
Rorty, Richard, 4–5, 201–205
Rousseau, Jean-Jacques, 9, 63
Russell, Bertrand, 2, 3, 47, 136, 138, 142, 239
Ryle, Gilbert, 138–142, 236

sacred texts, 9
Santos, Boaventura de Sousa, 158
Sargent, Lyman Tower, 75
Sartre, Jean-Paul, 54–58, 95, 236
Schelling, Friedrich, 9
Schiller, Friedrich, 9, 64, 66–67
Schlegel, Friedrich, 66
Schlick, Moritz, 138
scientific realism, 35
secondness, phenomenological
    category, 11
semantic realism, 36
Sen, Amartya, 221–225
Settlement House Movement, 8, 71
shamans, 113
situational realism, 37–38
Slagle, Eleanor Clark, 11, 70, 86, 88
Smith, Linda Tuhiwai, 158
social exclusion, 224–225
Social Gospel Movement, 17–19
social movements, momentum of, 64–65
socialism, Christian, 16–19
    Abbot, Francis Ellingwood, 18
    Addams, Jane, 17–18
    Bellamy, Edward, 16
    Bliss, W. D. P., 17–18
    Christian Labor Union, 17
    Christian socialism, 17–19
    de Saint-Simon, Henri, 16
    Engels, Friedrich, 16
    Fiske, John, 18–19
    Fourier, Charles, 16
    Gladden, Washington, 18
    Marx, Karl, 16
    Metaphysical Club, 18
    Owen, Robert, 16
    Peabody, Francis, 18
    Progressive Era, 19
    Rauschenbusch, Walter, 18
    Social Gospel Movement, 17–19
    Society of Christian Socialists, 17
    Spencer, Herbert, 18
    Strong, Josiah, 18
    "utopian socialism," 16
Society of Christian Socialists, 17
sociocultural perspectives, 101–109
    activity theory, 103–104
    Bakhtin, M. M., 102, 104–105
    concepts, 102–105
    dialogism, 104–105

impact, 105–106
implications, 106–108
    education, 106
    practice, 107–108
    research, 106–107
Leontiev, Aleksei, 102–107
    understanding, 105–106
Vygotsky, Lev Semyonovich, 101–104,
    106
zone of proximal development, 103
Socrates, 11
Solomon, Robert, 58
sorcery, 114
Spencer, Herbert, 18
Strong, Josiah, 17, 18
structural realism, 36
structural thinkers, 148–149
structuralism, 145–153, 181–182
    Barthes, Roland, 149
    concepts, 147–148
    culture, applications to, 147
    de Saussure, Ferdinand, 145–147, 149
    facets, 146
    goals, 147
    imaginary order, 148
    impact, 149–151
    implications, 151–152
        education, 151
        practice, 152
        research, 151
    Jakobson, Roman, 148–149
    Lacan, Jacques, 148
    Lévi-Strauss, Claude, 147–148
    real order, 148
    structural thinkers, 148–149
    structure of language, 145–146
    symbolic order, 148
    understanding, 149–151
Stumpf, Carl, 53
symbolic order, 148

Taylor, Graham, 17
teleological perspective, 45–52
    Bacon, Francis, 47
    Christian Humanism, 47
    education, 50
    Erasmus, 47
    impact, 49
    impact of humanism, 49
    implications, 50–51
    Maslow, Abraham, 47–49
    Mill, John Stuart, 46
    Petrarch, Francesco, 47
    practice, 51
    research, 50–51
    Rogers, Carl, 47–49
    Russell, Bertrand, 47
    Third Force Psychology, 47
temporality, structures of, 57
Third Force Psychology, 47

thirdness, phenomenological category, 11
Thoreau, Henry David, 9–11, 67–68, 70
transactionalism, 83–90
  Addams, Jane, 86
  Arts and Crafts Movement, 86
  Bacon, Francis, 85
  Chicago School of Civics and
    Philanthropy, 86
  Dewey, John, 85
  Hegel, Georg Wilhelm Friedrich, 85
  Hirsch, Emil G., 86
  Hull House, 86
  impact, 86–87
  implications, 88–89
    education, 88
    practice, 88–89
    research, 88
  James, William, 84
  Lathrop, Julia, 86
  Meyer, Adolf, 85–86
  Moral Treatment Movement, 86
  Peirce, Charles Sanders, 83–84
  Slagle, Eleanor Clark, 86
Transcendental Club, 10
transcendental social reforms, 69–70
transcendentalism, 9–11, 61–74
  Age of Reason, 9
  Arnold, Matthew, 67
  Arts and Crafts Movement, 71
  Bhagavad Gita, 9
  Byron, Lord, 9
  creative works, 65–69
  Descartes, René, 63
  Douglass, Frederick, 69–70
  Emerson, Ralph Waldo, 10, 67
  Enlightenment, 9
  Fuller, Margaret, 10, 70
  Goethe, Johann Wolfgang von, 9, 65–66
  Hinduism, 9
  impact, 71–72
  implications, 72–73
    education, 72
    practice, 73
    research, 72
  music, romanticism in, 69
  Native American tribe displacement, 10
  Newton, Isaac, 63
  painting, romanticism in, 69
  Peabody, Elizabeth Palmer, 70
  Romanticism, 10
  Rousseau, Jean-Jacques, 9, 63
  sacred texts, 9
  Schelling, Friedrich, 9
  Schiller, Friedrich, 9, 66–67

Schlegel, Friedrich, 66
Settlement House Movement, 71
social movements, momentum of,
  64–65
social reforms, 69–70
Thoreau, Henry David, 10, 68
Transcendental Club, 10
Unitarianism, 9
Upanishads, 9
Whitman, Walt, 68–69
Wordsworth, William, 9
Tutu, Desmond, Archbishop, 115

Ubuntu, 115
Unitarianism, 9
Upanishads, 9
"upper-case" philosophy, 4–5
utopia, 75–81
  Bacon, Francis, 76
  de Saint-Simon, Henri, 77
  dystopia, 75
  Engels, Friedrich, 77
  Fourier, Charles, 77–78
  implications, 78–81
    education, 80
    practice, 81
    research, 80
  intentional community, 78
  literary utopia, 76–77
  Marx, Karl, 77
  More, Thomas, 76
  Owen, Robert, 78
  Sargent, Lyman Tower, 75
  utopianism, 75–81
"utopian socialism," 16
utopianism, 75–81

Vázquez, Adolfo, 193, 196
Vienna Circle, 15, 138
Vygotsky, Lev Semyonovich, 101–104, 106

West, Cornel, 2
Whitehead, Alfred North, 128, 129, 130
Whitman, Walt, 68–69
"whole-ness of be-ing," 115
Wiredu, Kwasi, 2
witchcraft, 114
Wittgenstein, Ludwig, 137, 138, 139, 141,
  142
Wordsworth, William, 9
Wright, Chauncey, 9, 11, 14, 15

zone of proximal development, 103

Printed in the United States
by Baker & Taylor Publisher Services